The Original Holistic Health Series From Random House/Bookworks:
Edited by Don Gerrard

Fine Quality Paperback Editions

70685   **BE WELL,** Samuels, M.D. & Bennett

73470   **BREATHE AWAY YOUR TENSION** (rev.ed.), Geba

70937   Feminism As Therapy, Mander & Rush

70970   **GETTING CLEAR,** Rush

73166   **LIVING YOUR DYING,** Keleman

70770   **THE MASSAGE BOOK,** Downing

70648   Massage & Meditation, Downing

70939   Psychic Development, Porter

73115   **ROOTS OF CONSCIOUSNESS,** Mishlove

73113   **SEEING WITH THE MIND'S EYE,** Samuels & Samuels, M.D.

70793   **THE TOOTH TRIP,** McGuire, D.D.S.

73167   **TOTAL ORGASM** (rev. ed.), Rosenberg

70969   **THE WELL BODY BOOK,** Samuels, M.D. & Bennett

48948   **THE WELL CAT BOOK,** McGinnis, D.V.M. (cloth)

48946   **THE WELL DOG BOOK,** McGinnis, D.V.M. (cloth)

73052   Women Loving, Falk

73038   **THE ZEN OF RUNNING,** Rohe

THE CADUCEUS

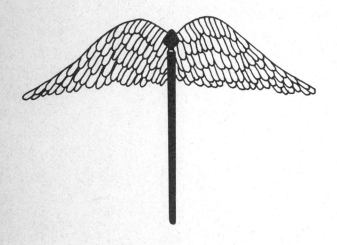

The caduceus symbol is many thousands of years old. The first part, pictured on the left, represents the staff carried by the Greek God Hermes, a guide of souls to rebirth.

The snakes entwined around the caduceus are symbols originating in China. They represent human energy rising toward spiritual enlightenment.

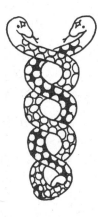

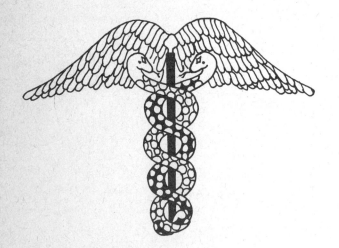

The placing together of the staff and the snakes represents, to us, the blending of eastern and western thought.

We have chosen the caduceus as a symbol for this book to re-introduce the ancient meanings of rebirth and energy as healing tools.

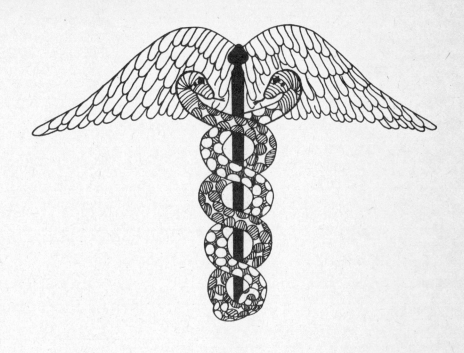

THE WELL BODY BOOK

by MIKE SAMUELS, M.D. & HAL BENNETT

illustrated by LINDA BENNETT

RANDOM HOUSE/BOOKWORKS

Copyright © 1973 by Michael Samuels, M.D. and Harold Zina Bennett
All rights reserved under International and Pan-American Copyright Conventions

First printing: March 1973	1,500 copies in cloth
	30,000 copies in paperback
Second printing: September 1973	1,000 copies in cloth
	14,000 copies in paperback
Third printing: May 1974	20,000 copies in paperback
Fourth printing: March 1975	10,000 copies in paperback
Fifth printing: June 1975	10,000 copies in paperback
Sixth printing: October 1975	10,000 copies in paperback
Seventh printing: July 1976	10,000 copies in paperback
Eighth printing: December 1976	15,000 copies in paperback
Ninth printing: August 1977	10,000 copies in paperback
Tenth printing: March 1978	10,000 copies in paperback
Eleventh printing: April 1979	10,000 copies in paperback
Twelfth printing: November 1979	10,000 copies in paperback
Thirteenth printing: December 1980	7,500 copies in paperback
Fourteenth printing: November 1982	5,000 copies in paperback

Typeset by Vera Allen Composition Service, Hayward, California
(special thanks to Vera, Dorothy, Betty and Gary)
Printed and bound by
under the direction of Peggy de Ugarte, Random House
Art Editor: Anne Kent Rush
Cover design and illustrations by Linda Bennett
Photos by Ted Benhari, Mike Samuels, and Linda Bennett
Editorial support by Nancy Samuels
This book is co-published by   Random House Inc.
201 East 50th Street
New York, N.Y. 10022
and   The Bookworks

Distributed in the United States by Random House, and simultaneously published in Canada by Random House of Canada Limited, Toronto

Library of Congress Cataloging in Publication Data

Bennett, Harold, 1936-
  The well body book.

   1. Hygiene.   2. Medicine, Popular.
I. Samuels, Mike, Joint author.   II.   Title.
RA776.B465   613   72-12651
ISBN 0-394-48405-3
ISBN 0-394-70969-1 (pbk)

Manufactured in the United States of America

Mike dedicates the book
"To Braxius, my imaginary doctor,
and
to Nancy and Lucas"

Hal and Linda dedicate the book
"To our children"

☆   ☆   ☆

I would like to thank Kurt Hirschhorn, M.D., who introduced me to medical research; John Berryman, my college writing teacher; David Cheek, M.D., who taught me some hypnosis; the people at Headlands Clinic — Irving Oyle, D.O., the director; Jesse Wexler, M.D., who teaches yoga; and Kevin O'Dea, who does massage. I would also like to thank Rolling Thunder, who taught me about healing; Fred Holschuh, M.D., who helped with the emergency medicine chapter; and Fred Miller, M.D., who helped with the diagnosis and treatment sections.

— by Mike

We would like to thank all the people who posed for pictures in the book: Jean Robertson, Alden Robertson, Wendy Robertson, Reynaldo Cortez, Luma, Don Gerrard, Eugenia Gerrard, Nancy Samuels, Mike Samuels, Hal Bennett, Linda Bennett, Nathan Bennett, Aaron Jellum, Helia, Maxine Stoddard, Larry Washington, Liz, Jorja Vliet, Betsy Warren, Ray Feichtmeir, and Jack Hughes. We would also like to thank Eugene Rush for his comments and suggestions. We all thank Jean Porter for her special help, advice, and support.

We would like to take the opportunity of a new printing to thank the thousands of people, both lay people and doctors, who have responded so positively to the book. We especially thank all of you who have sent us your well wishes and your suggestions for changes or additions, many of which we have tried to incorporate in this new printing.

To all of our new readers, as well as to all of you already familiar with the book, we extend our warmest wishes. May you all enjoy life in every way.

ABOUT THE WELL BODY BOOK

Many people, from everywhere in the country, have sent us letters to say how much they liked the first printing, and some sent helpful suggestions for changes and additions which we incorporated into this new printing. The following letter communicates a nice overall view of the book, and we have decided to print it here as a kind of introduction.

☆   ☆   ☆

It is exactly what its title states, and more — it is a "Well Being Book," inviting and often leading you before you are aware of it into some very tranquil spaces within your own consciousness and your own body.

It is a book that de-mystifies the practice of medicine and the drugs used in medicine ... But it is a book that pays respect and reverence precisely where such is long overdue — to the body as its own three million year old healer, to the individual's capacity to assume responsibility for the care and preventive medicine of his own body's health and well-being, and to those areas of medicine that are truly miraculous and helpful and require no "mystique" to be recognized and sought after.

It is a readable, practical, reliable *handbook* of diagnosis and treatment for the layman, a *workbook* towards well-being and the prevention of disease (covering suggestions about diet, clothing, meditation, sleep, muscle relaxation, massage, image control and non-control) a Consciousness III, age of Aquarius, non-linear *life style book* that speaks to everyone. It is a ... a ... well, look here, it is everything that it says it is — A *Well Body Book*. It goes on my waiting room table right now. May all my patients read it.

Sincerely,

William B. Goodheart, M.D.
Clinical Faculty Member
University of California School
of Medicine at San Francisco

SHORT TABLE OF CONTENTS

IF YOU ARE SICK

If you are using this book to diagnose and treat an illness which you now have, look upon that illness as an opportunity for you to put together a new approach to healing for yourself. There are several ways to do this:

Medical Encyclopedia Method: Most people do this out of habits established by standard home medical book formats. You look up the name of the disease which you think you have in the *Diagnosis and Treatment Index,* page 194.

Diagnosis By Symptoms: If you don't know what you have, or if the disease you looked up doesn't match the one you have, turn to the *Diagnosis and Treatment Index,* page 194, and look under *Organ Systems.* Turn then to the organ system where most of your symptoms appear: i.e. *Skin* is the organ system for a skin rash. Skim the symptoms of each disease that you find under that organ system until you find one that most closely corresponds to the ones you have. Or, look up your symptoms in the general index, page 347.

Traditional Doctor Approach: If you want to diagnose what you have in the way that your own doctor might do, start by doing a physical exam, pages 145 — 182. The p.e. report form, page 184, has page numbers after each finding that refer you to specific illnesses in the diagnosis and treatment section of the book.

Alternative Diagnostic Methods: If you want to develop other diagnostic skills, read pages 1 to 16. If you want to learn to read your body's messages, read pages 63 to 64, and 152. Remember that the entire *Preventive Medicine* section, page 69 to 142, tells you about numerous ways to get in touch with your body's messages, as well as how to change your life for health.

Alternative Healing Methods: If you are seeking new ways to help your body heal itself, read pages 1 to 14. An example of how these pages are used is described on page 15, *Disease As A Positive Life Force.* Look at pages 50 to 66. Exercises for bringing healing energy to your body are found on pages 65, 100, 105, 108, and 111. General healing exercises are described on pages 145, 181-182, and 284. Exercises for increasing the healing energies of drugs are given on page 319.

Doctor As A Resource: If you are using a doctor you will find pages 299 to 307 helpful, since they deal with patient lib techniques. If you are using drugs as healers, see page 308.

Emergency Medicine: For information about how to handle medical emergencies, see page 285.

HOW TO USE THIS BOOK

There are several different ways to use *The Well Body Book*. Before you start reading it you may want to look over some of the ways that we have foreseen. These are:

Read the book through and stop to do the exercises which we describe as you go along. This would be the most complete use of the book since you would then be participating at the level which will involve you the most. We have developed in the book a way to incorporate into your daily life a consciousness that will help you become more in harmony with your body. Doing the exercises as you go along is the best way to bring this consciousness into reality in your own life.

OR you can concentrate on particular chapters of the book. You can:

Use the *Diagnosis and Treatment* chapter to learn about diagnosing and treating common diseases, as well as to learn what is going on in your body when you have one of these diseases. If this is the way you intend to use the book, the *Index*, page 347 to 349, and the introduction to the *Diagnosis and Treatment* chapter, page 193, will be helpful to you.

OR

Read the chapter *Your Doctor As A Resource* if you want to know how to get the most from your doctor or clinic.

OR

Use the *Physical Exam* Chapter, page 143, to learn either how to do a physical exam yourself or what your doctor is doing when you get a physical exam from them.

OR

Use the *Preventive Medicine* chapter to learn how you can improve your health through food, relaxation, evaluation of your physical surroundings, or any of the other life situations which we discuss there.

If you want to use speed reading techniques, you can also:

Scan the book to get a fast overall understanding of the system of healing which we describe. To help you in this we've divided most chapters of the book into sub-chapter headings which are one line descriptions of the things discussed under it. In addition we have set key lines of the text in bold or italic typefaces. By scanning all of these you can get a *gestalt* of the entire book in an hour or less. Then later you may wish to go back and do the exercises or more carefully read chapters that interest you.

The Well Body Book is a basic tool for developing your own practical system of healing and preventive medicine. As such this book will replace the more traditional home medical encyclopedia for you.

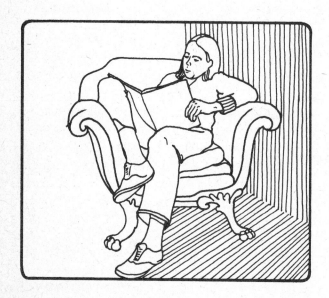

Editorial Notice: Throughout this book you will come across what may seem to you to be a rather strange use of the pronouns they, their, *and* them. *We have used these pronouns to avoid gendered pronouns such as* he *and* she *when referring to the doctor. We felt that making the sex of the doctor indefinite was worth the sacrifice of more proper grammar.*

LONG TABLE OF CONTENTS

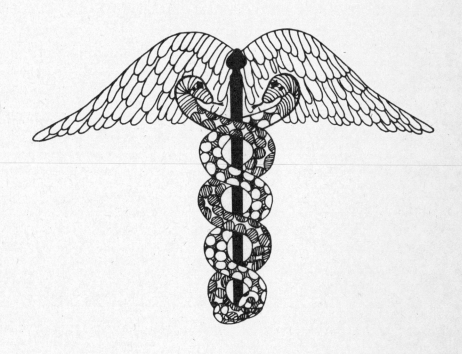

THREE MILLION YEAR OLD HEALER

Your body is a three million year old healer. Over three million years of evolution on this planet it has developed many ways to protect and heal itself. When you get a cut you do not have to think about healing that cut. Your body knows how to handle it. If you were asked to take a peanut butter sandwich and a glass of milk, and heal the cut with these things, there would be no way you could do that, but your body can easily heal a cut "without you", using the ingredients of these foods. In a similar way your body cures its infections, mends its broken bones, and heals its diseases.

You have all the knowledge, tools, materials, and energy necessary to keep yourself healthy. The way to allow your three million year old healer to heal you is to get out of its way. It is not a matter of teaching your body to heal and mend; it is a matter of first learning how you *prevent* your three million year old healer from working, then learning conscious skills to provide your three million year old healer with the space and energy it needs to keep itself well.

The things your body does to heal a simple cut are so complex that only the most advanced medical scientists are even beginning to understand them. Yet compared to the other healing processes that your body knows how to do, a cut is a simple job. It also knows how to analyze thousands of substances from the external environment that can cause disease, and how to protect itself from them by creating incredibly complex protein molecules, called *antibodies,* which neutralize these otherwise harmful substances.

In your blood are many different kinds of cells, each a unit of life in itself, and each with a specific job to do: some bring nutriment to other cells; some break down bacteria and carry it away; some carry away the waste produced by cells; some produce antibodies, etc. Each cell knows exactly what to do — without any conscious directions from you. *But you can stand in the way of these processes.* For one thing, if you tense your muscles, you prevent blood from freely circulating in the tense area. This means that that part of your body may not get the full benefits of these specialized cells.

In this book we look upon tension as a message from your body telling you to get into better harmony with Nature. If the message is ignored, that same tension will open your body to disease. We tell you how to recognize these first messages, so that once you recognize them you can choose between disease *or* changing patterns in your life to achieve greater harmony and health.

How do you choose between harmony and health on the one hand, and disease on the other? Let's take the example of a cut hand. *A choice for disease* might go something like this: You cut yourself while working in the garden. Immediately you become angry. You tense up in the area that's cut. You wipe the blood off on your work pants, and then you're back working again with your hands in the dirt. For a day or two you're mildly angry at your hand for hurting. Maybe you're also becoming a little worried about it. Then, two days hence, your're surprised when you discover that you're "struck down" by an infection where you cut yourself. You may feel, at that point, that you have been dealt a cruel blow. Now your body needs outside help to heal itself. That's when you go to a doctor.

A choice for harmony and health might go like this: You cut yourself while working in the garden. You realize the cut is a message telling you to pay attention to your work. You rest for a moment, you relax the area of the cut, knowing that your body knows exactly how to heal the cut. You help it a little by washing it off with clean water, and you protect it from the dirt as you work for the rest of the day. You might stop work a little earlier than you planned, to take a warm bath and relax in order to bring greater circulation to the area of the cut, further helping your three million year old healer to heal you. All of these things are what we call working for harmony and health. Put another way, it is *working in harmony with Nature.*

Your mind has a great deal to do with helping your three million year old healer. Medical scientists are now proving what Indian yogins and other healers from the eastern world have known and practiced for thousands of years: that by conscious control you can influence blood flow, heart beat, blood pressure, glandular secretions, and muscular tensions in all areas of your body. These are skills which can be learned in the same way that you learn to drive a car, play tennis, ride a bicycle, or anything else.

When the mind holds ideas such as worry, fear, anger, jealousy, hate, etc., your body manifests these feelings as muscle tension, decreased blood flow, and abnormal hormonal secretions. Eventually these states of consciousness result in disease. In this way people literally create their own diseases.

When your mind entertains ideas and feelings of love, joy, peace, harmony, and openess (knowing and understanding fear, anger, jealousy, hate, etc., but also understanding that you need not *hold onto* those feelings) your body manifests these feelings as relaxation, acceptance, radiance, alertness, and a natural flow of blood, energy and hormones. This is a healthy state. Through your thoughts and feelings you create your own well body.

So the choice for harmony and health is a choice of ideas and feelings. This book will help you to create a state of consciousness in which your three million year old healer can work to its fullest advantage by combining the tools of western medicine, and other forms of medicine, with these ideas.

When you let your body receive the energies of the universe, when you are open to them and not closed, when you are relaxed and not tense, when you have positive ideas and not negative ideas, the energies of the universe will flow into your body to keep you well or heal you. Your body's use of these energies is more powerful than any drug or herb, more powerful than any surgeon, than any healer known to man. All effective healing makes use of these energies. You can make use of these energies yourself. This book is a tool for opening your body to the energy flow of the universe, and for allowing the three million year old healer to heal you.

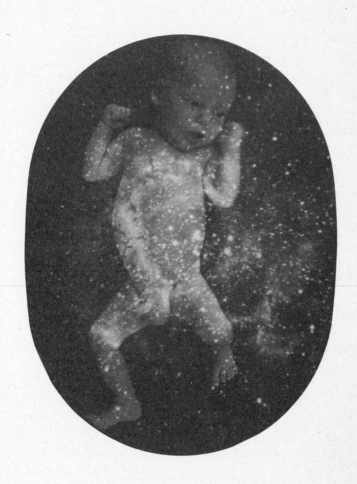

VISUALIZATION EXERCISE

Many of the exercises in this book depend on your ability to visualize actions, objects, and people in your mind's eye. We find that there are *visualizers* and *sensitives*. If you are a visualizer you can bring visual images quickly to your mind as actions, objects, or people are described to you with words. If you are a *sensitive* you may *feel* actions, objects or people in your mind, while you don't always *see* them in your mind's eye. Most people fall somewhere in between. You can become a stronger visualizer through the following exercise:

Sit in a comfortable chair, arms and legs uncrossed. Take three or four deep breaths. Exhale slowly and relax yourself.

 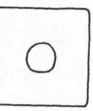 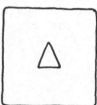

  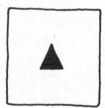

Close your eyes. Picture a home movie screen in your mind, or picture a plain, white sheet of paper about two feet square. You may find it necessary to get an actual piece of paper and fasten it on the wall; stare at it for five seconds, close your eyes and try to visualize it for five seconds, then open your eyes and stare at the paper for five seconds, and so on until you can actually see the screen (paper) in your mind's eye.

Change the color of the screen in your mind to red. Hold it in your mind for five seconds.

Change the color of your screen to blue. Hold it for five seconds.

Change the color of your screen to yellow. Hold it for five seconds.

Change the color of your screen to black. Then change it back to white.

Now picture a red square in the center of your white screen for five seconds.

Change the color of your square to yellow.

Change the color of your square to blue.

Change the color of your square to black.

Bring your white screen back.

Now picture a red circle in the center of your white screen for five seconds.

Change the color of your circle to yellow.

Change the color of your circle to blue.

Change the color of your circle to black.

Remove the circle entirely, leaving the white screen.

Now picture a red triangle in the center of your white screen for five seconds.

Change the color of your triangle to yellow.

Change the color of your triangle to blue.

Change the color of your triangle to black.

Now picture your screen white all over.

Change your white screen to black.

Open your eyes. You have now completed the visualization exercise.

Because of the large size of the visual cortex in the brain, the ability to visualize is a powerful tool for activating mental energy. It will expand the use of your mind in activities outside this book, but is also an essential tool for understanding many parts of the book.

If you have no problems at all doing this exercise, you probably need no further visualizing practice to do the exercises in this book. If you did have difficulty, practice the exercise until it is easy for you to do. You can do the entire exercise in less than five minutes, and will find yourself expanding your visualizing powers after doing it as few as three or four times. With practice you will develop the ability to create images of actions, objects, and people in your minds eye at will or as these things are described to you with words.

Everyone can learn to visualize. If it takes you a long time to learn it, the chances are that you are a *sensitive* and able to *feel* presences quite strongly. You will become a *sensitive* with strong visualizing powers if you are a *sensitive* practicing this exercise.

If you cannot, after several tries, do this visualization exercise very well do not let it worry you. Depend instead on your powers as a *sensitive*. Visualization may or may not eventually work for you. Do not feel that you are lacking in necessary skills if you cannot visualize since your skills as a *sensitive* can accomplish similar ends.

CREATE YOUR IMAGINARY DOCTOR

When you bought this book you got, in addition to the physical book, your own *imaginary doctor*. This character, who you will create by following the instructions in this chapter, will become your *alter ego, advisor,* or *helper* for using the *WELL BODY BOOK* to its fullest advantage. You will be able to turn to him or her whenever you feel anxious, confused, doubtful, or when you feel the need to consult with someone you can fully trust. In addition, you will find instructions for using your imaginary doctor in specific situations throughout the book.

If you do not stop here to create your imaginary doctor you are passing up one of the most useful tools in this book. The peoples of many cultures down through history, including some American Indians, created personal spiritual advisors to guide and assist them throughout life. Your imaginary doctor can be such a guide. The proper time spent on this exercise could benefit you for a lifetime.

If you have trouble creating your imaginary doctor with the instructions contained in the book, go back in memory to good times at play as a child. Remember those witches and saints you and your friends became? Even a darkened room held several imaginary people. Try to get in touch with this mood and spirit, letting your memory wander freely over the past. Did you have a favorite house as a child, perhaps the home of a relative or a friend, that seemed more beautiful, exciting, or secure than anything in the world? Re-explore that house in your mind. Perhaps your imaginary doctor will live there. Still having trouble? Get hints from someone you know who reports success creating his or her imaginary doctor. It's not difficult. The key to success is relaxation.

If you are working on the book with a friend, have them read these instructions to you as you follow them. The only special consideration would be that your friend be sensitive to you as you do the exercise. They should slow down, stop, or speed up the reading to allow you to complete each part of the exercise at your own rate. They can tell whether you are inhaling or exhaling by watching your mouth, chest and stomach as you do the exercise. When I am reading the exercise for a friend I also try to imagine how long it will take them to complete each step as I read it.

After you get in touch with your imaginary doctor, reverse roles with your friend, with you reading the instructions while they do the exercises. You can compare notes on your imaginary doctors. Those of us working on the book who have imaginary doctors really have fun exchanging information learned from our imaginary doctors. You can even discuss with your imaginary doctor ideas that you have learned from your friends' imaginary doctors.

If you are doing this section of the book alone, but with the help of a tape recorder, the procedure is slightly different. The first thing that you'll have to do is to record a tape of the instructions, using your own voice. As the instructions will tell you, record in a slow monotone. You will have to imagine yourself doing the exercise as you read so that your tape will be paced to your needs when you play it back to yourself. We recommend using a

90 minute cassette tape to do this recording. The entire exercise will not take that long, of course, but having the extra tape will give you plenty of time to complete the exercise, and then take care of shutting off the machine and rewinding the tape in a leisurely fashion after you are done.

If you want to do the imaginary doctor exercise, and you are doing the book alone and without a tape recorder, the problem is a bit more difficult, but not impossible. In this case, you will have to read the exercise through to yourself until you have the whole thing clearly in mind. Some people will do this by memorizing the instructions, others will do it simply by getting an overall sense of the many steps necessary for getting in touch with their imaginary doctor. This will probably take three or four readings before you are actually ready to follow the instructions.

If you are reading through the book without the intent of stopping to do the exercise, you will probably discover that a part of you will do the exercises automatically, and you may be able to use the experience as fully as others who do the instructions more deliberately.

It is essential to **do this part of the book in a place and at a time of day when you will not be interrupted for at least half an hour.** If you have young children in your home, this may prove to be difficult. But work out the best situation you can, even if it means getting someone else to look after your kids for an hour or two.

If, when doing the exercise and getting an imaginary doctor, you feel that you are *making the whole thing up* (and perhaps you even feel a little bit silly) understand that these feelings are exactly right. Most people do feel this way at first. But once you have him or her, your imaginary doctor becomes a very useful tool, and in that way, a reality.

You will find that you do not need to limit the use of your imaginary doctor to the contents of this book. Most of us who have them turn to our imaginary doctors for help in other matters — everything from figuring out ways to locate a leak in the roof to finding solutions to marital conflicts. Wherever you need to relax and work things out, wherever you feel that you would like to step back from feelings which may be blocking you from finding a solution to a problem, you will find the imaginary doctor helpful.

Finally, I want to point out that *everyone's imaginary doctor will be different.* They may or may not be someone in real life, such as the remembered fantasy of a doctor you had as a child. Most people are surprised to find that though they think they are going to get a certain imaginary doctor just before doing the exercise, when they actually do it, the imaginary doctor they get is quite different.

It has been important to many people doing this exercise for the first time to be told that the exercise was not aimed at stimulating the memories of a doctor who you knew in the past; the real point is to relax and *create* your own imaginary doctor. The exercise will help you to get to a state of consciousness where this will be possible. Beyond doing the exercise, you will not have to consciously think about how you will create this character, any more than you consciously worked, as a child, at creating your imaginary playmates.

Occasionally, though rarely, people get imaginary doctors who they don't like. If this happens to you don't worry about it. Simply do the exercise again until you get one you like. There is, incidentally, no need to do anything about the one you don't like. Leave them be, they'll do no harm and it may prove interesting and fun to have them around.

Everyone can get an imaginary doctor, though it takes more effort for some than others. You may have to try the exercise more than once, or even several times — even at different times in your life.

It may be helpful for you to know that your imaginary doctor will not necessarily appear in the guise of a medical doctor. People who have done this exercise with Mike or me report getting friends, parents, old teachers, famous religious figures, unrecognizably plain people, beings from outer space, primitive people, and various entities and non-human forms (light beams, spots of color, vague feelings, bells, etc.)

The imaginary rooms that people have reported range from clearings in the forest, to elaborate castles, chalets, plain houses in the suburbs, barns, amorphous spaces, antiseptic laboratories, and warm cabins. Anything is possible.

The imaginary doctors might have objective realities of their own; *several people report having met their imaginary doctors in real life after creating them in the exercise.* We found that the imaginary doctors act with their own personalities and idiosyncracies and not as though they were a part of your conscious mind. Whether they have objective realities or not the imaginary doctors provide a method of getting in touch with the part of you that has access to collective unconscious information.

The more frequently you use your imaginary doctor, the stronger and more meaningful this tool will become in your life. So have fun with it. Make a tape of the instructions so that your friends can get imaginary doctors too. We've found, in our own lives, that sharing our experiences with our friends has increased the richness and usefulness of our imaginary doctor for us all.

THE INSTRUCTION.

Read the following in a slow monotone, pausing between lines to allow your friend — or yourself if you are tape-recording this section to do by yourself — to do as each line instructs.

Preliminary: Sit in a comfortable chair, both feet on the floor, uncrossed, hands lying relaxed in your lap. If you wish you may also lie on your back on a flat, comfortable, but firm surface.

Close your eyes. Take a deep breath. Hold the breath for a moment; exhale slowly. Do this three times or more. Allow your body to become more and more fully relaxed.

Now breathe normally. Breathe in a comfortable, relaxed rhythm

As each part of your body is named in the instructions below, inhale, then imagine as you exhale that you are sending your breath to that part of your body. Practice this form of breathing for a moment if you wish: *Inhale. Then as you exhale imagine that you are sending your breath to whatever part of your body you wish to relax.* Your body will do the rest.

Detailed instructions begin here.

Inhale. Send your breath down to your toes and relax them. Send your breath to the soles of your feet . . . and to your ankles, and relax them.

Your feet are now fully relaxed.

Inhale. Send your breath down to the muscles of your lower legs from your ankles to your knees and relax them. First do your left leg . . . and then your right leg.

Inhale. Send your breath to the muscles of your thighs. Relax them. First do your left leg . . . and then your right leg.

You are now more fully relaxed from your toes to the tops of your legs.

Inhale. Send your breath to your buttocks . . . and to the muscles in and around your genitals, and relax them.

Inhale. Send your breath to your stomach muscles . . . and to the muscles in your lower back. Relax them.

Breathe very slowly and easily, allowing your breathing to match the rhythms of your relaxed body.

Inhale. Then send your breath to your chest muscles and then to your upper back muscles. Relax them.

Inhale. Send your breath down through your shoulders to the tips of your fingers, and relax them.

You are now fully relaxed from your toes to the tops of your legs . . . and from the tops of your legs up to the tops of your shoulders . . . and down your shoulders, along your arms, to your fingertips.

Inhale and then send your breath to your forehead . . . to your cheeks . . . to your eyelids . . . and to your jaw muscles, and relax them. Let your jaw drop. You will feel a comfortable *letting go* as you relax these muscles in your face and jaw. Let this feeling of deep relaxation spread to the muscles of your neck, throat and tongue.

You have now relaxed all these parts of your body. Your body is fully relaxed from your toes to the roof of your mouth. This state of consciousness allows more energy to flow freely to your mind. It is a quiet and relaxed flow of energy which you now feel moving to your mind.

If any part of your body still feels tense, inhale, send a breathe to that part of your body and relax it.

☆　　☆　　☆

Your mind is now in a healthy, open and very relaxed state of consciousness. But there is no threat to your being in this state of consciousness because you can bring yourself out of this state and back to your normal, everyday state of consciousness at any time that you wish. You need only to count to three and you will be back at this normal everyday state. Some people will be able to return to the normal, everyday state of consciousness simply by opening their eyes. But counting to three before you do so will make the process more comfortable.

☆ ☆ ☆

Now imagine a house. It can be any house you choose, and it may be anywhere in the world.

Imagine the size of the house, and the style of architecture.

Imagine the land surrounding it.

Now go up to the entrance of the house. Open the door. Go inside.

Somewhere in this house is a room which is entirely your own. Whenever you enter it you are completely at ease. Go directly to the door of this room. Open the door. You are now looking at the inside of your room. Before you enter do whatever is necessary to make yourself fully at ease in this room. Imagine furniture. Imagine a chair which you would like to sit in. Now go to the chair and sit down. Make yourself comfortable.

Imagine that somewhere in this room there is a special door opening into a space adjoining; it is the space in which your imaginary doctor moves and has (his or) her being. The door of this room opens in a peculiar way. It is a sliding door that opens from the top and slides down into the floor. The reason for the door opening in this way is to allow you to fully visualize your imaginary doctor, beginning with the top of his or her head and working down toward the feet. You are able to open this door by willing it to open. You need only to imagine it opening and it will open. You need only to imagine it closing and it will close. Since you created it from your imagination, only your imagination can open it or close it.

☆ ☆ ☆

You are now ready to create and meet your imaginary doctor. Remember, this person may be a woman or it may be a man. Here are the basic traits which your imaginary doctor will have:

Calm and Humane: He or she understands and cares about your feelings. He or she knows about having a well body, and their explanations fully satisfy you and calm fears or doubts that you might have.

Firm and Honest: He or she understands that your thoughts and feelings represent ways in which you use the energy created within your body. He or she knows that *you are* this energy, that thoughts, feelings, and the body are one. Thus they will be firm and honest in pointing out ways for you to use these things to create a fully well body. They will not be afraid to tell you information which you may find difficult to accept but which is necessary for your health.

Ironic: Your imaginary doctor has a sense of humor and does not get so involved with the game of being an imaginary doctor that they become inattentive to your health.

Now imagine that this doctor is in the imaginary space adjoining your imaginary room.

☆   ☆   ☆

You are now in your imaginary room, sitting in your chair. The door opening into the space in which your imaginary doctor stays is directly in front of you. In a moment you will see your imaginary doctor in your mind's eye. You are now ready to open the door, remembering that the door opens or closes according to your will, and that it is a sliding door that opens from the top and slides down into the floor.

Open the door until you see the top of your imaginary doctor's head. Imagine the color and texture of the doctor's hair, and whether or not (he or) she is wearing a hat.

Open the door until you see the whole face, stopping at the shoulders up. Is the face round or elongated? Note the color of the imaginary doctor's eyes, and the eyebrows. Note whether the nose is long, short, broad, or thin. Study the cheeks, mouth, and chin. Taken together, note what expression of feeling the face projects — happy, sad, warm, cold, indifferent, outgoing, withdrawn, or what?

Open the door until you see the top half of the imaginary doctor's body, stopping at the waist. Note the color and texture of clothes, and note the tailoring of the dress, blouse, shirt, or coat they are wearing, if any. Note how the clothes fit over the upper body, asking yourself to imagine also the flesh beneath the clothes. Is the doctor broad or narrow across the shoulders? Does the chest seem to be thin, well fleshed, or muscular? If a woman, note the size of her breasts and the shape. Note how the imaginary doctor carries his or her upper torso. Do they stand straight or are they slightly bent?

Open the door the rest of the way. You will now see the imaginary doctor's body from the waist down to the soles of their feet. You may also see their hands for the first time. Note the color and texture of the clothing — skirt, dress, pants, or other form of clothing — which they are wearing. Check to see if they are wearing a belt of any kind. If so, note the material it is made of, the color, and the design of the belt buckle, if any. Note the width and bulk of your imaginary doctor's pelvic area, and note whether they carry this area of their body tightly or loosely. For example, do his or her legs appear almost to hang from the hip sockets, or are they tightly held in at the hips?

You may now wish to study the imaginary doctor's hands for a moment. Note their general size: large, medium or small. Are the fingers long and graceful, short and fleshy, or somewhere in between? Note whether they are strong hands accustomed to hard labor, or delicate hands. Note any jewelry worn on the hands or wrists — a watch, a bracelet, rings. Are the hands hairy or smooth?

Now note the approximate bulk and muscular development of the thighs. Note the knees — their shape as well as their apparent strength, weakness, tightness, or looseness. Note the lower leg — its muscular development and shape. Now take a look at the shoes. If your imaginary doctor is not wearing shoes, look at the bare feet. Note the color and texture of the skin. If they are wearing shoes, are the shoes shiney and polished or dull and dusty? Note whether they are new or well worn. Note particularly how the bottoms of the shoes meet the floor. From this you can get a sense of the weight carried by the feet. If your doctor's feet are bare, it will be even easier to see how his or her feet carry their weight, by studying how the toes meet the floor, whether the toes are spread for balance or held in tightly and perhaps slightly curled. You will also be able to see the arch of the foot, and the way the flesh of the heel forms into the floor or ground.

Scan your imaginary doctor's entire body from head to foot until you have gotten a strong feeling of his or her bulk and weight, as well as their relative grace or clumsiness. Also note how you feel in your imaginary doctor's presence. Concentrate on *feelings* rather than on your intellectual interpretations of what the imaginary doctor represents to you.

You may wish to estimate your imaginary doctor's age, as well as other things about them, such as family situation, or past experiences in their life. You may be aware that they come from a different social background than your own, or a different culture, country, or even planet.

Look over your imaginary doctor to see if there is anything you have missed such as a necktie, a kerchief, a necklace or other piece of jewelry, a flower or a club pin in a lapel, a hankerchief in a breast pocket, etc. They may also be carrying something, which you missed the first time over.

You have now fully created your imaginary doctor. Have them step into the room with you if they have not already done so. You may wish to go up to them and shake their hand, embrace them, or simply walk around them to fully take them in. Others may wish to sit across the room and observe from a distance. However you do it is fine. Introduce yourself to him or her. Ask their name if you wish. Note that you and/or your imaginary doctor will communicate with your own language of the imagination. This language may be wholly, partly, or not at all verbal. You may, for example, communicate with your imaginary doctor by *telepathy,* symbols and images, body movements and gestures, music, or some other form of communication not mentioned here. However you do it is fine so long as it works for you both.

When you get to this point, you will probably discover that you have very definite things which you will want to discuss with your imaginary doctor. If you are worried that you may not have anything to discuss with her (or him), here are some suggestions based on what others have reported discussing on the first meeting:

Tell your imaginary doctor that you would like him or her to help you with this book in whatever ways are indicated in the pages to come.

Tell them that you want them to be close at hand whenever you feel anxiety, confusion, or doubt about anything concerning your health, and to help you work out solutions.

Tell them that you want them to act as a focal point toward which you will direct all knowledge for making and keeping your body well.

Discuss with him or her how they will help you to stand away from your feelings whenever these feelings are getting in the way of making an important decision that concerns your health. You and your imaginary doctor will try out different ways of accomplishing this until you find a way that works well for you.

Note that these are only suggestions. You do not *have* to do any of them. What you do in this first meeting with your imaginary doctor will be wholly up to you.

This conversation with your imaginary doctor may at first seem *silly* or *made up* to you. These feelings are quite normal for anyone raised in our society and doing the exercise for the first time. Most people who have succeeded in creating and using their own imaginary doctors have more than likely experienced these same feelings at first. Their attitude is usually that the imaginary doctor is a good tool that really works, so it doesn't matter that it seems *silly* or *crazy*.

☆ ☆ ☆

When you have finished this first meeting with your imaginary doctor, have him or her return to their space beyond the door through which they entered your imaginary room. Exchange goodbyes, if you wish, and then *will* the door to close between you and them, remembering that the door will close by moving from the floor toward the ceiling. Each time you meet your imaginary doctor it will be easier and easier, and they will appear more real to you.

You are now ready to leave your imaginary room.

Imagine yourself getting up from your chair, if you were last sitting there, or simply walking up to the door which leads you to the corridor. Open the door. Go outside your room. Close the door. Lock it if you wish to do so.

Walk down the hallway, and out of the house in which you found your imaginary room.

By counting from one to three, slowly, you will leave this state of consciousness and will return to your usual and every day state of consciousness, feeling rested and relaxed, healthier than before. One. Two. Three. Open your eyes. Now you are back in your normal, every day state of consciousness.

☆ ☆ ☆

Having once created an imaginary doctor by the above method, you will be able to return to your imaginary room and consult with them at any time that you wish, simply by closing your eyes and going quickly through the exercise alone and in your mind's eye. In time, and with practice, you may even be able to return simply by relaxing and imagining yourself there.

☆　　☆　　☆

Once you have created a strong impression of the imaginary doctor for yourself you may be able to see things as they see things, simply by asking yourself "How would my imaginary doctor see this?" This will provide you with a broad and objective point of view which will be valuable in making full use of the material contained in this book.

DISEASE AS A POSITIVE LIFE FORCE

Disease as a positive life force? This idea ran contrary to everything I had been taught about sickness. I had been working for nearly a month on this book: writing, studying, and trying to put together everything that Mike was teaching me about medicine. I was working ten to twelve hours a day, and Mike warned me that I was pushing myself too hard.

As I write these notes it all seems obvious that I would get sick. But it was not obvious to me at the time. I was simply not "paying attention."

One Friday evening I felt achey, weak, and vaguely sick to my stomach. After dinner I took my temperature; it was 101°. That night I slept badly, and woke up feeling worse. But I went to my study to work on the book. The irony struck me immediately — working on a book to show people how to stay well, and me with a temperature of 101°! About noon I called Mike.

I told him my symptoms and answered the few questions he asked. He told me that I had a cold with a sinus infection but insisted that I should look upon it as a positive thing. He said it was my body telling me to "pay attention." Furthermore, he said that my body would know both the cause and the cure of the illness. I had only to get in touch with it and these answers would come to me. How to do that? The answer was obvious. Use my imaginary doctor, Mike said.

This was the first time I had turned to my imaginary doctor to actually help me solve a health problem, and I was skeptical. My imaginary doctor was an outgoing German lady about 40 or 50 years old. She was a medical scientist who seemed to know about the sources of illness and what to do about them. She told me that the illness I now had was caused by something against which my body could easily have built its own defense, had that been the right thing for it to do. She said for me to acknowledge the fact that I had been using energy faster than my body could comfortably produce it. If I continued at the rate I was going, my body would begin robbing energy from vital organs (my kidneys, she said) which would cause damage not easily fixed. My present illness stopped me from going that far.

This explanation felt right to me from what I knew about my body. My brain and my emotions are the main tools I work with (being a writer and teacher) and getting the flu or even a bad cold, always makes me nearly unable to think, and barely aware of my emotions.

From working with Mike and learning his approach to medicine I had discovered that the back of my mouth, my nasal passages and sinuses were the most vulnerable areas of my own particular body. I also learned that my body ordinarily kept a balanced environment with bacteria and normal cells living in harmony in these areas. My imaginary doctor taught me that whenever I began misusing my body, it — perhaps deliberately — set about changing the temperature and moisture of these areas, therefore allowing whatever bacteria happened to be in the area to infect the surrounding tissue.

I put all this together piece by piece, and came up with the conclusion that my sickness was not just the simple presence of infection. My sickness was everything that led up to these areas becoming a suitable breeding ground for whatever was causing the infection. Mike confirmed the fact that there are always bacteria or viruses in the air, as well as in my own body, which can make me sick. But the environment inside my body, over which it (my body) has nearly complete control, is not always an ideal environment for bacteria to grow to a point that would cause disease. My body controls moisture and temperature of all its various parts, and this was all it needed to change the environment of my mouth and sinuses to a place that would be good for the bacteria or viruses to multiply.

I believe it to be no accident that my body gets sick in the particular organ it does. When I get a cold and sinus infection, it is as though the energy flow to my brain is suddenly blocked. Since my brain is one of the most important tools for putting sentences on paper, I have no choice but to slow down. Thus my body protects itself from further harm. An earache would not stop me. But an earache would most certainly stop a musician. And a stubbed toe would not stop me, but it would most certainly stop a dancer. As far as I can remember I have never had an earache, though a good friend who's a musician seems to get them as often as I get my colds. And I seldom stub my toe, but I have known dancers who frequently did.

I asked my imaginary doctor what I should do to cure my colds and sinus infections. *Stop working and let your body rest,* was her emphatic reply. She told me that I should sleep whenever I felt the least bit tired, and that I should not even think about the book for at least three days. She told me to consider my brain completely out of the action for this three day period and to take no medication.

All this may not agree with standard medical practice. But I do know that in terms of my own body the knowledge is very sound.

My imaginary doctor's cure really did work. I took no medication and found myself content to relax and thoroughly rest. I slept as many as ten hours a day. The knowledge and acceptance that my brain would be *shut down* for three days, no matter what I tried to do about it, more or less forced me to rest. After the prescribed period of time my brain felt rested, and I was refreshed and ready to go back to work on the book. Though not entirely over the infection, the symptoms no longer bothered me, and working at a leisurely pace helped me to get in touch with a rhythm of working that felt better to my body than my previously feverish pace.

This was quite a departure from my usual pattern of fighting the illness for days, sometimes weeks, forcing my brain to work in spite of it all. The past results have always been a prolongation of the illness and a scatter of little dabs of mediocre work.

Many people will see nothing unusual about my imaginary doctor's prescription for a "cure." As I reflect on it now I feel that it's the explanation of the cause that I value even more than the cure, since this knowledge has taught me to pace myself more sensibly — something I might not have worked out without my imaginary doctor.

I relate these things to tell you ways in which my imaginary doctor worked for me in a certain space and time in my life. I do not mean these things to be prescriptions that will work for all people. But, there may be some tools here that will work for you as well as they worked for me.

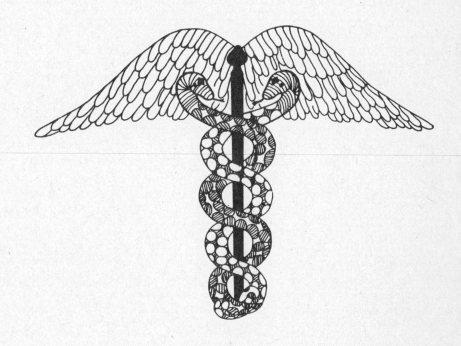

In this section you will find ways to help you focus on, and assess, your past and present health.

The chapter called *General Information* and the one called *Systems Review*, will tell you where your body *has been* in terms of health and illness. Most people will probably discover that they have been very healthy.

From the information which you collect you will make a *Health Colors* chart which will provide you with a visual mental image of all the information you have collected about your body. This will be your tool for knowing what parts of your body have been most prone to illness and what parts call for your extra attention for health.

Through doing what we call the *Bright Life* chart you will create another visual mental image of your body as healthy, vibrant, and full of life. You will learn how to use this as a healing tool.

The last chapter of this section, called *Mirror Mirror*, is a way of assessing your health in the present. It is a way to get in touch with your body on a day-to-day basis.

All these will work along with the rest of the book to help you develop a well body.

GENERAL INFORMATION

In your grandparents' or great grandparents' day, most people had a special page in the back of their family *BIBLE* where they kept information such as the dates of births, marriages and deaths, as well as relevant health information. Sometimes they passed the family *BIBLE* down through many generations, with each new generation adding its own entries. From a medical standpoint these pages were often rich in data and history. This chapter is an updated version of the pages in the back of the family *BIBLE.* Through it you will create an important tool for evaluating your health.

BODIES, SHOTS, HISTORIES, HAZARDS, AND DRUGS

In this chapter, you will learn about and make a permanent record of:

Your body type: Learn to accept and appreciate your own body even though it may not conform to the shape, size, texture and color of the body type currently upheld as the model of beauty for the society or culture in which you live.

Shots and immunizations you have had: Knowing which of these diseases and/or immunizations you have had can release you from unnecessary worry the next time you find yourself exposed to them.

Your family health history: A few diseases can be inherited. Others can be *learned.* Knowing what these diseases are and whether or not your family or you have had them, will put you in a position of being able to find ways to minimize or do away with the threat of that disease for you and your children.

Your occupational health hazards: This knowledge will put you in a position of being able to correct a job or home situation which is a threat to your body, or strengthen and aid your body to deal with those hazards.

Drugs to which you may have unhealthy reactions: Many people have allergic reactions to prescription drugs and patent medicines. This section of the book is a place to begin learning about these drugs and to keep a record of the ones that you have found are not good for you.

All the above information will be helpful when you are diagnosing an illness which you now have, or when you are working with other sections of this book. But we'll tell you more about these things later.

This chapter is easy to do. Just follow the directions which we give as you go along. The only tool you'll need (besides the ones built into your body) is a pencil or pen.

YOUR BODY TYPE

Medical scientists recognize three different body types: the *ectomorph*, the *mesomorph,* and the *endomorph.* From the point of view of health, the kind of body you have makes very little difference. It is, however, important for you to *know and accept the body type that you have,* so that you will not be tempted to try to change your body into a form it can never be. Think this sounds strange? We have only to look at the millions of books on weight reducing, and the millions of dollars spent annually in "body building parlors" for the evidence that a great many of us are disatisfied with our bodies.

Let's say you are a woman with an endomorph body, the body type that is naturally large-framed and fleshy. If you were that woman you might damage your health by attempting to slim down to the proportions of the wiry ectomorph whose streamlined body was pictured in the latest fashion magazines. It is equally unhealthy for the wiry ectomorph male to lift weights all summer in the hope that he can develop a mesomorph body with huge bulging muscles.

The fact is that you are working *against nature* by attempting to change your body type. Obey nature. Accept and get to know and love your body, and learn how to live with it in harmony.

Male beauty standards have their roots in the Middle Ages when the mesomorph had a certain practical value in being better able to survive the physical violence of the times. The muscular mesomorph was better adapted to that age than the other two body types.

Female standards are more flexible. Since the female body is exploited by the world of advertising, female beauty standards vary according to what's being pushed: clothes (ectomorph), sex (endomorph), sporting equipment (mesomorph).

The following are descriptions of the three body types:

Ectomorph: Shakespeare once described a character in one of his plays as having "a lean and hungry look." These words adequately describe the ectomorph. In addition to being thin and wiry, the ectomorph person is usually a very active person. If you are an ectomorph, you probably have relatively small bones, and your arms and legs tend to be long in proportion to your torso. Your chest is probably thin, and your ribs prominent. Your stomach is flat and your buttocks small.

Mesomorph: Charles Atlas was a mesomorph who over-developed his natural body traits. (Overabundant muscles can limit body movement and even cut down circulation.) If you are a mesomorph, you will have naturally well-developed muscles in your neck, shoulders, chest, stomach, buttocks, arms and legs. You probably will have large bones and a great need for physical activity. As children, mesomorphs often aggravate their parents and teachers because of their need for constant movement.

Endomorph: This body type is soft, and even has bulges in places. If you are an endomorph, your muscles may be as strong as the mesomorph's, but it is difficult to see the difference between your muscles and fat until you squeeze them. This is not to say that you need to be fat or overweight if you are an endomorph. But it does mean that your body appears soft, just as the mesomorph tends toward muscularness, and the ectomorph toward wiry-ness.

Understand that few people fit exactly one set of standards or another. You will probably only *tend* toward one type or another. The idea is to decide where in this scheme you feel that you best fit, and then learn to accept where you are. When you get to the section of this chapter where you do a family history, you may find it interesting to trace down the body types in your family, to see where you inherited the body type that you have.

SHOTS AND IMMUNIZATIONS

The following is a list of the shots and immunizations commonly given. Most of them give you lifetime protection from a single shot. The *tetanus* and *diptheria* are the exception to this. Most doctors now agree that you should get a *booster* every ten years.* Or if you get a deep cut or puncture wound, your doctor may want to give you one in a shorter interval.

Check off everything you can remember having gotten in the list below. Exact dates are not important for those things that require dates, but try to get them within a year or so.

INVENTORY OF SHOTS AND IMMUNIZATIONS

DPT (Diptheria, Whopping Cough-Pertussis, Tetnaus) _____ yes _____ no

Polio Immunization: Salk shots _____ yes _____ no

Sabin drops or cubes _____ yes _____ no

(Polio shots were later replaced by Sabin)

Measles _____ yes _____ no   German Measles (Rubella) _____ yes _____ no

Smallpox Vaccination _____ yes _____ no _____ date

Tetanus Booster _____ yes _____ no _____ date

TB Skin Test _____ yes _____ no _____ date _____ result

Chest X-ray _____ yes _____ no _____ date _____ result

Note any other shots you have had.

If you come across shots that you are not sure you had, and which you feel that you would like to or should have, go to your doctor or clinic and ask about getting them. Afterwards, record them above.

*1972 Medical data

There are two ways to become immune to certain diseases. One way is to deliberately introduce (immunize) your body to the disease by giving your body a small dose of the disease, usually a dose not large enough to cause symptoms that you will notice. The other is for you to actually get the disease. Also, you may have a disease but never notice any symptoms. Either way, your body builds *antibodies* against the disease, which protects your body should you be exposed to that disease in the future. Remember, though, not every disease works in this way. In some cases your body will build a partial resistance only; next time you are exposed to that disease you will be less likely to get it or it will be less severe.

In the inventory below you will find lists of diseases — some for which your body can build complete immunities, others to which it can build only partial immunities. Circle any and all diseases which you have had.

DISEASES WHICH YOU CAN ONLY GET ONCE

Measles   German Measles (usually)

Mumps   Chicken Pox

DISEASES WHICH YOU CAN GET MORE THAN ONCE

Mononucleosis   Pneumonia

Venereal Diseases (VD)   Tuberculosis

Rheumatic Fever   Syphillis

Gonorrhea   Hepatitis

Note here any diseases which you have had, and about which you want more information. Use the **Diagnosis and Treatment,** *and* **Preventive Medicine** *chapters to fill in anything you need here:*

☆   ☆   ☆

This information will be helpful to you in filling in your knowledge about your body's immunities, and will also help you in diagnosing any disease by using this with the chapter called *If You Are Sick.*

YOUR FAMILY HEALTH HISTORY

The health histories of your parents and children may hold information to help you keep your body well. The reason for this is that doctors have found some diseases to be *familial* — meaning that they tend to show up generation after generation in the same family. As with many other things familial, it is often difficult if not 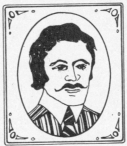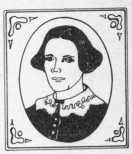 impossible, to say whether these diseases are learned or are passed on through the genes. To complicate matters, researchers are now speculating that the genes can carry knowledge to guide behavior, in addition to determining body traits. This means that you can either learn or inherit the knowledge to control the circulation, temperature, mosture, and body chemistry for each part of your body, in the same way that you learn to walk and run as a child. With these powers you control your health. In the section called *Preventive Medicine* we tell you about techniques you can learn to increase your control of your own body and health: to improve your health or prevent disease from being manifested in your body.

Here is a list of diseases which Mike believes to be familial — genetic or learned:

Allergies: eczema, asthma, hay fever, etc.

Heart diseases; strokes and high blood pressure

Cancer (sometimes)   Diabetes

Ulcers   Suicide

Glaucoma   Migraine headaches

Sickle Cell Anemia   Alcoholism and drug use

As you do your family health histories on the following pages, it will be helpful to you to keep the above list in mind. Be sure to note any of the diseases above if they have occurred.

FAMILY HEALTH HISTORY
FOR
YOUR PARENTS

Describe their general health, record their ages, and if they are dead tell why they died. Tell about any health problems which they had and which you feel may be important in terms of your own health. Try to describe your feelings toward any of the health problems your parents have had.

If you suspect that you may have learned or inherited a disease that your parents had, use this space to make notes to yourself about learning ways to prevent further occurrences of those diseases in your body. Use this book as your reference.

Remember, just as disease can be a positive life force in your own life it can also be a positive life force in the lives of every member of your family. When you learn ways to improve your health you can pass this information on to other family members. Especially important with familial diseases!

FAMILY HEALTH HISTORY
FOR
YOUR BROTHERS AND SISTERS

Describe the general health of each brother and/or sister, and record their ages. If any have died, tell why. Tell about any problems which they had which you believe might affect your own health. Write down your feelings about any health problems that they have which you believe might affect you.

If any of your brothers or sisters have had any of the diseases on the list of familial diseases, check back to see if your parents also had these diseases. Make any notes that you feel are relevant to this in the above space.

FAMILY HEALTH HISTORY
FOR
YOUR CHILDREN

Describe the general health of your children. If any have died, tell why. Record any health problems which they have which you believe might relate to your own health.

If your children have diseases on the familial disease list, and these are diseases which you or your parents have had, make notes on this here.

Sometimes when you are attempting to diagnose an illness using the *Diagnosis And Treatment* chapter, you will find that we refer you back to this section. So you will find the information that you record here useful to you throughout the rest of the book.

OCCUPATIONAL HAZARDS

What you do at your job or at home is also a health factor for you to consider. Some factors are very obvious, like the obvious danger of cave-ins to miners, or grease burns to house people. But many hazards are less obvious. You may be constantly under pressure to meet deadlines or to keep other people working; your body has to cope with stress which may be detrimental to your health. How much or how little you are able to communicate your feelings to family members or fellow workers may also be a source of stress, and thus a health hazard. These are at least as important to your health as being subjected to toxic chemicals that might poison your system. How you *feel* about the work you do will probably affect how you feel about your body.

OCCUPATIONAL HEALTH HAZARDS

Describe how you feel about your job or home. Describe anything such as stress, fumes, dust, or mechanical dangers that you feel are detrimental to your health. Don't overlook things like lighting, noises, smells, and conflicts with family members or fellow employees.

DRUGS AND SENSITIVITIES

This is the place to go over any drugs toward which you have any kind of allergic reaction. It is especially important that you have this information about *antibiotics* — penicillin, sulfa, tetracycline, etc. A minor allergic reaction, such as a skin rash, can tip you off to the possibility that the next time you take that drug you might have even more severe reactions, such as difficulty breathing.

Allergic reactions can be rash, itching, stomach ache, nausea, dizziness, anxiety, heart pounding like a drum, or other things.

Whenever a doctor gives you a prescription for drugs, tell them about the drugs to which you have had allergic reactions. Make certain they are not giving you one of these drugs, or a drug with elements of that drug in it. **Do not assume that the doctor will read the part of your medical records which would tell them about your allergic reactions to drugs.** Remind your doctor of your drug allergies each time he gives you a prescription.

The following list will help to remind you of drugs which you may have taken, and to which you had allergic reactions.

DRUGS WHICH SOMETIMES CAUSE ALLERGIC REACTIONS

*circle drugs to which you have had
any kind of allergic reaction*

Aspirin	Benzedrine or Dexedrine
Hay Fever medicine	Iron or anemia medicine
Penicillin	Tetracycline
Sulfa drugs	Other antibiotics
Pain medications	Phenobarbitol or barbiturates
Serum or antitoxins	Tetanus shot

*Write in the names of any other drugs or shots to which you have
had any kind of a bad reaction:*

If you do not know the name of a drug to which you had an allergic reaction, use the space below to describe that drug: why it was then given to you, its shape, size, and color. Pills, and other forms of medication, are color coded. *Your doctor can help you identify any pill you've taken.* Most doctors have a catalog of drugs manufactured in the United States which describes each drug by color, brand name, shape, size, and content. (See *Going Further*, page 333, *Physicians Desk Reference*.)

NOTES ON IDENTIFYING CERTAIN DRUGS

*Use the pictures below
to help you in your
descriptions.*

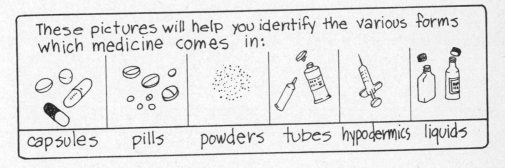

These pictures will help you identify the various forms which medicine comes in:

| capsules | pills | powders | tubes | hypodermics | liquids |

One last but important note: Many times doctors do not tell their patients the names of the drugs which they prescribe for them. But this is information which we think you should have. *Always ask your doctor the name of any drug which they prescribe for you.*

SYSTEMS REVIEW

In Mike's medical practice he has found that people keep coming back time after time with the same organs or systems of organs manifesting disease. It is possible for you to locate those organs of your body most prone to disease and to discover how these diseases come about. It is also possible for you to discover why your body selects these organs for illness while others are never affected. Your search for this knowledge can start with the tools we present in this chapter.

In the pages that follow we'll show you how to use a tool called *Systems Review.* With it you will locate the organs in your body in which disease most often occurs. Mike calls these organs "target organs." The first thing to know is that the healthiest people in the world have target organs. Discovering which organs they are takes you closer to the knowledge of how to stay well, since once you have located your target organs you can begin developing skills to keep them and all other parts of your body healthy.

By learning about your target organs you can watch for and can pay attention to situations and your own actions which might aggravate those particular areas of your body. You can learn to not aggravate them. If for example, you found that your skin was a target organ, you could turn your most positive attention to keeping it in the best possible shape, bathing it with soaps that would not irritate it or remove the protective surface oils, and avoiding contact with rough clothes, or chemicals which might be in the make-up, hair spray, or deodorant that you use. (We tell more about this in the chapters **Preventive Medicine** and **Diagnosis And Treatment**) In other words, you would learn to pay more attention to, and express more love toward, your skin than toward some other areas of your body that might need less attention.

On the following pages you will find a number of boxes, one for each organ or system of your body. You can use the contents of each of these boxes in three ways. (Turn to page 32 if you want to see the kinds of things you'll be dealing with.)

The drawing in each box shows you what that particular organ or system looks like. In most cases these drawings also show you where each organ or system is located in your body. **To use these drawings** first look at each one carefully, and then picture where these organs or systems are located in your own body. If you wish, touch yourself in the place indicated by the pictures. After you have done this for every drawing you will have completed what amounts to a mini-course in practical anatomy. The drawings you will find in this section will be used as symbols throughout the book where it is important for you to locate that organ in your body.

The list of symptoms in the center of each box is the *Systems Review* for the specific organ named. This inventory of common symptoms will be useful to you in two ways: to provide you with knowledge about your own body and its target organs, and to aid you in doing a thorough diagnosis of a present illness when you are sick. We will tell you more about these things further into the book.

To the right of the *Systems Review,* in most boxes, you will find some page numbers. These page numbers will refer you to either the *Preventive Medicine* section of this book or to other sections which tell you how to keep that particular organ or system in the best shape possible. It is *your guide to preventive medicine techniques* for each part of your body.

DOING THE SYSTEMS REVIEW

In going through these lists of symptoms, some people will find that they have experienced a large number of the symptoms noted. Others will feel that they have not had any of the symptoms *to a degree serious enough to note.* You will want to know how mild or severe these symptoms should have been for you to circle them. Here are some guidelines to follow that will help you decide:

Put a circle around symptoms for which you have sought any kind of treatment from a doctor or healer.

Put a circle around symptoms that have caused you discomfort — in the form of irritation, pain, or worry — enough to cause you to consider getting treatment or medical advice of any kind, even if you did not actually get this treatment or medical advice.

Put a circle around anything for which you had to go to a hospital, or which forced you to adjust your usual life style for an extended period of time.

Put a circle around anything for which you turned to the Diagnosis and Treatment section of this book.

You may wish to stop and consult with your imaginary doctor on any questions which may arise.

Some people become nervous when they begin circling symptoms, perhaps because they feel they are discovering that their body is not well. If you find yourself feeling this way, understand that it is normal to circle symptoms in several boxes. So relax and withhold your judgements about your body until you have completed this entire chapter.

You, like most other people, will end up with a more positive attitude toward your body and your health than you may now think is possible.

SKIN AND HAIR

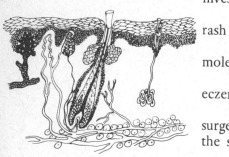

hives

rash

moles

eczema

surgery to remove any growth on the skin

_____
any other complaint?
_____
_____

athletes foot

dandruff

dry hair

oily hair

Pages 87-97, 111, 155-156, 201-217

EYES

wear glasses or contact lenses

eyes tear a lot

color blindness

night blindness

eyes sensitive to light

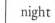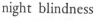

treatment for injury to eye or adjacent area

_____
any surgery?
_____

any other treatment?
_____
_____

any other complaint?
_____
_____

Pages 111, 115, 156, 157, 220-223

EARS

earache

drainage from ear

loss of hearing, either full or partial

punctured ear drum

surgery or treatment of
any kind

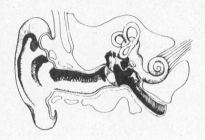

Pages 111,
158-160,
223-226

_____

_____

any other complaint?

_____

_____

NOSE

discharge from nose

head colds

sinus problems

nose bleed

allergies

nose running or sneezing

any treatment or surgery?

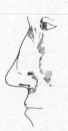

Pages 111,
160, 161,
227, 233-236,
239, 243, 292

_____

_____

any other complaint?

_____

_____

MOUTH

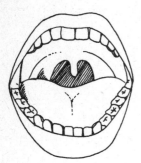

toothache	abcessed teeth	Pages 111, 161-163, 228, 233-239
false teeth	partial plate	
sore tongue	sore cheeks (inside)	

sore roof of mouth

sore gums   difficulty chewing

difficulty swallowing

sore throat   tonsillitis

tonsils removed   dry mouth

salivate so much it bothers me

change in the way things taste

any surgery?

_____

_____

any other complaint?

_____

_____

BREASTS

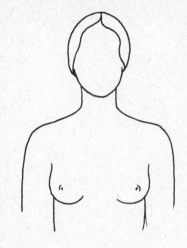

soreness   tenderness

problems with nipples

lumps in breasts

any treatment or surgery?

_____

_____

any other complaint?

_____

_____

Pages 193-197,
111, 163, 164,
230-231

LUNGS

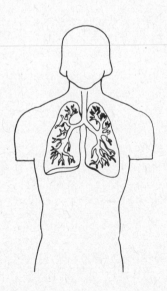

cough

coughing up a lot of phlegm

coughing up blood

difficulty breathing

chest pains   wheezing

pneumonia   bronchitis

congested lungs   tuberculosis

any treatment or surgery?

_____

_____

any other complaint?

_____

_____

Pages 98-118,
164-168,
233-247

HEART

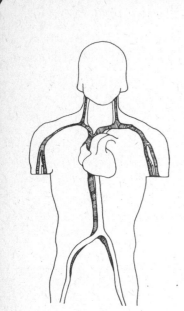

get short of breath	nausea	Pages 67-142, 168-169, 180-181, 299-307, 320-326
pounding of heart	palpitations	
high blood pressure	pain in chest	
low blood pressure	heart murmur	
I get swollen ankles		
vomiting of blood		

any treatment or surgery?

_____

_____

any other complaint?

_____

GASTROINTESTINAL

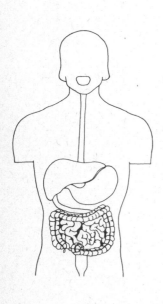

loss of appetite	indigestion	Pages 72-86, 111, 169-171, 248-263
stomach pains	nausea	
vomiting	belching	
excessive farting	use laxatives	
take a lot of antacids		
blood in bowels	hemorrhoids	
difficulty moving bowels		
vomit up blood	bleeding from rectum	

recent change in bowel movement habits

any treatment or surgery?

_____

any other complaint?

_____

GENITOURINARY

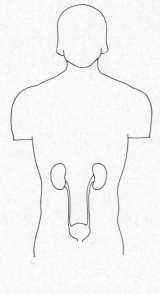

difficulty stopping or starting the flow of urine

Pages 87-92, 100-103, 171-176, 264-274

sores in genital area

pain when urinating

urgency to urinate

bothered by need to urinate frequently

wake up in the night to urinate

blood in urine   urine looks cloudy

urine dribbles when I don't want it to

discharge from penis or vagina

past history of kidney trouble

past history of bladder trouble

past history of unusual findings from urinalysis

sugar in urine   venereal disease

any treatment or surgery?

_____

_____

any other complaint?

_____

_____

EXTREMITIES

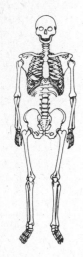

pain in knees, elbows or any other joints

swollen joints   rheumatism

arthritis   muscular weakness

numbness   difficulty walking

tingling sensations in fingers or toes

difficulty with any body movements

any treatment or surgery?

_____

_____

any other complaint?

_____

_____

Pages 98-118,
176-179,
275-279

REPRODUCTIVE ORGANS
Women

pain during menstruation

pain directly before menstruation

cramps   spotting

any treatment or surgery?

_____

_____

any other complaint?

_____

_____

(See
Genitourinary)

REPRODUCTIVE ORGANS
Men

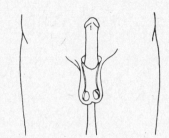

hernia   rupture   (See
                                                     Genitourinary)

circumcision after infancy

any sores

any treatment or surgery?

_____

_____

any other complaint?

_____

_____

NERVOUS SYSTEM

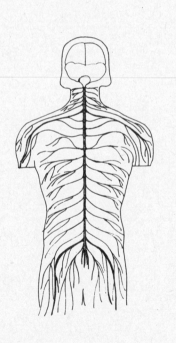

headache   dizziness   Pages 98-142,
                                        176-179,
weakness   convulsions   192

nervousness   paralysis

sensory changes

feeling pins and needles

use drugs daily (alcohol, marijuana
opiates, tranquilizers, uppers, downers,
etc.)

any treatment or surgery?
_____

_____

any other complaint?

_____

_____

ENDOCRINE SYSTEM

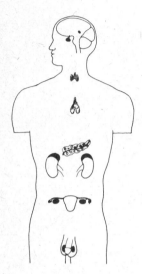

Unquenchable thirst or hunger

urination so frequent as to aggravate you

thyroid disorder

any other glandular problems that you know of

any treatment or surgery?

_____

_____

any other complaints?

_____

_____

Pages 315, 342

AURA

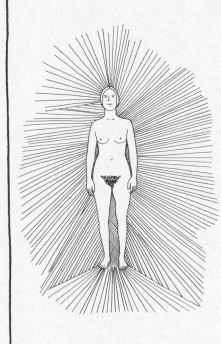

In western medical terms the nerve net of the body produces a magnetic field just as the wire circuit of a radio transmitter produces a magnetic field. This field extends out from the body and expresses its overall condition. The magnetic field that makes up the aura of the body can be visualized in terms of colors. Imagine that your body is surrounded by a field of color which reflects its condition. Now imagine the colors of the field as they extend from various parts of the body as mentioned in the *Systems Review* above. Do the colors of the auras over parts of your body appear: absent, muddy, dark, bright, weak, ethereal, or vibrant? Each organ or system has its own aura that goes to make up the whole aura surrounding your body. We will tell you more about this in the directions for doing your *Bright Life* chart. In the meantime, become accustomed to considering the aura as one of the *systems* of your body. In the space below, briefly describe the color and condition of your aura.

Pages 50-53, 64, 113

If you got this far but were not sure what you were circling, go back to the instructions (page 31) and note that there are *four separate* instructions for what to circle. Read each of the four instructions over again, and then go through the entire review four times, once with each separate instruction in mind.

☆　☆　☆

People who circle many things for which they have *never* sought treatment from a doctor or healer, often have an unrealistic image of their body as "sick." People who circle nothing even though they have received treatment or have seen a doctor for some of the symptoms listed, also have an unrealistic appraisal of their health. If you find yourself in either one of these groups we advise you to develop a more moderate picture of your health, based on the instructions for doing the *Systems Review*. As you get further into this book you will discover some of the positive aspects of disease. But in order to make full use of these positive aspects you will first need to have a clear picture of your target organs.

DOCTOR DIAGNOSED DISEASES AND OPERATIONS

Go through the following list and circle any disease which you have had diagnosed by a doctor. Use this list as a reminder to you of diseases which you have had but which you may not have noted your first time through the Systems Review. *If you find that you've forgotten anything go back to the* Systems Review *and make additions.*

Heart disease, stroke or high blood pressure

Strep throat   Ulcers

Glaucoma   Epilepsy

Pneumonia   Tuberculosis

Asthma   Hepatitis or Liver disease

Kidney disease   Bladder Infection

Gallstones or gall bladder trouble

Veneral disease (V.D.)

Syphilis   Gonorrhea

Any other disease you have which you consider important enough to note.
Specify_____

_____

OPERATIONS WHICH YOU HAVE HAD

Make a list of any operations which you have had. This list should include even relatively minor operations such as appendix and hernia surgery.

1.   3.

2.   4.

In doing this list you may be reminded of symptoms which you had either before or after an operation. If you discover anything that you forgot to note in the *Systems Review* go back and make these additions now.

43 .

HEALTH COLORS CHARTS

The Health Colors Chart which follows is a tool for condensing into a single image all the information and knowledge which you have collected when you did the *Systems Review*. The image you create here will give you an immediate visual reference to your target organs and systems. Because it is visual, the *Health Colors Chart* works within the visual memory centers of your mind, and thus does not limit your body knowledge to a verbal list such as the original *Systems Review* list that you have already completed.

The *Health Colors Chart* works best when you choose your own colors to "code" it. Because of the detail and the size of the charts we provide in the book I'd suggest that you get a set of colored pencils to do the job. Here are the guidelines for coloring the chart.

Study the *Health Colors Chart* (page 45 for women 47 for men) until you feel comfortable with it.

Examine your colored pencils. **Scribble small patches of color** on a piece of paper. Then **ask yourself how each color makes you feel.** You will probably find, as we did, that some colors evoke strong feelings while others seem to evoke no feelings at all.

Go through the *Systems Review*. Stop at each symptom that you have circled. Ask yourself **which color best expresses the way you feel toward the organ in which that symptom occured.** Then turn to the *Health Colors Chart* and fill in that color in the corresponding body part. Do this for the entire *Systems Review*. You may also wish to draw in, on your *Health Colors Chart,* such things as **surgical scars and eyeglasses.**

Choose a color for each part of your body on the *Health Colors Chart.* However, if you feel that some organs should not be colored in, trust that feeling and leave them blank.

You will notice that the **Nervous System** *is shown on the Health Colors Chart as a space around the body between the skin and the Aura.* Color this area using the same guidelines as for coloring any other organ or system of your body. Do the same for coloring the *Aura.*

Remember as you do your *Health Colors Chart* that you want to choose colors that will have personal meaning for you. It is important here to allow your feelings to dictate your actions.

HEALTH
COLORS
CHART

45

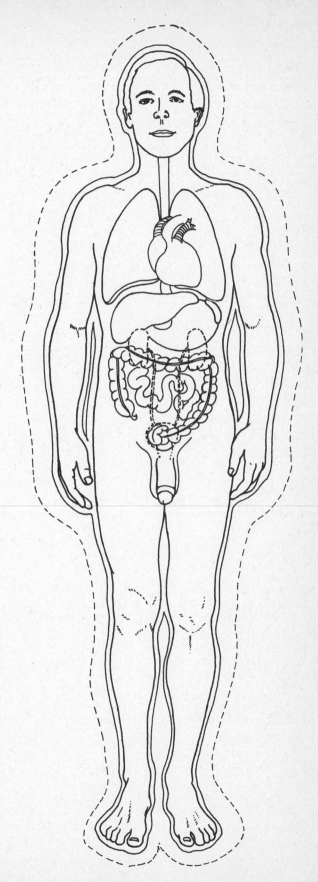

HEALTH
COLORS
CHART

FINISHING UP

After you have completed your *Health Colors Chart*, sit in a relaxed position and gaze at it until you have a clear image of the chart in your mind's eye. To further commit the chart to memory, do the following:

Do the exercise for getting in touch with your imaginary doctor. But before you have your imaginary doctor enter your imaginary room, imagine that you are putting your *Health Colors Chart* on the wall. This chart can be as large as you wish. In my imaginary room I have a life-sized *Health Colors Chart* of my body. No matter what size you make it, be sure the information it contains is accurate.

Have your imaginary doctor enter your imaginary room. Then show him or her your *Health Colors Chart.* Discuss the chart with them if you wish.

A friend of ours who did this part of the book for the first time reports that her imaginary doctor, after studying her *Health Colors Chart,* went into her body and massaged her stomach. The woman had a history of ulcers. As a result of the experience she learned how to fully relax her stomach for the first time. This new skill allows her to avoid her previous difficulties caused by her "nervous stomach."

You have now completed the *Systems Review* and *Health Colors Chart* section of the book.

BRIGHT LIFE CHARTS

On the pages immediately following, you will find charts to color, similar to the *Health Colors* charts which you already did after the *Systems Review.* With the *Bright Life* charts you create an image of your body as completely healthy, alive, vibrant, and energetic. By doing the *Bright Life* chart you activate millions of brain cells around this very positive body image, thus sending out signals of health and energy to every part of your actual body, increasing your own energy and health measurably. Here are the instructions for coloring your own *Bright Life* chart.

Get out your colored pencils and choose colors which express health and vibrant energy to you.

Ask yourself what color best expresses the way you feel toward your healthiest organ, and begin coloring your *Bright Life* chart that color. Then improvise freely. Use many colors. Send colors radiating out from that organ in all directions.

Color each organ of your body in the brightest, most beautiful ways that you can imagine. Decorate the chart freely. Decorate the target organs, making them all radiate absolute health, strength, beauty, and energy.

Pick the most vibrant colors and do the aura around your body until it glows and vibrates with color. Create an image of your body that glows and sparkles like the most beautiful thing you can imagine.

When you are done, stare at the image you have created, in bright, indirect sunlight if possible, for half a minute or so. Then close your eyes. You will now see your *Bright Life* chart duplicated in your mind's eye. Keep your eyes closed. Take a deep breath. Exhale, imagining that your breath is sending out greater energy to your mental image. Take another deep breath, exhale, and imagine that this breath is magnifying both the size and the intensity of the image you see in your mind's eye. Take another breath, and exhale. Send still more energy to your image — the colors of your body image glowing, shimmering, becoming more and more intense. Enjoy your body image as a bright new planet in the universe. Bask in its brightness for as long as you wish. Now open your eyes and go away, with the knowledge that you can create this image of your body at any time that you wish.

On the next starry night you may wish to pick out a star or other body in the universe which will become your cosmic body image. Choose one that represents to you the same kind of vibrant health and energy that you discovered in doing your own *Bright Life* chart. Meditate on this image whenever you wish to improve your health, increase your energy, or improve your feelings about your life.

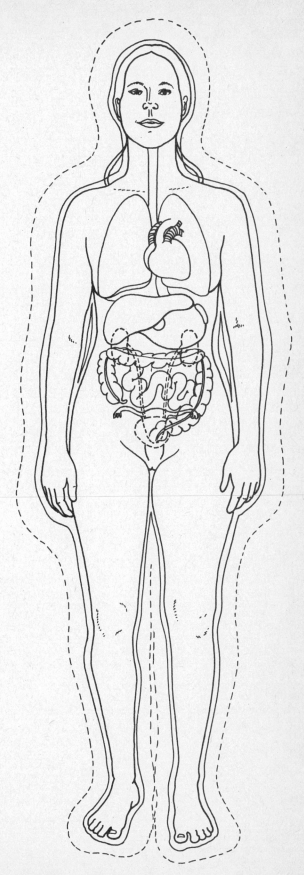

BRIGHT
LIFE CHART

51

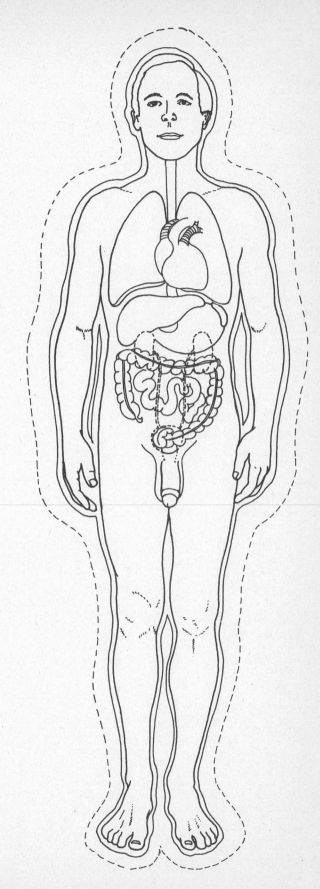

BRIGHT LIFE
CHART

53

MIRROR MIRROR

Mirror Mirror is a simple exercise for getting acquainted with your body by:

Communicating with each organ and system of your body in order to read its relative health.

Giving yourself a light massage.

Teaching yourself to visualize the image of your body in your mind's eye.

Keeping in touch with the shape, size, tension, texture, and sensitivity of all the areas of your body.

Using the information you collected in the *Health Colors* chart to visualize target organs of your own body.

Translating the image you created in the *Bright Life* chart to the reality of your own body.

This exercise can be done once (now) or it can be done daily. How often you do it is up to you.

GETTING READY

You will need two mirrors for doing this exercise: one hand mirror six inches or more in diameter, and one full-length mirror. Mount your full length mirror on a wall in a room where you will feel comfortable being naked and where you will not have to think about being disturbed as you do the exercise. (At present prices — 1973 — you can buy the best plate glass mirror, measuring 18 x 36 inches, at a glass store for about $15.00.)

GETTING ACQUAINTED

Many people have a mental image of the way they wish their body looked: thinner, fatter, taller, shorter than it actually is. Take off your clothes and jewelry, and stand in front of your full length mirror. As you look at the image of your body, are you satisfied with what you see? If you are, that's healthy. Are you dissatisfied? Then you may be blinded by your mental image of how you wish your body would look. If so, indulge yourself with a comparison for a moment. Talk to your body. If, for example, you wish that your legs were thinner:

Look at your legs in the mirror and say, "Legs, I wish you were thinner." You may also imagine yourself as your legs talking back; "I would be thinner if you would give me more exercise." If there are any parts that you'd like to have different, tell those parts exactly what you feel about them, and tell them how you would like them to be. Then listen to them talk back to you.

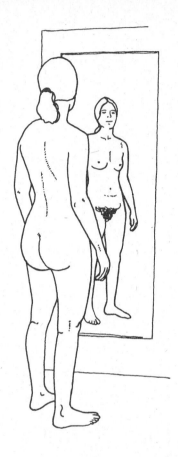

Now drop your wishes. Put them out of your mind, and try to find the beauty of your own body as it now appears before you. Here are some suggestions to help you to do this:

Understand that most **concepts of physical beauty are arbitrarily established** by the advertising world. You do not need to accept those standards. Your own body has its own beauty.

Imagine that your body is the only one in the world. There are no others, and so your body establishes the only standards for physical beauty in existence.

If a loved one has been telling you that you should be fatter or thinner than you are, quietly suspend your feelings about those wishes. Understand that you are not permanently rejecting those thoughts, nor are you rejecting the person who voiced the wishes that your body was different than it is.

Imagine that your imaginary doctor is telling you that you have a beautiful body. It is sound and in good health — or you can make it so — feel free to enjoy having the body you have.

If you are unable to accomplish these things on the first try, keep at it until you can look at your body and be happy with it as it is. **Learn to see and accept the image of your own body. There is none other like it in the world.**

Now begin exploring your body from angles you may have never seen:

Take your hand mirror and use it to look at your back and sides in the full length mirror.

Put the hand mirror on the floor, and then stand over it. Look down at the image of your body that you see from that vantage point.

Dance naked in front of the full length mirror. Then suddenly stop as though to freeze your motion. Look at your image in the mirror. Study how the muscles look. Stop yourself in many different motions.

Pick up your feet and study the soles in the mirror.

Turn your back to the mirror. Then bend over as though to touch your toes. Look back at your image in the mirror.

If you have long hair, lift it up and look at the back and the sides of your neck, using the mirrors to accomplish this.

Play with your image. Explore the possibilities that the mirrors hold for seeing your entire body. Play until you feel completely comfortable doing so.

HOW TO USE THE MIRRORS FOR HEALTH

There are several ways to use *Mirror Mirror.* First read *Mapping the Tour of Your Body.* After you have learned the *body tour,* you can use it for: giving yourself an over-all massage (both for pleasure and to stimulate circulation); to visualize your own body in your mind; to read the body's messages; to project an image of perfect health and high energy to your body. In the following pages we will show you how to do these things.

MAPPING THE TOUR OF YOUR BODY

This is the general route to follow when doing *Mirror Mirror.* Use it as a guideline to cover your entire body, from head to foot. Do as much of the exercise as possible without losing fingertip contact with your body.

HEAD: Begin with your hair. Touch it. Feel it with all your fingers.

Move your fingers down the back of your head to the base of your skull.

Draw your hands forward, around the sides of your head to your ears. Feel your ears using all your fingertips.

Now move your fingers to your temples. Caress your temples lightly.

FACE: Move your fingertips to your forehead. Caress your forehead lightly.

Close your eyes and allow your fingertips to brush lightly over your eyebrows, and then feel your eyeballs under your closed eyelids.

Move your fingers to the highest part of your cheeks. Massage them lightly.

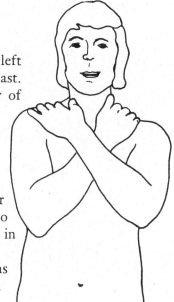

Move your fingers to the center of your forehead, in the place called the "third eye." Rest there for a moment, then move these fingers down your face, slowly one finger on each side of your nose. Follow the line down each side of your nose and out to the corners of your lips.

Trace your mouth with your fingertips in whatever way feels good to you.

Let your jaw relax. Press your cheeks just enough to feel your teeth through your cheeks. Feel your gums and teeth in this way from front to back.

Drop your hands to your sides. Relax.

NECK: Now tip your head back. With your left hand, caress the right side of your neck, starting just above the shoulder and working around to the center of your windpipe. Then do the other side of your neck with your right hand. Do one side at a time.

CHEST: Begin as shown in drawing.

Slowly move your right hand down over your left breast, and your left hand down across your right breast. Massage your breasts for a moment. Stop at the center of your rib cage.

Drop your hands to your sides for a moment. Relax.

With your right hand, reach around to the left side of your body, feeling your ribs as far back as you can reach. Move your hand around, massaging as much of your body as you can feel. Then massage and caress around to the center of your rib cage. Do both sides of your body in the same way.

Find your *sternum* — that hard flat bone that runs down the center of your rib cage. Massage your sternum lightly from top to bottom.

ABDOMEN: First imagine your abdomen as illustrated:

Place your hand in the center of the upper right quadrant. Move your hand in a slight circular motion, pressing firmly but gently. Do this in each quadrant of your abdomen.

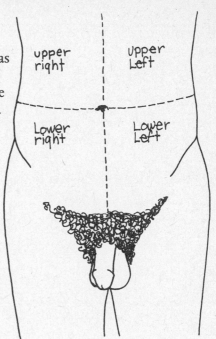

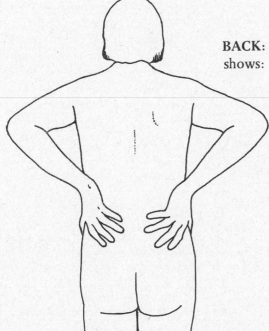

BACK: Reach as far back as possible, as the picture shows:

Feel and rub as much of your back as you can reach in this way, working all the way down to your buttocks.

GENITALS AND LIMBS: Start as drawing shows.

Press gently and move your fingers in small circles, doing a light massage.

Move your hands lightly over your genitals.

Move your hands to the upper part of your left thigh, one hand on the inside of your thigh, the other on the outside. Massage up and down from top to bottom. Do both thighs in this way.

Move your hands to your knee, one hand on the inside, the other on the outside of your leg. Feel your kneecap and the entire area all the way around the knee joint.

Move your hands down the calf of your leg, using your hands the same way you used them to massage your thigh and knee.

Feel your ankle all the way around. Do both ankles.

Lift your foot and feel it top and bottom. Feel each toe, and feel between each toe.

Do both legs from top to bottom.

Now do your shoulders and arms. Begin at the top of your shoulder. Give your shoulder muscles a good rub.

Feel the muscles of your upper arm, all the way around.

Feel your elbow with all its little knobs and bumps.

Feel your forearm. Stop at your wrist and feel it all the way around.

Do the palm of your hand and the back of it.

Finish up by doing each finger and thumb.

Do both arms in the same way from top to bottom.

FINISHING UP

Upon finishing the body tour, or any of the other *Mirror Mirror* exercises, you may find that it helps to do the following:

Place your hands on your buttocks and do this:

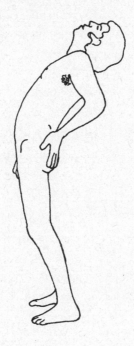

Do not stretch or force your muscles. Go easy. Be good to yourself.

Lean forward and touch the floor with your finger tips.

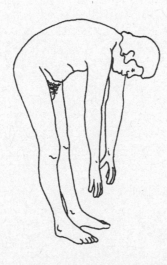

Reach as high as you can, standing on tiptoes. Stretch upwards as high as you can.

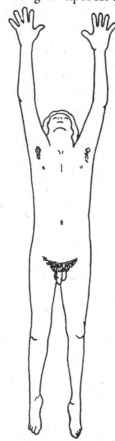

Drop your hands to your sides. Then *scissor* out your legs. Stretch your arms out from your sides as far as you can reach.

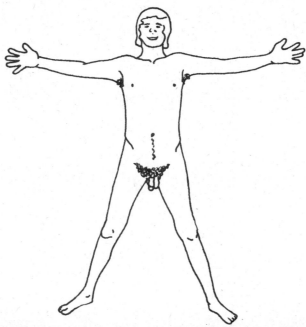

Return to a normal standing position. Visualize your body as in the paragraph above, *BRIGHT LIFE AND YOUR BODY*. You are now in great shape to start the day.

WAYS TO USE THE BODY TOUR

Now that you know the basic *body tour* there are several ways to use it. In the next few pages we describe some of those ways.

You will find that each exercise does a different thing. I'd suggest that you read them through to get acquainted with what's there. Then keep them in the back of your mind as "tools" that are available to you any time you need them. You may find uses in your own life for all of them, one of them, or none of them. You might find that one of the massage techniques offers you a way to relax your body and increase circulation after a long, tense day at work. Or, you might find that one of the *Bright Life And Your Body* exercises works well for you as a way to start your mornings on positive grounds.

Go wherever you want with these exercises. Work out your own ways to use *Mirror Mirror* — either as a daily routine, or as an occasional exercise to help you over the rough spots. Become familiar with what we offer here, and then improvise on these exercises, or invent your own ways of doing the body tour.

GIVE YOURSELF A MASSAGE

This is the easiest and most pleasurable way to do *Mirror Mirror.* Just follow the regular body tour as described above, but use your fingers caressingly as you go. Or, move your hands vigorously and in firm circular motions as you go over your body. The first method will stimulate sense receptors in your skin and will increase the flow of energy over your whole body. The second method will help you relax and open small capillaries under the skin, thus increasing the circulation of blood throughout your body. Watch your image in the mirror as you do the massage, and enjoy the sight of your hands moving over your flesh.

A third method of massage is to use firm pressure with your fingertips, pressing deep into muscles to relax them. Imagine that your fingers are sending energy and life to the areas you are massaging, to relax your muscles, increase circulation, and bring new energy to your body.

All these self massage methods are healthy and pleasurable. Work with combinations of these techniques for the greatest benefit to you. When you are sick, massage will help you to open capillaries to areas that may be sick. **By opening these capillaries you make it possible for health-bringing nutriments to get to cells more quickly, you increase the speed at which waste products excreted by the cells are carried away from the cells and thus out of your body, and you make it possible for antibiotics to get to the site of the infection.**

READ YOUR BODY'S MESSAGES

Do the body tour with light fingertip pressure. But this time imagine that your fingertips have the ability to pick up signals sent out by all the parts of your body. Here's a model to help you with this:

Each cell that helps make up each organ of your body, **contains a radio transmitter. Your fingertips are receivers** which pick up every signal sent out by each cell. These receivers have direct lines to your brain. Each cell transmits information about its health.

Here's a second model:

Each organ of your body has its own aura. **When healthy, every organ projects bright colors.** When unhealthy, the colors are dull. Each of your **fingertips possesses an eye** which sees the aura of each organ. These eyes connect to your brain in the same way that your regular eyes connect.

Here's a third model:

Each cell in your body possesses a magnetic field. When a cell is fully healthy this magnetic field is strong. When a cell is unhealthy the magnetic field is weak. Imagine that your **fingertips are sensitive to the strong or weak pulls from the magnetic field** projected by each cell.

Use any of these models, or invent your own, as a way to read the relative health of each part of your body, as you do your self-massage.

Stand in front of the mirror and study the image of your body for a moment. Then, using your *Health Color* chart as a reference, picture an organ or system in your body. Allow your feelings and intuition to dictate this choice. Then move your hands over that area, reading the relative health of that area by whatever reading model you wish to use. After you learn where the organs and systems fit in your body you can read your entire body from head to foot very quickly.

In doing a reading, **pay attention to the shape, size, texture, tension, and sensitivity of all areas of your body.** Pay attention to what you see and what you feel. By doing the body tour every day or week you can learn to recognize changes in your relative health days or maybe even weeks before any disease symptoms appear. With this kind of forewarning, you can apply techniques described in the *Preventive Medicine* and *Diagnosis and Treatment* sections of this book to prevent disease from becoming manifested in your body.

HEALTH COLORS AND YOUR BODY

Stand naked in front of your full-length mirror. Now visualize your completed *Health Colors* chart. When you have it visualized, open your eyes to the image of your body in the mirror. Go back and forth between your visualized *Health Colors* chart and the mirror image of your body. After a few moments you will be able to visualize how all the information recorded in your *Health Colors* chart applies to your body. The ability to do this will prove valuable to you in doing readings of target organs as well as for many of the exercises described in *Preventive Medicine* and elsewhere in the book.

To project an image of absolute health to your mind's eye, follow up this exercise with *Bright Life and Your Body*, described below.

BRIGHT LIFE AND YOUR BODY

Stand naked in front of your full-length mirror. Close your eyes and visualize your completed *Bright Life* chart. When you have visualized it, open your eyes to the image of your body in the mirror. Close your eyes again and visualize your own body taking on the colors of the *Bright Life* chart. Visualize the colors radiating out from your center. Imagine the colors becoming brighter and brighter. Feel the colors as energy permeating every cell of every organ of your body. Imagine the color and energy filling your body, extending outward in all directions.

Close your eyes very tightly. Inhale deeply, then exhale slowly, imagining the colors radiating out from the center of your body, becoming brighter and brighter, with each breath exhaled, expanding further and further into the space around you. Do this for 15 seconds or more.

Once you have learned this exercise the **choice will be in your hands to create an image of your body as "sick" or an image of your body as "well."** Mike and I fully believe that the vibrant image of your body, in your mind's eye, promotes health. Whenever you detect even the smallest signs of disease or fatigue in your body, do this visualization exercise, either with or without the mirror. It is a basic technique for taking control of your body's health.

At different times in your life you may have had a mental image of yourself as small and unable to meet a challenge. For most people it happens before going to a job interview, or before taking an examination, or in any number of high stress situations. Your mental image often affects the way you come across in the interview or exam. We've found that by doing the above exercise before going to such a situation, your chances of success will be improved tremendously.

Here's a second exercise to help you, one that can be done any time of the day and nearly anywhere you happen to be.

Close your eyes and imagine your body in your full-length mirror. Imagine yourself clothed or naked, whichever you wish. Now imagine, and *feel* yourself, becoming bigger and bigger, brighter and brighter, healthier and more alive. Keep your eyes closed and meditate on this image for fifteen seconds or more, and with each exhalation of your breath imagine yourself becoming larger and brighter. If you wish imagine yourself in the interview or test succeeding tremendously. Keep this image working in your mind when you go into the job interview, examination, or other stress situation. You will discover that you will feel stronger and better able to succeed each time you do this.

AN INSTANT HEALING EXERCISE

Here's an instant healing exercise which you can do when you want to bring extra healing energy to a part of your body that feels tired, tense or ill. You can do it no matter where you are, so it's a nice skill to have:

Relax for a moment. Take several deep breaths. Form a mental picture of your body. (Look at the Bright Life chart if you need a simple image to work from.)

Scan your mental picture until you naturally stop at a part of your body that you feel needs healing energy. Trust your own decision in this. It may be a part of your body that has been sick, that is sick, or that just needs energy.

Now imagine your own favorite color, or a color that makes you feel alive, vibrant, and energetic. Imagine the color on the picture of your body in the area that you wish to heal. Then imagine a feeling of health, which the color represents to you, moving into your actual body.

Breath in and out. As you exhale, imagine your breath is increasing the intensity of the color and the feeling of health that your chosen color represents. Imagine that the colors are glowing, shimmering, becoming more and more intense.

Imagine the area of your body that you wish to heal becoming relaxed, pulsing with life, and vibrant — more and more healthy.

☆   ☆   ☆

By doing this exercise you activate millions of brain cells which send out signals for healing energy. You increase blood flow and bring your body's healing antibodies, hormones, cleansing fluids, and nutriments to the part of your body that you wish to heal. Scientists can measure this process in action.

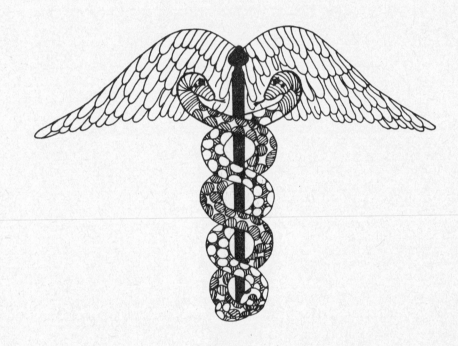

PREVENTIVE MEDICINE

PREVENTIVE MEDICINE

This chapter tells you how to stay well. Here we describe a number of skills for you to use to get in touch with your body's messages. That means learning to detect the often faint messages which your body sends out before it actually gets a disease. The messages are signals to your consciousness that you need more rest, different foods, relaxation, sleep, exercise, a change in your environment, or something else to improve your life. When you learn how to read these messages you are able to take positive actions, on your own, to bring yourself back to harmony and health.

With the information in this chapter you can reclaim your own body's health. You can fully participate in improving your present health and preventing yourself from getting ill. You can also use these skills to help your body heal itself when you are sick, and to prevent minor illnesses from becoming serious ones.

Parts of this chapter deal with areas of life that many people ordinarily overlook because they involve minor details, each of which, taken by itself, may seem insignificant. It is important to understand that the small details accumulate, each one sapping just a little bit of energy, but the sum total expending alot of energy. Health problems which require a huge amount of the body's energy for healing are often caused by things which most people don't give a second thought to, since they are so much an accepted part of their life. Rashes and bacterial infections caused by clothing that is too tight, or clothing made of a fabric that does not breathe, are examples of this. (More on this in the clothing section.)

In Aldous Huxley's book, *Island,* the island where the story takes place has many "mynah" birds which were taught to call out, "Attention. Attention. Here and now, boys; here and now." It was a wise man's idea to remind people to take note of their lives and the world around them at all times. That might well be the theme of this chapter of the book, which is essentially an operator's manual on conserving energy within your own body, and directing this energy where you want it to go. Paying attention to the smallest details in your life is the central path toward improving and maintaining a high quality of life within each living cell in your body. And that means having a well body.

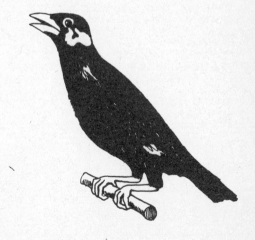

The tools which we describe in this chapter are fun. They are filled with positive energy. They are ways to feel happier, more at peace with yourself and your environment, and can elevate your feelings (get you high) in addition to helping you achieve a well body.

☆ ☆ ☆

The instructions in this section are detailed, and in a few cases rather lengthy. For this reason, don't ask yourself to assimilate everything here in one reading. You can read it straight through if you wish. Or you can follow your feelings, or your intuition, and start with the subject which you feel most strongly drawn to, because it interests you, because it is a part of your life which you would like to improve, or whatever.

Sit down in a quiet place with the book and imagine yourself in whatever situation the book discusses. For example, if the book is talking about bathing, imagine yourself bathing; if it's a food trip you're doing, imagine yourself in the kitchen, or eating. In this way, the instructions will have direct bearing on your imagined state of being, and so will become directly applicable to the moment.

You can use your imaginary doctor to help you with whatever parts of *Preventive Medicine* you want. The imaginary doctor may prove particularly helpful when you are doing instructions which ask you to evaluate your present situation. Also, a friend may be helpful to read you sections which ask that you do some activity with your eyes shut.

WHAT THIS CHAPTER CONTAINS

Eating Becomes You: Ways to get in touch with your own particular food needs. Also contains therapeutic diets and nutritional charts. Page 72.

Skin, Bacteria, And Chemistry: Tells you about your skin's interactions with chemicals and bacteria, and how to keep your skin healthy. Also tells about specific hygiene methods to prevent the spread of disease when someone is sick in your household. Page 87.

Clothes: How to use clothes to increase your body's energy, and how to evaluate how your own clothes affect your body. Page 93.

Exercise: How muscular activity can release energy blocks and bring muscles into harmony with surrounding organs. Also contains instructions for exercises to accomplish this easily. Page 98.

Relaxation Exercises: In many ways this is a key section of the book. In it we present a number of exercises to relieve tension and increase the flow of energy throughout your body. Page 105.

Rest-Work Cycles: Tells you how to get in touch with your own body's rest needs, and how to prevent fatigue. Page 119.

Sleep: How to get in touch with your sleep needs, and how to improve your sleep patterns. Page 125.

Dreaming: How to recall, understand, and participate in dreams. Page 128.

Life Rhythms: How universal rhythms and cycles affect your life. Page 134.

Where You Be: A way to get in touch with your inner vision of what you would like your external environment to be, and how to help make this vision a reality. Page 138.

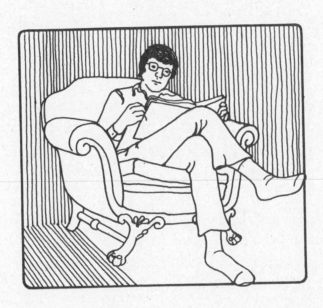

EATING BECOMES YOU

The quality of food which you take into your body will do a great deal to determine the quality of life that goes on in each cell of your body.

People are becoming discriminating about what they feed their bodies, wanting to know what the food actually contains: like how many and what chemicals, and what nutriment they contain. On the other hand, the fadism surrounding the subject of diet can become, in subtle ways, negative. There's a potential error in becoming so committed to one diet or another that you begin to tune out your body's messages; you ignore what your body is telling you that it wants or needs, and you insist that it stick with one diet or another which you have intellectually decided is the right one. And so you get out of rhythm with your body. You get into a conflict between your mind and your body, and the result is energy blocked or diverted from your use.

Food habits can be radically changed by trying different diets, and this in itself can be worth the effort. Like traveling to places you've never been before, trying out different diets presents possibilities that are difficult to imagine. From that experience you can learn how your body interacts with a large variety of foods.

At the moment, Mike and Nancy grow their own fruits and vegetables, bake their own bread, and have a small flock of chickens to provide them with eggs. They eat a moderate amount of meat, supplementing their protein needs with eggs, cheese and nuts.

Linda and Hal, being urban dwellers, have no land suitable for growing their own food, so they buy most of their food from a natural foods store, and from the local supermarket. They avoid processed foods, and are careful about where their food comes from, preferring food grown within a 150 mile radius of their home, food from small farms rather than from giant Agro-business complexes, and food from stores run by people who appear to have good feelings toward food.

GENERALIZATIONS ABOUT FOOD

There are numerous theories about food, some of them based on practices which are thousands of years old, such as Yoga diets, while others are more current, such as the work of George Ohsawa or Adelle Davis. You can shop around for their books in any large book store. Some themes which appear to be common to most food theories are:

Your body is best able to digest the food you take in, and is most able to use the energy which the food contains, when you eat slowly, chew completely, and eat the amount that is most comfortable for your body.

Foods which are free of fats — especially animal fats — cause your body less energy expenditure than foods which are heavy in fats.

Foods which are free of chemicals — sprays and preservatives — are probably better for your body than foods which have those chemicals in them.

Eating with a calm, relaxed attitude aids digestion.

Protein foods — meats, cheese, eggs, whole grains, nuts, and legumes — are a more stable energy source than foods with a high sugar content.

But here agreement ends. The kinds of foods you eat, and how they are prepared and served, individualizes all the diets we know of.

GETTING IN TOUCH WITH FOOD

Food involves, or can involve, one or more of the following:

Nourishment: At its most basic level, food provides the stuff your body needs to keep going — vitamins, minerals, protein, bulk, trace elements, water, etc.

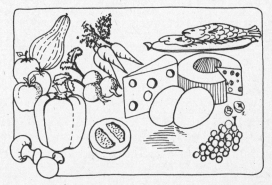

Life Rhythms: Everyone's body has individualized standards as to what, how much, and when to eat. This is most obvious in *quenching* your thirst — being one of the last remnants the adult in our society has of satisfying his body's food needs according to its messages. The newborn infant is, for example, completely in touch with his body rhythms — crying for food when his body is in need of it. As he or she grows older, the child is taught to adjust his life rhythms to rhythms which are more convenient for the family or for society. Imagine what would happen to the parents of three or more children if these social rhythms were not imposed on the infant. The parents would have to spend all their time preparing food and feeding the kids. Food *cravings*, like quenching your thirst, reflect your body responding to basic life rhythms, an example of this being the pregnant mother's *cravings* for foods with calcium, since her body uses almost twice as much calcium during pregnancy as it does when she is not pregnant.

Habit And Tradition: You tend to eat what your parents ate and prepared for you. Thus whole cultures can be identified by the foods they eat. Food habits and traditions are not easily changed since they involve a complex of activities, such as shopping and preparation, as well as the style of serving, and the sensations of touch, smell, taste, and sight which are involved. Digestion too, is different for different foods. To change food habits and/or traditions, you may need to deal with all of these things.

Social: Food often brings people together, sharing either the same food or the same space and time. This aspect of eating is reflected in the fact that most societies and families establish certain hours of the day to eat, a time for people to gather together.

Entertainment: Gourmet foods epitomize eating as entertainment. It is a way to be entertained, eating even though you may not be hungry, in the same way that dancing can be a form of entertainment when your body does not particularly need the exercise.

Substitution: People eat many foods not because their bodies need the nourishment they contain, nor for any of the other reasons listed above, but because the experiences of eating those foods satisfy an otherwise non-food related need. The ice cream cone that brings you up when you are feeling down belongs in this group, as does eating the box of chocolates when what you really want is for your absent lover to be near you. Not that these are the only reasons for eating ice cream cones or candies. Other people may eat meat or vegetables for the same reasons, too. Food substitution is a completely individualized thing.

Food As Medicine: The use of food to cure health complaints belongs in this group. Treating symptoms also belongs here. This includes everything from camomile tea for calming a nervous stomach to wine and other alcoholic beverages or narcotics for "loosening up."

Unless you are a very holy monk living on white light on a mountain top in India, and free of all distractions, your food habits will probably include elements of all of the above.

FOOD AND THE BODY'S MESSAGES: CREATE YOUR OWN DIET

The point of eating, simplified to its essences, is this: how do you get the highest quality of energy to each living cell of your body, enjoying it the most and expending the least amount of energy getting it? Instead of suggesting one diet for you to follow, we suggest that you create your own. You can use the following paragraphs as guidelines to help you in this:

Sit down in a quiet place and work out a day's menu by asking yourself what your body feels that it needs for that day. Do this with your family or your mate, if you wish. Use the food guide — page 81 — to help in this if you feel that you would like to use that information. Trust your intuition. Listen to food *cravings* even though they may seem silly.

When you shop for the food for this menu, find a store in which you feel relaxed, where you do not feel dazzled or confused by the number of choices available, by the decor, or by the activities around you. If you can't find such a place in your community, do the best you can and shop during the least busy time of the day. Take time choosing this food. Smell it, feel it, read the contents on labels, and as you are doing these things, remind yourself that you are going to incorporate that piece of fruit, or that potato, or that can of tuna fish, into the life within your body. It will determine the quality of energy available to you. It will become you.

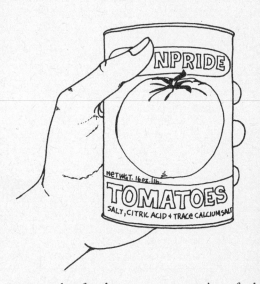

Prepare the food with love. If you feel tense before doing the preparation, stop what you are doing, clear your mind by doing one of the relaxation exercises. Get as close as you can to the food you are preparing; feel it, smell it, taste it, look at it as though you had never seen it before. For example, if you are cutting vegetables, pick up a slice of carrot, or tomato, or potato, and study the grain of its core, or the way it grows. Most vegetables appear to grow from the center out and in something like a star pattern.

Carefully observe what happens to a vegetable or fruit after you cut it. Some become drier, and some wetter on the surfaces just cut. All foods are now or once were living. Look upon each food with these things in mind: YOU ARE

75

GOING TO BE TAKING ANIMAL AND VEGETABLE CELLS FROM THE UNIVERSE TO COMBINE WITH LIVING CELLS OF YOUR OWN BODY. Your feelings about the food and the people you are preparing it for will play a large part in how well the interaction between the food and the cells of the eater's body works. One way to look at it is that your emotions are like herbs influencing the taste and quality of the food you prepare as much or more than do such things as thyme, oregano, cinammon, etc.

Serve the food in serving bowls so that each person can choose how much and what kinds of food he wants, rather than putting the food on each plate for each person.

Sit down to eat. But before you eat or put any food on your plate, pause and relax. Clear your mind of the day's tensions and troubles. If you feel that you would like to do so, do one of the relaxation exercises from this chapter.

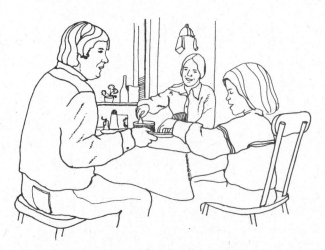

There is a physiological basis for this moment of relaxation. If you are tense, capillaries open in your muscles and constrict in your digestive organs. By relaxing and preparing yourself to eat you bring more blood to your digestive organs — meaning more energy going to the places it's needed the most.

Immediately before eating, pause and ask yourself if you are hungry. If you are not really hungry, ask yourself why it is that you are sitting down to eat at this time. It may be because everyone in your family is sitting down to eat, or because it is "time" to eat. Other reasons: dinner appointment with friends or business associates, etc.

Serve yourself only the *kinds* and *amounts* of food which your body tells you that you need. It may help you to remember this: most people are taught as children to "clean your plate." If this happened to you, you may have lost touch with your body's messages about what and how much it wants or needs to eat. Simply having this knowledge will help some people to free themselves of the *plate cleaning* impulse. But if that doesn't work, putting the food in serving bowls and serving yourself only what you feel that your body wants, will allow you to get in touch with real food needs and to clean your plate, too. If you have children in your family, they can get back in touch, or keep in touch with their body's individualized food needs if you become good at encouraging them to choose their own portions. It may take several weeks but they will eventually start eating foods which their bodies need, assuming, of course, that a full range of food choices are available.

Look at your food and ask yourself what feelings you get from it. Does it make you feel happy, sad, angry, disappointed, elated, indifferent, or what? Imagine that these feelings are part of the *nourishment* which you'll be incorporating into your body, just as the feelings of the cook during preparation become part of the food. You can choose which feelings to take into your body, or, if you are extremely hungry, you may have to choose between these feelings and the straight nourishment which your body needs.

As you begin eating, notice how the food tastes, its texture, and how it works in relation to your teeth, your tongue, and the roof of your mouth. There are many sensations involved with food, and most people are aware of only one or two. Awareness of them will eventually give you added criteria for judging food.

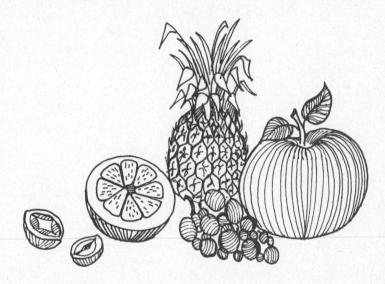

As you swallow, make note of how the food feels in your throat. Throats are much more than simple chutes — they actually push food to your stomach. Thus, your throat interacts with your food in its own particular way. Be sensitive to the messages that it gives off.

Notice the speed at which you are eating. Are you chewing fast or slow? Are you finishing before most of the people around you have finished, or after them? Are you talking alot during the meal? Does your mind wander as you eat? Is it hard for you to think about eating?

Food remains in your stomach from 2 to 4 hours after eating a full meal. Whatever messages you get from your stomach during that time will tell you about the food you have just eaten and how it is getting along with your body. If you are more or less unaware of your stomach, or if it feels good to you, then the chances are that your body got what it wanted or needed for that meal. If, however, your stomach is uncomfortable, locate the reason for its complaints. For example, if you're too full or still hungry you'll either feel "stuffy" or have "hunger pangs." Those, of course, are the most common complaints, ones that most people experience. If you are having discomforts other than these — indigestion, or gas — you will have to do a bit more work to locate the cause. Here's how: As you are feeling the discomfort, go down thru the list of foods which you have just eaten, and ask yourself, or your stomach, if any of them is the cause of your complaint. In most cases, and with a little bit of practice, you'll feel a change in the feelings or sensations in your stomach at the mention or thought of the offending food. Once you have located such foods, it is a simple matter to either limit the amounts of them which you eat in the future or eliminate them from your diet altogether.

Take note of your energy levels between meals. If you have a great burst of energy soon after eating, followed by a sudden decrease in energy a couple of hours later, evaluate your diet for sugar content. Anything sweet, of course, has sugar in it, so that much is easy to assess. Sugar gives you tremendous energy at first, due to the fact that your body can make use of it almost immediately. But sugar, and the energy it gives, is used up very quickly, and the *come down* is sudden, coming down to a body energy lever lower than before you ate — accounting for the feeling of depression which many people who eat alot of sugary foods have.

Protein, on the other hand — contained in nuts, fish, meats, eggs, milk, cheeses, and whole grain cereals — is broken down into useable form by the body very slowly. Though you may not feel the sudden burst of energy with protein that you get on sugar, the energy slowly builds up to a level at least as high as the sugar, and the energy level stays high. By adding protein to your diet, and decreasing your sugar intake, you can get a more even energy flow throughout the day. If you're a slow starter, but have good even energy, you may want to increase your sugar intake slightly by adding such things as fresh fruits to your diet.

A certain amount of burping and farting is a healthy — if not necessarily socially acceptable — body response. The amount you have will be directly related to the kinds of food you eat. If you are at all concerned about these things, turn to the *Gastro-intestinal* section of the *Diagnosis and Treatment* chapter.

VITAMIN DEFICIENCIES

Vitamin deficiencies are difficult to assess. Many vitamins are destroyed by food processing techniques, and a person eating only processed foods is often undernourished. Labels on such foods may tell you that vitamins have been added, but they are added before processing and cooking, and some vitamins, such as vitamin C, are destroyed by heat.

The act of processing food often removes most of the vitamins the natural food started with. Manufacturers add vitamins, but in many cases they add only *some* of the vitamins which they have removed. B-complex vitamins in flours used in white breads are an example of this phenomenon. Only part of the nutriments removed are later replaced.

There has been much controversy and confusion over the vitamin issue. In one government bulletin on processed foods, the authors claimed in one sentence that *food processing did not remove nutriments*. In the next sentence, explaining what the word "Enriched" meant on flour and bread wrappers, they said that *a manufacturer enriches a food product by replacing some of the nutriments removed in the processing*.

After being involved in developing food programs and trying many diets on our own, we feel that if you eat mostly processed foods you have a high probability of being deficient in vitamins A, B-complex, E, as well as protein. If you are interested in fully evaluating your own diet in terms of vitamins, minerals, and other food values, study the books listed on foods in the *Going Further* chapter. We tell you there which of these books contain food charts showing nutritional values.

It is very probable that disease is frequently due to dietary deficiencies. A person may look alright on their physical examination by a doctor, but be deficient in all vitamins, minerals, protein, and iron. Moderate deficiencies produce general, vague discomforts, and losses of energy which most doctors find extremely difficult to pin down. Consequently *you* and not your doctor are in the best position to evaluate your food needs.

FOOD RHYTHMS AND MOODS

Everyone has their own rhythms in eating, and the three-meals-a-day routine is largely arbitrary, imposed through social necessities such as "business lunch hours," and family efficiency. However, if you are at a place in your life where you can experiment with your eating rhythms, why not get into trying a larger number of meals throughout the day, each one lighter and simpler than your usual midday and evening meals?

Seasonal rhythms are also important in diet. Fresh fruits and vegetables, for example, are more scarce in winter than in summer. Also, the nutritional contents are lost, often times, in foods kept in cold storage, frozen, or canned. Vitamin "C" is most suceptible to these changes. So, you may want to use a good *natural* vitamin "C" supplement in the winter in order to ensure that you get enough. Because fruits are harder to get in the winter, you may find yourself craving a food you can't get, and, in the case of fruit, trying to satisfy that craving with sugar. Become aware of how the availability of foods in your area changes with the seasons, and then watch your diet, and how you feel, supplementing your vitamin intake where and when it seems appropriate.

Your body receives the *moods* in which the food you eat was grown, harvested and prepared.

Cooking prayers and eating prayers, practiced by many peoples, are beneficial. The cooking prayer, at the very least, gets the cook in a generous and open frame of mind, and this, rather than anger of indifference, goes into the food they prepare. The eating prayer gets your stomach ready for the food; it is a signal to your body to direct energy to all areas of your body involved in eating and digesting. If you don't believe in prayer, consider a quiet period after sitting down at the table; pause, open yourself to the food before you and start in eating. Any of the relaxation exercises in this book can be adapted here. We suggest doing one of the *Instant Relaxation* exercises which take less than a minute to do. See page 112.

Sometimes your body tells you that it does not want to eat. If you are in touch with your body and you trust its messages to you, feel free to fast. There is little medical evidence to indicate that limited fasting is not good for your body if you are otherwise healthy. Many people believe that occasional fasting promotes health by ridding your body of impurities.

APPROXIMATE DAILY NUTRITIONAL REQUIREMENTS

	Calories	Protein gms.	Calcium mgs.	Iron mgs.	A Units	B$_1$ mg.	B$_2$ mg.	Niacin mg.	C mg.
Average Man	2,900	70	800	10	5,000	1.2	1.7	19	70
Average Woman	2,100	58	800	15	5,000	.8	1.3	14	70

TABLE OF THE NUTRITIVE VALUE OF FOODS

	Calories	Protein gms.	Calcium mgs.	Iron mgs.	A Units	B$_1$ mg.	B$_2$ mg.	Niacin mg.	C mg.
Dairy Products									
Whole milk, 1 c.	160	9	288	.1	350	.07	.41	.2	2
Skim milk, 1 c.	90	9	296	.1	10	.09	.44	.2	2
Cottage cheese creamed, 1 c.	260	33	230	.7	420	.07	.61	.2	0
Cheddar, 1 oz.	115	7	213	.3	370	.01	.13	Trace	0
Swiss, 1 oz.	105	8	262	.3	320	Trace	.11	Trace	0
Processed cheese American, 1 oz.	105	7	198	.3	350	.01	.12	Trace	0
Ice cream, 1 c.	255	6	194	.1	590	.05	.28	.1	1
Yoghurt, 1 c.	150	7	272	.1	340	.07	.39	.2	2
Eggs									
Boiled, poached or raw, 1	80	6	27	1.1	590	.05	.15	Trace	0
Scrambled, 1	110	7	51	1.1	690	.05	.18	Trace	0
Fats and Oils									
Butter, 1 T.	100	Trace	3	0	470	—	—	—	0
Margarine, 1 T.	100	Trace	3	0	470	—	—	—	0
Vegetable oil, 1 T.	125	0	0	0	—	0	0	0	0
Mayonnaise, 1 T.	100	Trace	3	.1	40	Trace	.01	Trace	—
Meats									
Bacon, 2 slices	90	5	2	.5	0	.08	.05	.8	—
Beef, Hamburger, 3 oz.	245	21	9	2.7	30	.07	.18	4.6	—
Roast, 3 oz.	375	17	8	2.2	70	.05	.13	3.1	—
Steak, 3 oz.	330	20	9	2.5	50	.05	.16	4.0	—
Liver, beef, 2 oz.	130	15	6	5.9	30,280	.15	2.37	9.4	15
Pork, chop 3.5 oz.	260	16	8	2.2	0	.63	.18	3.8	—
Lamb, chop 4.8 oz.	400	25	10	5.0	—	.14	.25	5.6	—
Hot dog, 1	170	7	3	.8	0	.08	.11	1.4	0
Chicken, ½ breast fried	155	25	9	1.3	70	.04	.17	11.2	—

TABLE OF THE NUTRITIVE VALUE OF FOODS   Vitamins

	Calories	Protein gms.	Calcium mgs.	Iron mgs.	A Units	B$_1$ mg.	B$_2$ mg.	Niacin mg.	C mg.
Fish and Shellfish									
Salmon, 3 oz.	120	17	167	.7	60	.03	.16	6.8	—
Shrimp, 3 oz.	100	21	98	2.6	50	.01	.03	1.5	0
Tuna, 3 oz.	170	24	7	1.6	70	.04	.10	10.1	0
Dried Beans and Nuts									
Navy, 1 c. dry	225	15	95	5.1	0	.27	.13	1.3	0
Almonds, 1 c.	850	26	332	6.7	0	.34	1.31	5.0	Trace
Peanut butter, 1 T.	95	4	9	.3	0	.02	.02	2.4	0
Vegetables									
Bean, green, 1 c.	30	2	63	.8	680	.9	.11	.6	15
Broccoli, 1 c.	40	5	136	1.2	3,880	.14	.31	1.2	140
Carrots, raw, 1	20	1	18	.4	5,500	.03	.03	.3	4
Corn, ear, 1	70	3	2	.5	310	.09	.08	1.0	7
Lettuce, 1 head	60	4	91	2.3	1,500	.29	.27	1.3	29
Peas, 1 c.	115	9	37	2.9	860	.44	.17	3.7	33
Potatoes, 1 med.	90	3	9	.7	Trace	.10	.04	1.7	20
Potatoe chips, 10 average	115	1	8	.4	Trace	.04	.01	1.0	3
Spinach, 1 c.	40	5	167	4.0	14,580	.13	.25	1.0	50
Squash, summer, 1 c.	30	2	52	.8	820	.10	.16	1.6	21
Sweetpotatoe, 1 boiled	170	2	47	1.0	11,610	.13	.09	.9	25
Tomato, 7 oz.	40	2	24	.9	1,640	.11	.07	1.3	42
Fruit									
Apple, 1 med.	70	Trace	8	.4	50	.04	.02	.1	3
Applesauce, 1 c.	230	1	10	1.3	100	.05	.03	.1	3
Banana, 1	100	1	10	.8	230	.06	.07	.8	12
Cantaloupe, ½	60	1	27	.8	6,540	.08	.06	1.2	63
Grapefruit, ½	45	1	19	.5	10	.05	.02	.2	44
Lemon, 1	20	1	19	.4	10	.03	.01	.1	39
Lemonade, 1 c.	110	Trace	2	Trace	Trace	Trace	.02	.2	17
Orange, 1	65	1	54	.5	260	.13	.05	.5	66
Orange juice, frozen, 1 c.	120	2	25	.2	550	.22	.02	1.0	120
Peach, 1	35	1	9	.5	1,320	.02	.05	1.0	7
Raisins, 1 c.	480	4	102	5.8	30	.18	.13	.8	2

TABLE OF THE NUTRITIVE VALUE OF FOODS

	Calories	Protein gms.	Calcium mgs.	Iron mgs.	A Units	Vitamins B₁ mg.	B₂ mg.	Niacin mg.	C mg.
Grain Products									
White bread, 1 slice	70	2	21	.6	Trace	.06	.05	.6	Trace
Whole wheat bread 1 slice	65	3	24	.8	Trace	.9	.3	.8	Trace
Cornflakes, 1 c.	100	2	4	.4	0	.11	.02	.5	0
Oatmeal, 1 c.	130	5	22	1.4	0	.19	.05	.2	0
Pancakes, 1 med.	60	2	27	.4	30	.05	.06	.4	Trace
Rice, 1 c. cooked	225	4	21	1.8	0	.23	.02	2.1	0
Spaghetti, cooked, 1 c.	155	5	11	1.3	0	.20	.11	1.5	0
Sugars, Sweets									
White sugar, 1 T.	40	0	0	Trace	0	0	0	0	0
Honey, 1 T., strained	65	Trace	1	.1	0	Trace	.01	.1	Trace
Jam, 1 T.	55	Trace	4	.2	Trace	Trace	.01	Trace	Trace
Desserts									
Pie, apple, 1 slice	350	3	11	.4	40	.03	.03	.5	1
Cookies, commercial 1	50	1	4	.2	10	Trace	Trace	Trace	Trace
Cake, Devil's Food 1 slice	235	3	41	.6	100	.02	.06	.2	Trace
Miscellaneous									
Yeast, brewers 1 T.	25	3	17	1.4	Trace	1.25	.34	3.0	Trace

ADDITIONAL RECOMMENDED NUTRIENTS

The following are nutrients for which recommended daily requirements have not been established (in some cases) but which are known to be necessary in human nutrition. Under each nutrient are the foods which are good sources for that particular thing. We suggest that you include some foods from each group in your daily diet.

Vitamin B_6

Bananas
Whole grain cereals
Chicken
Dry legumes
Egg yolk
Most dark-green leafy vegetables
Most fish and shellfish
Muscle meats, liver, and kidney
Peanuts, walnuts, filberts, peanut butter
Potatoes and sweet potatoes
Prunes and raisins
Yeast

Magnesium

Bananas
Whole-grain cereals
Dry beans
Milk
Most dark-green leafy vegetables
Nuts
Peanuts, peanut butter

Vitamin B_{12}

(present in foods of animal
   origin only)
Kidney
Liver
Meat
Milk
Most cheeses
Most fish
Shellfish
Whole egg and egg yolk

Folacin

Liver
Dark-green vegetables
Dry beans
Peanuts, walnuts, filberts
Lentils

Vitamin E

Vegetable oils
Margarine
Salad dressing
Whole-grain cereals
Peanuts

Vitamin D

Vitamin D milks
Egg Yolk
Salt-water fish
Liver

Phosphorous

Whole-grain cereals
Cheese
Dry beans
Eggs
Meat
Milk
Peanuts, peanut butter

Iodine

Iodized salt
Seafood

REVEALING OUR SOURCES

Our source for the food charts and nutritive requirements above is the U.S. Department of Agriculture. We tell you where to get more complete information of this kind in our chapter called *Going Further*.

BLAND THERAPEUTIC DIET

This is a therapeutic diet to use when you want or need a diet that minimizes irritation of the digestive system: such as, gastritis — acute indigestion, ulcers, or as a bridge back to your usual diet after a period of fasting.

Protein: Eat recommended daily requirements of lean meats, fish, poultry, eggs, cottage cheese, and milk. Boil or broil meats.

Fats: Eat only moderate amounts of butter, margarine, cream, and cream cheese. (To suppress gastric secretions.)

Polyunsaturated Fats: (As in soft margarines) Use these in place of saturated fats.

Carbohydrates: Eat only potatoes, white or sweet, and applesauce if desired.

Other Foods: Restrict irritants to your stomach, such as alcohol, caffeine, cocoa, cola beverages; no chili powder, curry, nutmeg, black pepper or other spices.

Chew your foods very slowly and thoroughly. Eat frequent small meals, instead of the usual three large meals. Eat nothing that is not specifically listed above. We suggest supplementing your diet with a good multiple vitamin while on this diet.

HIGH PROTEIN, HIGH VITAMIN, HIGH CALORIE THERAPEUTIC DIET

This is a therapeutic diet only, to be used in cases of Hepatitis, or during periods of high physical activity or stress when extra nutritive energy is needed.

In general, increase your intake of calories 25-50% over the recommended daily requirements. Increase protein to about 100 grams per day. Eat foods of high vitamin content, especially B complex foods. Eat in small, frequent meals, as much as 6 to 8 times a day.

Protein: Drink up to one quart of milk per day. Eat one or more eggs. Eat cheese for snacks or added to other foods. Eat 2 to 3 portions of meat, fish, or poultry per day, with each serving at least 2 to 3 ounces.

Fats: Eat 2 to 3 tablespoons per day of butter, margarine, cream, mayonnaise or oil.

Carbohydrates: Eat 4 to 8 servings of whole grain cereals or breads.

Fruits or Fruit Juices: Eat or drink 4 to 6 servings per day, with added sugar.

Vegetables: Eat 1 to 2 servings of raw, fresh vegetables, with mayonnaise or dressing, plus 1 to 2 portions of cooked green, white, or yellow vegetables per day.

Starch: Eat 1 or 2 servings of potatoes or rice, with added sauces, butter, gravy, etc.

Soups: Cream Style or thick, rich soups as desired.

Deserts: Ice cream, sherbets, custard, pudding, plain cake, fruit deserts, gelatin, and cookies. Two or more servings per day.

Sugars: Eat 2 to 4 tablespoons of jams, honey, syrups, etc.

Beverages: Cut down on any beverages with caffeine: cola drinks, cocoa, coffee, tea, etc. No alcoholic beverages.

SKIN, BACTERIA AND CHEMISTRY

The cells on the external surfaces of your body — your skin — are living in balanced harmony with many helpful bacteria. These bacteria remain helpful only so long as this delicate, co-existing balance is maintained. For the most part the cells and the bacteria work out this delicate balance for themselves. But when you add chemicals, or bacteria that don't ordinarily live there, to your skin, your body often needs extra energy to maintain the healthy balance. And that demonstrates one of the basic principles of the well body: **You are in a position to choose how your body is using energy — for your own trip or for healing infections, which is the trip that bacteria and viruses will force upon you.**

DON'T BE TOO CLEAN

Your skin is alive. Cells inside your body are always surrounded by fluids, to cleanse them, cushion them, and carry nutriment to them. Outer cells (your skin) are no exception. To keep skin healthy it will need careful bathing, and it will like you to protect it from chemicals and certain bacteria.

A part of every doctor's practice is spent seeing people with rashes and skin infections directly caused by the chemicals they put on their skin. Your skin is not an impenetrable and insensitive wall. It is sensitive and alive. It is that which lives in the area between the life inside your body and the world outside. It is your border. It is living and breathing, sensitive to pressure, temperature, and the texture of the world.

87

Certain things can and do pass from the external world through your skin cell membranes to affect the life force within each cell in your body. *Hexachlorophene* was considered safe for many years, and was used in soaps, deodorants, and cosmetics. It was taken off the market when traces of the chemical were found in the blood streams of infants.

Discover what chemicals you put on your body and find out what they do. **Read the labels on everything you put on your skin and hair.** Some commonly used things that contain chemicals are: toothpaste, hand soap, deodorants, hair dies, hair setting lotions, douches, shaving soaps and lotions, hair sprays, feminine deodorants, make up, foot powders, mouth wash, clothes washing detergents that eventually get to your skin, dishwashing detergents, household cleaners, etc. As you go over these things, ask yourself if your skin is happy with them. How does your skin feel when you use these things?

Do the things that you use on your skin increase or decrease your energy? If you feel that they do not increase your energy, figure out why you are using them. It may be social pressure, or it may really be because you like them. If you are worried about smells, are you sure your body smells "bad" when you don't use the chemicals? Find out by discontinuing their use for a day or two.

All animals have a natural odor to which other members of the species respond for identifying one another, and also for sexual attraction. Mankind is no exception. This odor is normal, and in deodorizing yourself, you may well be taking yourself out of harmony with Nature. Examine the possibility that you may have been *taught to fear* your body's natural odors by advertising techniques aimed at getting you to buy deodorizing chemicals. These ads may not have been aimed at helping you; they may have been aimed solely at making money for the chemical companies.

SUGGESTIONS FOR KEEPING CLEAN

Here are some general guidelines for developing your own alternatives to using chemicals on your body:

Hair: Use a mild pure soap or castile shampoo, or a preparation that isn't filled with antibacterial chemicals. Many so-called *dandruff treatment* shampoos really aggravate the dandruff problem by removing protective oils and upsetting the normal bacterial balance of human hair. Daily brushings stimulate the flow of oils produced in your own body, exercise each hair shaft by stretching it (they're very elastic) and clean each strand at least as well as a good shampoo. Use a *natural* bristle brush, or one of the new metal bristle brushes with the bristles mounted in sponge rubber, designed for long hair. Most *synthetic* bristles fray the ends of hairs and are quite damaging.

Mouth: You can find out everything there is to know about your mouth in a book called *The Tooth Trip*, which we tell you about in the chapter called *Going Further.* But here's a summary on brushing:

Use a natural bristle brush.

Avoid *brightener* toothpastes. They contain strong abrasives, which wear out the enamel of your teeth.

Brush all surfaces of your teeth in the direction that they grow.

Brush, rinse your mouth thoroughly with water, or eat crisp raw vegetables or fruits as soon as possible after meals.

Massage your gums daily, either by lightly brushing them, or with your fingers, or both.

Clean between your teeth with dental floss.

According to many dentists you should never have to use a mouth wash to combat bad breath. If your breath smells bad it is either because you need to get work done on your teeth or because of something you ate. Anti-bacterial chemicals in some mouth washes can upset the balance of life worked out by the cells and the helpful bacteria in your mouth. If bad breath worries you, eat fresh parsley leaves. Natural chlorophyl "cleans" your breath and is an excellent source of vitamin A.

Underarms: Mild soap and water are enough here to keep these areas clean without disrupting natural odors and bacterial balances. Chemicals in deodorants plug up hair follicles and are known to cause boils. This condition is, in fact, so common that doctors have actually given it a name: *Hidrandenitis Suppurativa.* Understand that this does not mean that you have to smell "bad." Contrary to what most of us have been taught, it is possible to smell good without spraying yourself down with chemicals. If you have been using deodorants for a number of years, however, it may take several days or weeks for the normal bacterial balance to restore itself after you discontinue the use of deodorants. You may have to bathe your underarms more frequently, using mild soap and water only, during this period. But this will become less necessary as the bacterial balance is restored.

Genitals: Men, bathe your penis and testicles the same way you do the rest of your skin. But remember that the skin here is thinner, softer, more sensitive than in other areas of your body. If you are uncircumsized, pull back the foreskin and wash the surfaces there whenever you bathe. Dry thoroughly afterwards so that you won't create a moist environment that may upset bacterial balances. Avoid the use of chemicals.

Women, bathe the labia carefully with mild soap and water, treating your skin here as the sensitive area it is. Avoid douches, and all chemicals in this area. Avoid *feminine deodorants.* Your vagina is a place where the cells of your body live in *delicate* harmony with helping bacteria. Don't upset this balance with chemicals. (We tell you more about this in the *Vaginitis* section of *Diagnosis and Treatment.*

Feet: If you wash between your toes, and thoroughly dry in these places every time you bathe, you will have no need for foot powders. Go barefoot whenever possible to give your feet air.

(If you have complaints such as rashes, itches, and sores, turn to the *Skin* section of the *Diagnosis and Treatment* chapter.)

MATCHING YOUR SOAP TO YOUR SKIN

Many people are now finding that skin problems which they have had are being caused by the soaps they use! They have found that by changing soaps, their skin can regain its natural protective oils, smoothness, and health. In most areas of the country you can now buy preparations for bathing which contain no soap but which do contain natural or organic oils, which you may find to be more compatible with your skin.

One manufacturer suggests that you can test the things you use on your skin to find out if they are compatible with the acid balance of your skin, measured as the "pH factor." They say that the pH factor of skin is 4.5 to 5.5. You can test the acid balance of your bathing preparations with test papers which you can buy in most any drug store for about a dollar and a half. Ask the clerk for *test papers to test the full range of the pH factor, or at least from 4.5 to 9.* These papers turn different colors according to the pH factor of the thing you're testing. (Drug stores sell them for urine tests, so they probably won't know what you're talking about if you say you want to test soap.) They're fun to use.

We believe that the best way to test your bathing preparation is to

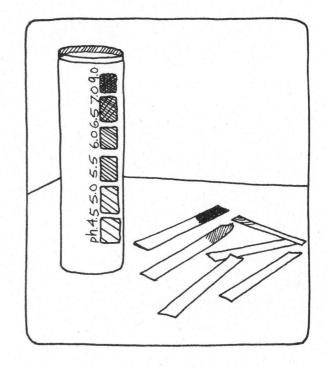

get in touch with how your skin feels after you bathe. Rub your fingers over the skin areas toward which you feel most positive before you bathe. Healthy skin is smooth, slightly oily, elastic, and feels good. If your skin does not feel this way try changing bathing preparations, using the mildest you can find. After a week or so of using this mild preparation check out your skin again. Most people will begin to notice changes after as few as three bathings. Follow the same procedures for your hair.

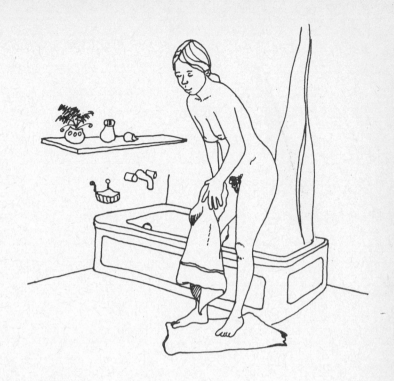

CLEANLINESS DURING ILLNESS

Many diseases can be transmitted from one person to another. Simple cleaning (if someone in your house is sick) can often prevent the spread of these infections. In this book we tell about *four ways by which infection is spread.*

Fecal-Oral: Bacteria or viruses are carried out of the sick person's body in their feces. If you are sick and you wipe yourself following a bowel movement, your hands come close enough to the feces to pick up the bacteria or viruses which it contains. Understand that you do not have to actually touch the feces itself. Later you may touch other areas of the house where people prepare food or eat. The viruses and bacteria will then be left on the surfaces which people touch and which food touches, and they will then make their way to those other peoples' mouthes. A common disease spread in this way is Hepatitis.

To prevent fecal-oral spread: If someone is ill in your house, everyone should carefully wash their hands directly after going to the bathroom. When possible the person who is sick should have use of a different bathroom than the one used by other members of the house. Make a special effort to keep the bathrooms very clean during this time.

The person who is sick should have their own glasses, plates, and eating utensils which should be separately washed. You should wash bedsheets separately, too. They should not share cigarettes with others, nor share anything else through which oral contact is possible. They should have their own washcloth and towel.

Kitchen and eating areas should be kept especially clean during illnesses which are spread through the fecal-oral route. We tell you how diseases are spread in each of the diseases we describe in the *Diagnosis and Treatment* chapter, when this information is applicable.

91

Skin To Skin: (Or person-to-person) Bacteria or viruses on the skin or on mucous membranes are passed from one person to another by physical contact with the affected areas. Examples of diseases spread in this way are: Impetigo, Gonorrhea, and Conjunctivitis (pink eye). If you have an infection which can be spread in this way the responsibility is yours to prevent contact of affected areas with other people. Keep your body especially clean during this time. Use your own towel and wash cloth.

      To prevent skin-to-skin spread: Avoid physical contact with others until you are fully healed. Understand that infections can still be spread while you are taking antibiotics or other medications.

Airborne: Bacteria and viruses are carried in droplets of saliva and are spread when you cough or sneeze. These tiny droplets can travel several feet. Examples of diseases spread in this way are Strep throat and Bronchitis.

      To prevent airborne spread: Cover your mouth when you cough or sneeze. Dispose of any tissues you use carefully, and wash your hands before preparing or handling foods that other people will eat.

Bugs: Bugs are spread by person-to-person contact, and contact with clothing, bedclothes, furniture, sleeping bags, etc. Examples are: lice and scabies.

      To prevent the spread of bugs: First heal yourself of the infection. (See *Diagnosis and Treatment*.) Make sure to wash all your clothes at high temperatures. Dry clean blankets and sleeping bags. If necessary spray furniture with anti-bug sprays which are available at drug stores.

      Understand that you do not have to do these things regularly. The point is to take special care of yourself, and those around you, when you or a member of your household are sick.

CLOTHES

A Chinese friend told me about her grandmother who advised her children to "dress always in the color of the season: black in winter, white in summer, and with the colors of the forests in the months between." This advice has its scientific basis in the fact that black absorbs heat and so would help keep you warm during the cold winter months; white, of course, reflects the light and thus the heat of the sun, and so keeps the wearer cool in the summer. As to the colors of the forest in the months between, they would be as good a guideline as any to choose reflecting colors fitting to the warmth of the season.

The color and weight of clothes are obvious factors in keeping your body warm. In addition, the texture and chemical makeup of clothes, as well as the way they are washed, will affect your skin. Colors and patterns will affect your emotion — or be a reflection of them.

Clothes can be a way to get yourself into a very high and joyful place. Get in touch with yourself in the most joyful state you can imagine. And then visualize the kind of clothes you'd be wearing at that moment. Remember how the clothes look and feel, and then get yourself real clothes to wear that look and feel like that. You might find it fun to take castaside clothes and cut, dye, and embroider designs on them until they express the feelings you would like them to express.

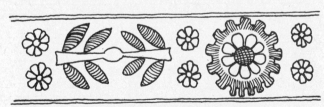

Clothes can elevate your feelings or bring you down, and in this respect they clearly affect the energy level of your body. Even on a scientific level it is known that colors have the power to excite or depress you. Though it is a subtle thing, color should certainly not be overlooked. Expressing your innermost feelings, whether through your clothes or through words and caresses to people you love, does good things for your body and brings your energy level up.

Different colors produce different vibrations which you can use to bring in specific energy levels that your body needs. When you filled out your *Bright Life Chart*, you got in touch with the colors which your body needs for maximum energy and health. You can now go back and study that chart to help you choose clothing colors to either heal specific parts of your body or bring greater energy to the parts that need extra energy.

You can also use decorations made of precious metals and stones to concentrate large amounts of energy on parts of your body. These stones and pure metals have particular molecular structures of great symmetry which represent high energy forms. There are whole systems of medicine in other cultures which use gems and metals for healing. You may wish to consult with your imaginary doctor to find out which gems and metals will work best for you.

PREVENTING ENERGY DRAINS: There are common medical complaints that doctors see every day which can very often be traced to clothing: heat rashes from clothes that are too hot; allergies related to the fabric the clothes are made of; allergies related to the detergents left in the clothes from washing; mechanical chafing from tight clothes or the elastic in clothing; "jock rot" from wearing pants that are too tight and fabrics that don't breathe; vaginal infections from wearing nylon underpants that don't breathe; rashes and chafing from coarse- textured clothes on delicate skin surfaces such as the genital areas, underarms, breasts and neck; fungus infections of the feet from wearing non-breathing socks and tight, non-breathing shoes; blisters and infections from blisters on the feet as a result of badly-designed or ill-fitting shoes.

The principles involved here are: *chafing,* which rubs off and kills living cells of your body; *allergy,* which is your body recognizing substances as a threat to it; *fungal growth,* which is a result of normal bacterial balances of your body being disrupted by abnormally moist and warm environments created by your clothes.

All these conditions can be prevented by paying close attention to the clothes you wear. Evaluate your own clothes to find out if they are now causing, or could cause, any of these complaints: bend over and touch the floor; reach over your shoulder and scratch your back; move your head from the extreme right to the extreme left. If any of these movements chafes, binds, or restricts your movements in any way, it can cause skin irritations in that area.

Check the cuffs of your sleeves. If you can slide two fingers between the cloth and your skin, they are okay. If not, they are tight enough to cause skin irritations and/or restrict the circulation of blood to and from your hands. Check for elastic marks around the tops of your socks, waist, and the legs, armholes, and neck of underwear. If you see any marks on your skin from the pressure of the elastic, that area is prone to rash and restricted blood circulation.

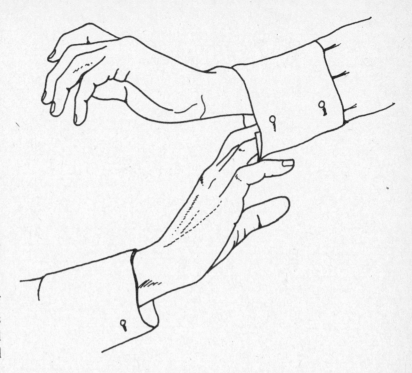

Go over your favorite and most-often-worn clothing; read the labels and check for fabric content. Many synthetic materials do not breathe due to the fact that the fibers are non-porous. This means that your perspiration and body heat are held in, creating an overheated skin area where the balance of normal organisms is disrupted. Leather garments, especially those worn next to the skin, can have the same effect. If you want to know more about this, read the *Vaginitis* section in the *Diagnosis and Treatment* chapter.

Common names of synthetic fabrics are nylon, dacron, acrylic, polyester fibers, manmade fibers, and almost anything else that isn't specifically labeled cotton, wool, or silk. Most clothing manufacturers who use synthetic materials now blend them with cotton so that the clothing it is made into can breathe and is absorbent. The standard seems to be 50% cotton and 50% "manmade fibers." These are good things to keep in mind when you're out buying new clothes, or buying material to make your own.

If you find large patches of skin anywhere on your body which are red or sensitive to the touch, this could be your body reacting to the laundry detergent which you use to wash your clothes. For more information about this, you may want to read the section on *Contact Dermatitis* in the *Diagnosis and Treatment* chapter. If you suspect detergent reaction, try changing to pure laundry soaps the next time you wash your clothes. Common "pure" laundry soaps are *Ivory Snow* and *White King.*

Look at your feet. If you find red places or "welts" on your feet or ankles, your shoes are either too tight or your socks are made of synthetic materials that don't breathe.

CHOOSING CLOTHES FOR THE WELL BODY: From the standpoint of having a well body and keeping your energy focused toward health, choose clothes that feel good — how they fit and how the material they're made of feels next to your skin; choose styles and colors that make you feel good toward your own body; choose clothes made of fabrics that breathe. Wash your clothes in non-irritating soaps. Wear shoes that fit well and let your feet breathe. Make certain that any elastic in your clothes is loose enough not to cause a mark on your skin.

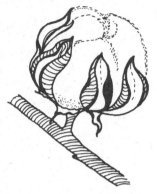

CLOTHES TO COME HOME TO: Tight clothes not only can chafe and upset the normal balance of your skin, they also slow down the circulation of blood in your body by pressing against, and constricting, small blood vessels and capillaries. It's a good idea, if you have to wear tight clothes on your job during the day, or for other social reasons, to have loose fitting clothes to come home to. If you're a man, take off your necktie and loosen your belt; if you're a woman, remove your girdle if you wear one. Find something that really feels good next to your skin, clothes that are loose and which please you aesthetically.

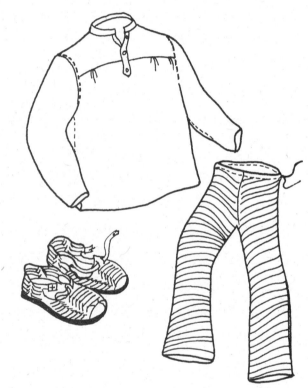

MOVEMENT, FOCUS, AND KARMA: Clothing can limit a person's activities tremendously, and can even get you to thinking and feeling that you can't do things that your clothes won't let you do. For example, most of the shoes that have been sold in the common shoe stores in our society for the past fifty years aren't walking shoes. They're for putting under a desk, or for showing off at a party. They're not made for leaving the pavement. People are buying hiking boots these days, and that's a healthy change. People can walk again. Their feet can leave the pavement. And women are freeing themselves of high heels. The bone structure of the foot, in most people, really isn't made to work well with anything higher than about a 1½ inch heel. A high heel restricts movement and limits what you can do and where you can go, causing both pain and physiological damage.

People probably choose clothes which focus attention to one part of their body or another. This emphasizes one area of their body more than others, bringing or taking energy away from it, and thus disrupting the body's organic balances. This is especially true in sexually associated areas: breasts, buttocks, legs, and crotch. On the other hand, clothes that emphasize a part of your body that you feel needs energy probably help to bring you harmony and energy. During illnesses, wear the most comfortable and beautiful clothes you can find, in order to focus as much healing energy as possible on your body.

If you're into the *karma* of things, consider the karma of the material in the fabrics of the clothes you wear: i.e. cotton = vegetable; dacron, nylon, etc. = chemicals; silk = silk worms spinning cocoons; wool = fur from sheep. Choose materials that are compatible with your own karma.

Clothing is like a second skin. Like feathers to the bird, or fur to the animal. If it feels really good, the person feels really good and healthy. If you look good, good coming from your *inner self*, you project much more positive messages, and people around you feel good. Your clothing is the care you are taking for yourself; your whole body will become healthier for that.

EXERCISE

Tension can be caused by neglected muscles. A muscle is meant to be elastic, capable of contracting and stretching many times the size of its relaxed length. An unused muscle becomes less elastic, less able to stretch. If it's forced to stretch after months or years of inactivity, it will have a tendency to tear rather than stretch, causing mild or extreme pain, depending on the extent of the injury.

Supple, elastic, good working muscles hold the organs of your body firmly, yet caressingly and lovingly — supporting them and giving them a gentle massage as you move around. The hard, unused, and inflexible muscle has an entirely different relationship to organs: more like a hard fist than like open fingers. Essentially, the inflexible muscles hold the body in a tight, static position at all times. There is no tension (contraction); neither is there relaxation. The body remains at an in-between state.

The rhythms and thus the interchange of energy between the supple and alive muscle and its neighboring organs, and the rhythms and interchange between the hard, unused muscle and its neighboring organs, are vastly different. The first is dynamic and everchanging, since the flex and tension of the healthy muscle is extremely variable; the second is static because the range of flex and tension is greatly limited. Because the unused muscle has less blood flowing to it, the cells which live in that area are more prone to infection, and they take longer to ward off disease, or to heal, than do muscles which are receiving a large flow of energy and blood.

If you increase the exercise a muscle gets, slowly over a period of several days or weeks, you can stimulate the growth of capillaries in that area, bringing that muscle and its neighboring organs more nourishment and energy.

CHOOSE EXERCISES THAT PLEASE YOU

Exercise should be a pleasure, not a chore. If exercise seems no more than an arduous task to you, the chances are that you won't stick with it for long. And then you'll be right back where you started.

If you are going to increase the amount of exercise you are now getting, remember not to do it all at once. Work up gradually. Otherwise you might end up in the doctor's office with the very thing the exercises were meant to prevent — a strained muscle.

Exercise which is vigorous enough to provide most of the benefits that we've described in the above several paragraphs are bike riding, swimming, hiking, jogging, dancing, skating, water skiing, canoeing and kayaking, tennis, snow skiing, horseback riding, backpacking — and, if done regularly and along with other exercise, handball, basketball, tetherball, etc.

Healers since the beginning of recorded history have found that sunshine and fresh air make people feel healthy. If you can, do your exercising outdoors.

POSTURES FOR HEALTH

There are ancient body postures, called asanas, developed and perfected by Indian Yogis, which can relax your body and mind, strengthen muscles, and release areas of tension and energy blocks. These postures have proved effective for thousands of years and are powerful medical tools for preventing illness and healing your body.

In the pages that follow we show you some of these postures and tell you what each can do. Then you can choose which of them will be best for you. There are many books on *Hatha Yoga* which tell you in detail how to do more of these postures. (See *Going Further* for more information on these books.)

Some general instructions for doing these postures are: start with easy ones and do them for short periods of time. Never strain yourself. Done properly, the posture feels good; it doesn't cause discomfort or pain. You will not be able to do the more difficult postures completely at first because your muscles need exercise to become more elastic and supple. With a small amount of practice each day even the more difficult postures become easy and comfortable to do.

To begin with these postures, pick one which you feel you will enjoy. Hold it for as long as you wish. Five minutes is a goal to work toward. After holding a posture, do the "Corpse Asana" for the same amount of time that you did the posture. This allows your body to rest.

Every posture will increase your energy. Done regularly, they will improve your life tremendously. These postures are used for everything from medical treatment to spiritual enlightenment.

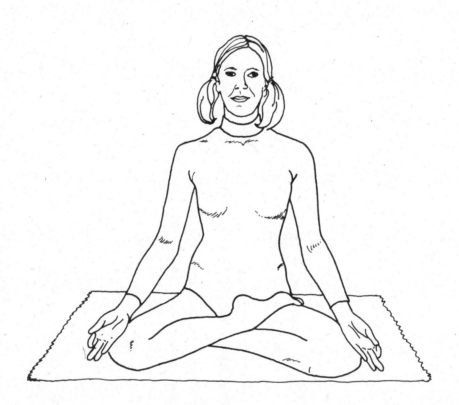

Lotus Asana

Relaxes the body and develops equilibrium.

Increases blood supply to the pelvic area.

Strengthens abdominal muscles.

Shoulder Stand

Stimulates thyroid gland. Increases circulation in genitals.

Helps relieve indigestion, constipation, and other abdominal conditions.

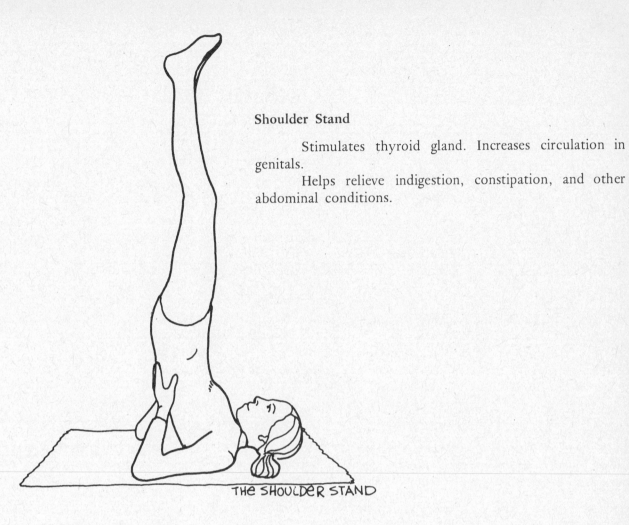

THE SHOULDER STAND

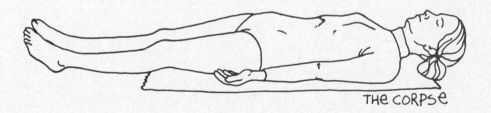

THE CORPSE

Corpse Asana

Relaxes body and mind. Rests nerves and muscles. Increases blood return to heart. Reduces high blood pressure. Reduces nervous tension.

101

Bow Asana

      Stretches abdomen
and hip muscles.
      Relieves stomach
gas. Reduces abdominal fat.

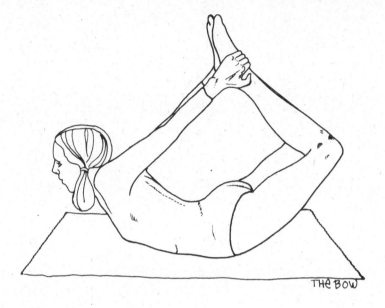

THE BOW

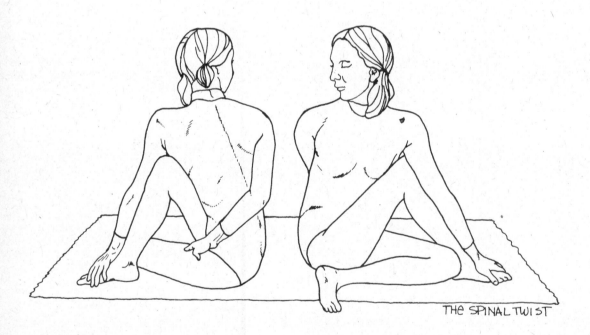

THE SPINAL TWIST

Spinal Twist

      Helps prevent back strain. Strengthens spinal muscles. Relieves constipation and indigestion.

Fish Asana

Strengthens back and neck muscles.

Helps sexual and abdominal muscles.

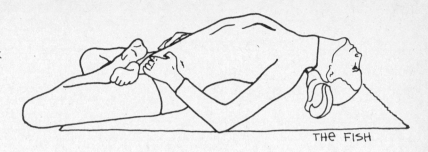

THE FISH

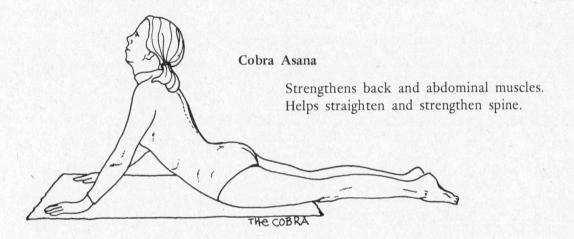

Cobra Asana

Strengthens back and abdominal muscles.
Helps straighten and strengthen spine.

THE COBRA

While doing any of these postures you may have thoughts enter your mind. Let these thoughts pass into and then out of your mind. (See the exercise for *Sitting and Counting Your Breaths* in the *Relaxation* section of this chapter for more on this.)

BREATHING EXERCISES

Breathing exercises are usually done after asanas. Learning how to do them, and how they make you feel, will no doubt lead you to discover many uses for them.

Breathing exercises strengthen muscles in your abdomen and chest. For this reason, these exercises will be of great benefit to anyone with respiratory problems.

Each time you exhale, impurities are sent out of your body. Each time you inhale energy from the universe is brought into your body.

FILLING THE BOTTLE

Sit in a comfortable position and imagine that your pelvis is the bottom of a large bottle and your mouth is the top. Now inhale slowly. As you inhale imagine that you are filling the bottle from the bottom up. When you get to the top, hold your breath long enough to feel your fullness. Then exhale slowly and imagine the bottle becoming empty. Do this exercise for as long as you wish. You will become

103

light-headed and may feel a tingling sensation throughout your body if you do this breathing exercise very many times. That's perfectly okay.

This exercise awakens the entire nervous system and checks the restless mind and senses.

ALTERNATING NOSTRILS

As before, sit in a comfortable position. Take two or three deep breaths with your mouth closed, breathing through your nostrils.

Inhale, hold one nostril closed, then exhale through the open nostril.

Now inhale through that same open nostril.

When you have achieved a full inhalation, close that nostril and open the other.

Exhale through the nostril you have just opened. Inhale. Then close that nostril and switch to the other side, repeating the same pattern.

This exercise does everything that *Filling The Bottle* will do for you. It also encourages people who tend to breathe from only one nostril to breathe from both. In addition, *Tantric* (Indian) healers believe that you can balance the acid-alkaline state of the body by learning to breathe from both nostrils. They say the right side is acid, the left alkaline.

RELAXATION EXERCISES

Often driving your car, doing your job, or simply walking down the street may require particular kinds of attentiveness, watchfulness, or apprehension. In most cases this means that your muscles are constricted in one or more parts of your body. It means that your muscles are in *readiness* — getting ready to perform an action which may be forthcoming. You may, for example, be ready to apply your automobile brakes suddenly to avoid disaster on the freeway, necessitating that certain muscles in your body stay tense for long periods of time. You may not *actually* have to apply your brakes in this way more than once a month, but that once a month experience is enough to convince you that you must be ready at all times.

The problem is that many people go around in a state of readiness at all times: ready to apply their brakes, ready to fight or defend themselves, ready to solve a problem, ready to run, etc. This readiness causes their bodies to be in a constant state of tension, which is not good for their health. Nor does it truly prepare them for the things they are getting ready for; it distracts and burns up energy. Complete relaxation, on the other hand, promotes mental alertness and allows you to act spontaneously and efficiently whenever situations in your life actually require you to act.

While a muscle is tense, capillaries constrict, actually slowing down or stopping circulation of blood. At the same time the cells in that area are producing energy;

eating, digesting, and excreting wastes. Available nutriment is being used up and the toxic wastes excreted by cells are building up around them. Thus, if cells in and around a muscle or an organ are to get their full benefit of a steady flow of blood, the muscle needs to go through a full cycle of tension, release of energy, and relaxation. Unless it completes the cycle, those cells end up being undernourished, and even *drugged* by the toxics which build up around them. In this state your body is more prone to disease; this is why we feel that relaxation is a key to preventing illness.

Different people tense up different areas of their bodies. You might, for example, carry a large amount of tension in your stomach while another person might carry tension in their neck. These tension areas can produce *energy blocks* which prevent energy from moving freely to other areas of your body. Mental tension, such as anxiety, doubt, or worry are *always* manifested as muscular tensions in various parts of your body.

Understand that your muscles are controlled by your mind. **Just as you can cause your arm to lift food to your mouth to eat, you can also cause your muscles to completely relax.**

You may not realize that parts of your body are tense, but after trying the exercises we describe here your body will feel quite different than when you started. People doing these exercises for the first time have reported that they discovered themselves relaxing more than they had relaxed since they were children. Look upon these exercises as tools to relax your muscles whenever you feel they are tense. They are a way to give each cell of your body a full flow of blood — energy and care — throughout the day, every day of your life.

BREATHING FROM YOUR ABDOMEN

The relaxation exercises described in this book work best if you learn how to breathe from your abdomen rather than breathing from high in your chest. Abdominal breathing is what you do when you're sleeping, and by breathing this way you ensure a smooth flow of energy to your vital organs and to every part of your body. Breathing from your abdomen may or may not come naturally to you, since "high production" people tend to breathe high in their chest during their working hours. Here's how to breathe from your abdomen:

Stand in front of your full length mirror, undressed, and place your hands on your abdomen. Turn sideways so that you can see your profile in the mirror. Then draw air into your lungs and note whether your chest or your abdomen rises as you inhale. This will tell you what kind of breather you are: an expanding chest means you're a chest breather, an expanding abdomen means you are breathing from your abdomen.

Practice breathing to your abdomen in front of the mirror until breathing in this way comes easily for you. Understand that you are not being asked to breathe this way all the time, but that breathing in this way is useful in doing relaxation exercises.

If you wear tight clothes during the day, or even wear a belt that is tight, you may find breathing from your abdomen difficult if not impossible. If you want to learn to fully relax and to use breathing from your abdomen as one of the techniques in accomplishing this, you'll have to wear clothes that are loose enough to accomodate the free rise and fall of your abdomen.

In all breathing and relaxation exercises, pay particular attention to *exhaling*. It is during the exhalation cycle that the lungs get rid of the cells' waste products in the form of carbon dioxide. One of the first things that people doing breathing exercises learn is that they normally place most of their emphasis on *inhaling*; because of this they sometimes don't empty their lungs enough to get a full breath of fresh air when they inhale again.

DISCOVERING HOW TENSION FEELS

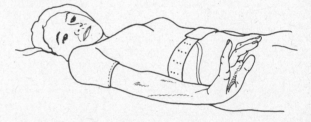

Lie down in a comfortable position. Raise one hand at the wrist. Raise just the hand, not the arm. Hold it there. Concentrate on the sensations on the top part of your forearm. The sensations that you feel will be *tension*. Now tell your hand to let go, and relax. The sensation which you now feel in your arm is *relaxation*.

If you wish, you can try this on any area of your body. Tense it, and then relax it. Note even the smallest changes in sensations that you feel. In this way you can have knowledge of your total body in terms of tension and relaxation. Start at your toes and work up to your head.

If you are unable to feel the sensation of tension as you tense a particular part of your body, you can touch the area with your hand and the tense area will feel hard to you. Interesting areas to try are your jaw, neck, and eye muscles. Most people are tense in these areas without being fully aware of it.

This exercise is a basic tool in learning to relax every part of your body. Take the time to explore yourself with it.

RELIEVING SIMPLE TENSIONS

This is an exercise that you can do any time and any place. It is especially good to relieve strain or minor aches and pains in the shoulders, neck and back, even as you are working.

Breathe from your abdomen and as you exhale, imagine that *you are sending your breath to the part of your body that you feel is tired or sore.* By thinking that you are breathing to that point you open capillaries, thus increasing circulation of blood. This is not so surprising when you stop to consider that most people can be caused to "blush" at the mention of a few words which embarrass them. Blushing is a form of verbally-induced capillary action. In the same way that you are able to tense your muscles through mental suggestion, you can also relax them.

For many people this exercise will begin working almost immediately; for others a bit more practice will be necessary. In either case it is a matter of getting in touch with any and all parts of your body where tension shows up, and then increasing blood flow and energy by relaxing the area, and thus opening capillaries. Slow and gentle suggestions are your tools. This is not like taking a pill. It is clearly building skills through practice.

Take advantage of moments when you are waiting in line somewhere, and use these moments to practice this exercise. Practice as you are waiting at the checkout counter at the grocery store, while waiting for appointments, while waiting in heavy traffic, and so on.

CENTERING

A very simple technique for getting in touch with yourself, as well as calming and relaxing yourself, is to concentrate on your *center.* Your center is literally your center. If you measured half way up your body you would touch a point a couple inches below your naval. Whenever you are nervous and tense, and especially if you feel pulled-in-all-directions-at-once, pause, if only for a moment, and concentrate on this point. Send your thoughts and feelings to your center. Feel it mentally. Feel it with your whole body. Send your breath to your center. Many people who do this for the first time feel tingling, tickling, or *magnetic* sensations emanating from a point below their naval. Others feel no sensations.

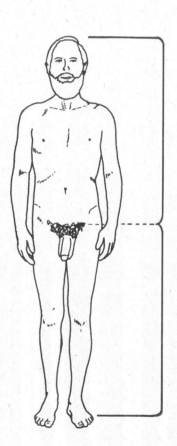

Concentrate on your center whenever you feel the need to bring yourself together, or whenever you are nervous or tense. It doesn't take more than a few seconds and you'll be quite surprised at the benefits.

TOTAL BODY RELAXATION

We have already described one way to get total body relaxation in the chapter on getting your imaginary doctor. Here's another one.

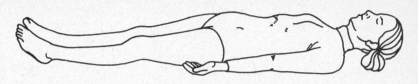

Lie down on your back with your legs uncrossed, arms at your sides or lightly resting on your chest. Close your eyes. Take several deep breaths in and out. With each breath you will be more relaxed. Then breathe as you normally do.

Tell your feet to relax. Do this mentally. Say to yourself, "I am relaxing my feet. They are becoming more and more relaxed." Now rest for a moment. Allow your feet to become relaxed. You may find it difficult to find the sensation of relaxation at first. Understand, however, that your feet are actually relaxing. After several times of doing the exercise you may feel this sensation of relaxing as tingling, numbness, warmth or cold, pulsing, or *magnetic* feelings.

Go on to relax your ankles. Tell them to relax. Say, "I am relaxing my ankles. They are becoming more and more relaxed." Rest a moment and let them relax. Let yourself feel the sensations of relaxation..

Now relax your lower legs. Use the same method described above. Then relax your knees. Your thighs. Your buttocks. Your pelvis. Your genitals. Your lower abdomen. Your upper abdomen. Your chest. Your back. Your neck. Your shoulders and upper arms. Your elbows. Your lower arms. Your wrists, hands, and fingers.

Now relax your jaw. Let it drop. Relax the muscles around your mouth. Relax your cheeks. Your eyes. Relax the muscles around your eyes. Relax your forehead and your scalp.

Allow the feelings of relaxation to flow throughout your body. **To deepen this feeling, count backwards from ten.** Say to yourself, "Ten. I am relaxed. Nine. More relaxed. Eight. Feeling deeper relaxation spreading through my body. Seven. More and more fully relaxed. Six. Etc." When you get to one you will be deeply relaxed, and will feel healthy and calm.

After you have done this exercise several times you will notice that your breathing (during the exercise) may become slow, deep, and rhythmically relaxed. It may be audible to you in the way that a sleeping person's breath is audible. This is a good sign of deep relaxation. You may also feel the sensation of *losing* or *going out of* your body. Do not be afraid of these feelings. Your body does not need your conscious control to keep functioning. Your heart beat will continue and you will breathe comfortably. These sensations, though perhaps strange to you at first, are signs of deep relaxation. With practice, you will feel how natural they are.

If you want to deepen your state of relaxation even further, imagine yourself on an elevator. Visualize the inside of the elevator completely. Imagine that it will be going from the tenth floor to the first floor. Watch the numbers of the elevator flash from ten to one as the elevator drops. Feel it drop. When you reach the bottom you will be deeply relaxed. Count each floor to yourself as you go down, in the same way that you counted to yourself in the first part of this exercise: "Ten. I am relaxing. Nine. Relaxing further. Etc."

You can also imagine that you are **pushing the image of your body to the edge of your consciousness**. To do this, visualize your consciousness as the edge of an ocean horizon. Allow your body to move out over the edge of your consciousness (the ocean) and then drop off the edge. Watch it fall, becoming smaller and smaller until it is out of sight.

Or you can imagine yourself drifting out into space, drifting weightlessly and able to move your consciousness wherever you wish to move it.

The first time you do these exercises, you may feel that nothing is happening. But doctors can measure *actual relaxation* in everyone who does this exercise. They can see muscles relax in most people even though the person may not fully recognize the sensations themselves. You can check this out by having someone touch your muscles as you relax, to feel the difference in the tension level as you do so.

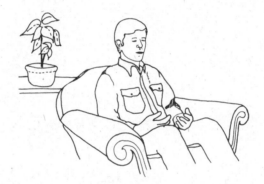

WAYS TO USE RELAXATION

Relaxation exercises are skills which once learned become easier and easier to do. After doing them a few times the process becomes automatic and you will discover yourself applying your skills unconsciously as you go through your daily routine. You will probably find that you can do even the total body relaxation exercise while sitting in a chair or during a short lull in your work. Total body relaxation can be used to:

Relax your whole body when you feel fatigued.

Relax your mind and body when you feel anger, emotional conflict, anxiety, grief from loss, or emotional upset of any kind.

Relax your body in order to increase circulation when you feel the first symptoms of an illness. This will help prevent disease.

Relax your body when you are ill to increase circulation and to send nutriment to the parts of your body that are ill, and to carry away wastes, thus allowing your body to heal itself.

Relax your body and mind to help you prepare for sleep.

Relax your body and mind in order to remove distractions and increase your alertness, to handle emergencies.

Relax your mind to reduce your *ego overlay* (see page 149) in order to help you get in touch with your imaginary doctor, your inner self, etc.

Relax your mind and body for spiritual enlightenment, extrasensory perception, seeing auras, achieving *alpha*, projecting your cosmic body, etc.

WHEN YOU ARE REALLY WIPED OUT

Sometimes people are so tired or tense that they feel they just don't have the energy to do a relaxation exercise. But this is probably when you need to do it the most. If you ever find yourself in this position, we suggest that you have a friend read you the total body relaxation exercise. Have them read in a slow, gentle, quiet voice, giving you plenty of time to relax after each instruction. This allows you to do the complete exercise without having to spend your own energy. All you have to do is listen to your friend's voice, and your body will do the rest. At times when your body is most fatigued and tense, you will be most open to relaxation suggestions presented in this way.

RELAXING A SPECIFIC PART OF YOUR BODY

The total body relaxation exercise can be modified to relax just one part of your body. First do the total body relaxation exercise as described. Then concentrate on the particular part of your body which you want to relax even more. Let's say you have a sprained wrist. After relaxing your whole body say to yourself, "I am relaxing my wrist. My wrist is becoming more and more relaxed. It feels warm, numb, feels so soft and relaxed that I can hardly move it, feels that is is pulsing with blood, feels that it is receiving energy from all over my body." Wait several moments and allow your wrist to completely relax. Do this exercise as many times as necessary for you to totally relax your wrist. With practice you may not need to do the total body relaxation exercise before you relax a part of your body. This partial body relaxation can be used to:

Relax a part of your body which is injured.

Bring increased blood flow and antibiotics (if you are taking them) to a part of your body that has an infection of any kind. This can work for anything from a boil to an infected fallopian tube.

Partially or completely anesthetize a part of your body which is feeling pain.

Relieve tension in fatigue target points of your body.

Relax muscles around blocked tubes, such as lung bronchi.

Increase blood flow to mucous membranes, allowing them to shrink, in the nose, Eustacian tube, throat and sinus areas, etc. This helps to relieve and heal those areas wherever they become inflamed.

Help a woman relax muscles around her uterus during labor in childbirth. This will make uterine contractions completely comfortable.

Once you have developed these skills you can apply them in any way that you wish.

INSTANT RELAXATION AND ENERGY

These exercises can be used to relax you and bring you energy in less than a minute. They are especially helpful at work, during arguments, before going in for an interview or exam, or in any situation where relaxation and mental alertness are important to you. We have included four exercises, one for each *element:* Fire, Air, Water, and Earth. You may find that you will be better able to receive energy from one of these elements than from any other. Most people do.

The benefits of these exercises can last up to four hours — or even a whole day.

Breathing Light: *(Element=Fire)* Close your eyes. Take several slow, very *deep* breaths, breathing from your abdomen. With each inhalation imagine that you are taking in energy from the universe. As you exhale imagine your whole body becoming more and more relaxed. Now imagine that the inside of your body, from your center out, is becoming brighter and brighter, radiant and illuminated. Let yourself fully enjoy this feeling for several moments. You are now relaxed and full of energy. Open your eyes and go about your business.

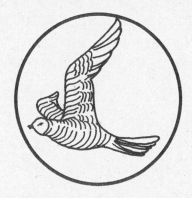

Expanding Aura: *(Element-Air)* Close your eyes. Take several slow, very deep breaths, breathing from your abdomen. With each inhalation imagine that you are taking in energy from the universe. As you exhale imagine your whole body becoming more and more relaxed. Now imagine that a thin aura of light surrounds your entire body. It can be any color you wish it to be. With each exhalation of breath imagine this aura becoming brighter and brighter, more and more colorful, and extending out from your body further and further. Imagine the aura pulsing and flashing with magnetic energy. Imagine the aura filling the space around you, and extending out as far as you wish it to reach. You are now relaxed and full of energy. Open your eyes and go about your business.

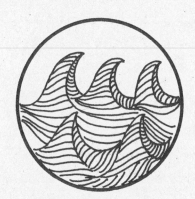

Diminishing Ripples: *(Element=Water)* Close your eyes. Take several slow, very deep breaths, breathing from your abdomen. With each inhalation imagine that you are taking energy from the universe. As you exhale imagine your whole body becoming more and more relaxed. Now imagine that you are standing on a ledge overlooking a quiet pool. Imagine that you are lifting a large, heavy ball over your head and then dropping it into the pool. Watch the ball as it enters the water. Imagine the splash in slow motion. Then watch the ball slowly sinking. As the ball disappears below the surface, visualize the water closing in around it. Visualize the rings of water rippling out over the surface. Watch until all the ripples have become completely still once more. You are now relaxed and full of energy. Open your eyes and go about your business.

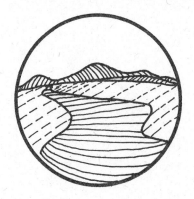

Energy From The Earth: *(Element=Earth)* Close your eyes. Take several slow, very deep breaths, breathing from your abdomen. With each inhalation imagine that you are taking energy from the universe. As you exhale imagine your whole body becoming more and more relaxed. Now imagine that you are sitting on the ground at a place you love. Visualize your body as beautiful, radiant, and healthy. Visualize the place you are in such as the beach, the forest, the mountains or the desert, as beautiful, radiant and healthy. You are fully in harmony with Nature. Now imagine that the energy of the earth is flowing up into your body, and you are becoming stronger, healthier, and more relaxed. You are now relaxed and full of energy. Open your eyes and go about your business.

You may find that some of the above work better for you than the others. Learn the ones which you like best and from which you experience the greatest benefit. Understand that these exercises will work better for you the more you use them.

You may wish to invent your own instant exercises, basing your inventions on scenes or memories in which you feel comfortable, relaxed, and full of energy.

Understand that when you get into a positive, relaxed, and energetic state of consciousness, your feelings will extend to people around you who may be less relaxed and energetic than you. This will improve your own feelings of relaxation and energy by easing sources of tension in the external environment.

A QUICKY EXERCISE FOR RELIEVING SIMPLE TENSION

At the first sign of fatigue in any part of your body, or when you first become aware of tension, stop whatever you are doing for a moment and imagine that your *Imaginary Doctor* is gently touching that spot. Imagine energy flowing from your imaginary doctor to that spot.

EYE RELAXATION

Eye strain can be at least as uncomfortable as a tension headache. Note too, that the eyes may be a fatigue target point for you. Palming is an excellent exercise for relieving this kind of tension:

To Palm: Place the palms of your hands directly over your eyes so as to block out all light. Do not press so hard that you feel pressure on your eyes. But you do want to block out all the light. Now let your eyes *remember* the color black. Many people will not see pure black at first. You may see pink, gray, green or most any color in the rainbow. You may also see shapes, colored clouds, flashes, etc. If this happens, and it probably will if you are palming to relieve eyestrain, find an object which is pure black and gaze at it for a moment; then go back to palming and try to remember black again. If you do not have a pure black object close by, imagine one. It may be a black coat, or a black chair, a black suitcase, etc. Most people remember *black fur* very easily. Black velvet is also easy to remember for many people.

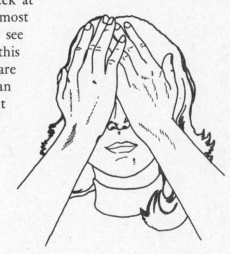

Your eyes will be resting completely when they can remember pure black and experience it in this way. Palm for periods of 2 to 3 minutes or until you get relief. Don't *strain* to see black. Simply relax your eyes and allow them to remember black.

Other benefits are often experienced in palming. By relieving tension and relaxing your eyes, you can actually improve your eyesight in many cases. Aldous Huxley claims to have improved his eyesight tremendously in this way. You can also feel other parts of your body relax as your eyes relax. Some people achieve total body relaxation with this method.

You can increase the effectiveness of palming, and also help your vision further, by relaxing the muscles in the back and sides of your neck. Other relaxation exercises in this chapter will help you in this.

A very few people find it very difficult to get pure black with palming. In fact, they may increase their eyestrain by working too hard at trying to get it. If you feel yourself straining in this way you should probably discontinue this exercise and try one of the others in this chapter.

SITTING AND COUNTING YOUR BREATHS — MEDITATION

Most people feel controlled by the thoughts that enter their minds. This exercise will free you from this feeling of *being controlled* or *victimized* by your thoughts.

Find a place where you will not be disturbed for ten minutes or more. Say to yourself that you are taking this time and devoting it to improving your life. (Many people feel they are unable to find time in their day to do this. They also feel that they want to improve their lives. If you find yourself in this position, realize that this exercise is as important as anything else you feel called upon to do.)

Sit on the floor, cushioned by a thin pillow or a rug, with your legs crossed, your back straight, and your hands resting palms up on your lap.

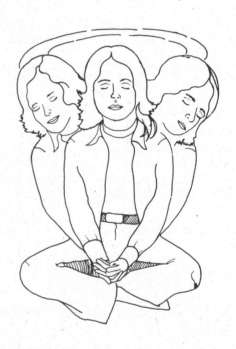

Close your eyes. Take several slow, deep breaths, breathing from your abdomen. Rock your body from your pelvis to the top of your head, making a full circular motion. Feel your body from the bottom of your spine to the top of your head as a whole unit. Rock in large circles at first, then rock in increasingly smaller circles until you feel your body coming to rest, centered, with your back straight. This is an equilibrium or rest position.

Now breathe in and out through your nose, taking breaths that are normal for you. Count "one" as you inhale, "two" as you exhale, "three" as you inhale, "four" as you exhale, and so on until you reach ten. Then go back to one and start all over again.

This completes the physical part of this exercise. *The idea here is to establish equilibrium and concentrate completely on counting your breaths.*

As you count your breaths, thoughts will enter your mind. Most people feel they have no control over these thoughts. You will feel that you do not consciously or deliberately think them or feel them. The thoughts may enter your mind and interrupt your counting without your asking them to come. You may be counting and you suddenly realize that you have stopped counting; you are thinking. When this happens, let the thought go. But don't try to resist it or stop it. Visualize your thoughts as birds flying toward you, flying freely into your mind, and then flying out of your mind again. When a

116

thought comes, note that the thought is there like a bird, let it fly freely through, then go back to counting your breaths.

The idea here is to **let your thoughts go.** Ordinarily a thought will stimulate you to think further. Relinquish the temptation to do this. Just let the thought pass. Then go back to counting your breaths. (An example of this process is: You have counted up to seven and you hear a car go by in the street. You find yourself thinking, "I wonder where the car is going?" Normally you might continue thinking about this for several minutes. During this exercise, however, say to yourself, *"noise of a car, wonder where it's going?"* Breathe in. *"Number eight."* Breathe out. *"Nine."* Etc.)

Although this exercise sounds very easy to do, it actually takes intense effort to succeed in counting breaths without interruption by your thoughts. Five minutes of this exercise is plenty at first. You can extend this time as you develop increasing skills.

☆   ☆   ☆

Use this exercise to:

Give yourself a complete **vacation from the pressures,** tensions, and duties of your daily routine.

Build a peaceful place in your mind, a personal space in your life where you are free from worrisome or negative thoughts and feelings.

Prove to yourself that **you do not have to act on every thought or feeling** which enters your mind. If you wish to do so you can let these thoughts and feelings pass as freely as you do in this exercise, leaving your mind alert, relaxed and energetic.

Understand that **you can control which thoughts or feelings you will hold onto and act on.** You have the choice of where to use your energy.

Choose thoughts to achieve health and promote healing if you are sick. This will relax muscles in your body, increase blood flow, and release energy blocks. Thus you can prevent disease in yourself when you first feel symptoms, and allow your body to heal itself if you are sick.

Remove causes of diseases, such as the mental tension which causes an ulcer.

Relax your mind and body for spiritual enlightenment, extrasensory perception, seeing auras, achieving **alpha,** projecting your cosmic body, etc.

Look upon the relaxation exercises here as key skills in preventive medicine and as basic tools for healing. Most people prefer to learn these exercises slowly and deliberately with the understanding that **it will take time and practice to fully** incorporate them into their lives. We suggest that you pick out one exercise that particularly appeals to you, and learn that one well before going on to learn others. Once your body and mind becomes familiar with these techniques, more complex exercises, or exercises which you invent yourself, will come easily.

REST-WORK CYCLES

Everyone's body converts food to nutriment at a different rate of speed. Likewise, your blood carries nutriment to the cells, and wastes away from the cells, at a different rate. In addition, every activity requires a different amount of energy. Things like the size and particular construction of your body, and the efficiency with which you work, will also affect the rates at which your cells eat and excrete. All this indicates that the amount of activity which you do in a day, and the amount of rest you need, will be highly individualized. Throughout your day, how much you can do at one stretch, before you must rest, and how much rest you need before more activity, will not be the same for you as for other people.

You can determine the quality of life for each cell in your body by getting in touch with the rest and work cycles which best match your body and the activities that you do. In the paragraphs that follow, we will tell you more about how to do this.

EVALUATING YOUR REST-WORK CYCLES

As a group, laborers, craftsmen, and people who use their muscles extensively in their work, are more in touch with their rest-work cycles than are office workers, professional people, house wives and house husbands, and teachers. Doctors see more house wives or husbands, and professional people suffering from fatigue than any other group. This is probably because the symptoms of body fatigue in people who use their bodies alot in their work, are usually much more straightforward and easy to *read*. Mental fatigue, or nervous fatigue, on the other hand, is more subtle and indirect for most people. The myth is that there is no reason to get tired unless you are doing physical labor, but we know now that *mental and emotional efforts take an equal amount of energy as, say, a carpenter building a house*. The only difference is that different parts of your body are doing the work.

To evaluate your own particular rest-work cycles, *locate the place in your body which shows the first signs of fatigue*. Nearly everyone has one or more *fatigue target points* but they are different for everyone. It may be soreness in your arms or across your shoulders, or in your lower back. It can be the eye muscles, the muscles in your neck and throat, or your stomach muscles. Mental fatigue often shows up as lack of concentration, worry, daydreaming, hallucinating, "edginess," irritability, mind-wandering, headaches, and so on. The way to get in touch with that is simple. Just note what part of you feels worse, or most tired, the next time you get overly tired. That will be one of your fatigue target points.

As you go through a normal day, pay particular attention to your fatigue target point or points. *Note the time of day when you first become conscious of these points*. This does not mean when it first gets sore. It means when your attention is first drawn to it: maybe it's a slight strain, maybe it's a very minor and subtle "ache," maybe it's when your mind begins to wander. These are messages from your body telling you to rest. If you rest at this point you will stay in harmony with your body's needs. Working while you are fatigued means that cells in some parts of your body may not be getting the nutriment they need and that they may not be getting rid of their wastes. This keeps them at a low energy level, where they provide excellent environments for growth of bacteria and viruses. So by controlling your level of fatigue, you can help control your level of health.

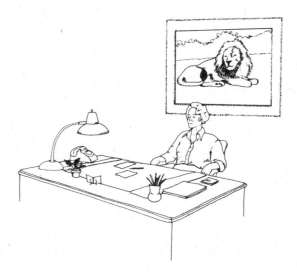

When you are fatigued, rest will allow the cells of your body to get rid of wastes and take in nutrients to restore their energy. There are many ways to get this rest. We show you some particularly effective ways of getting complete and beneficial rest in a very short period of time, as short as a few seconds or a few minutes. You'll find instructions for these in the section called *Relaxation* in this chapter.

After a rest or relaxation period, work at a pace that feels natural to you. Again be sensitive to your fatigue target points. When you again feel fatigued, stop and rest again. In this way you can keep your body at a healthy energy level throughout the day. Keeping track of rest-work cycles in this way is a deliberate and conscious act at first; but your body rapidly learns to take care of these things automatically. You are teaching your body a new skill to keep it healthy and well.

SPEED TRIPS

Many people experience the feeling of *over-revving* — the sensation that your body is going faster than your mind, or that your mind is going faster than your body. To synchronize your body with your mind, stop whatever you are doing and do a shortened version of any relaxation exercise in this chapter. You can do it while standing or sitting; either will work for this. Usually no more than 30 seconds will be necessary to re-establish the marriage between your body and your mind.

If you find yourself having a particularly "out-of-sync" kind of day, pause every hour or so to do a 30-second breathing exercise. You will discover that your energy level will increase and your body will become more comfortable.

EVALUATING WHERE YOUR ENERGY IS GOING

Tension and nervousness burn up alot of energy. So do other activities connected with work, but which may or may not be directed at getting the work done. The following can help you locate where your energy goes.

Someone looking over your shoulder: causing you to worry about your work, how you dress, how you look, how you get along with others, how you get along with him or her, and so on. The worry takes energy.

Time limits: worry about getting your work done on time consumes energy.

Production limits: worry and pressure about producing a quantity which you or someone else expects of you consumes energy.

Worry about home: your mind on family, relatives, neighbors, or friends, paying bills, doing repairs, and so on. These take energy.

General work discomfort: if you are doing work which is boring to you or which is uncomfortable for you, those factors will take energy.

Social dynamics and gossip: complaining about the boss, complaining about fellow workers, flirting with co-workers, and so on, takes energy.

Understimulation: if your work or environment asks less of you than you are capable of giving, or want to give, your energy output may be inhibited.

Senses overstimulated: loud noises, high levels of activity around you, noxious smells, provocative smells, too bright or too dim a light ... all these consume your energy.

Crowdedness: bumping into objects or people because of a bad arrangement of space, or simply that the average space between you and other workers or things is too close or too far away for your comfort, may be aggravating for you and will consume your energy.

Order and disorder: if things are never where you last put them, or if everything must be returned to an exact place, you will be spending alot of energy just looking for things or keeping them in order.

Competition with co-workers: Striving for promotions, pay raises, or simply praise from supervisors or fellow workers, requires alot of energy.

Everything you stop doing which you do not want to continue doing will bring you increased energy for the things you do want to do. *Understand that you can control your attitude in all of the above situations.* Note your worry whenever you feel it. Recognize that it is draining your energy and is not contributing to getting your work done. To reduce the worry, consider the things we discuss in *Other Alternatives* below.

OTHER ALTERNATIVES

If you are unable to rest or do relaxation exercises when you are tired, and are unable in other ways to establish rest-work cycles which are comfortable for you, consider alternatives:

Work slower from the beginning of the day, pacing yourself at a rate that feels right for you.

Quit the job and get one that works better for you.

Check up and see if there is anything you can do to increase your energy by doing something in one of the other parts of preventive medicine: sleep, bathing, clothing, exercises, etc.

Talk to your boss about exercise, relaxing, and work cycles. And show them the rest-work section of this book.

Point out to your boss that your efficiency level goes down at a certain time of the day, and that you've found you can bring up your efficiency level by taking a break for a short rest, or to do relaxation exercises.

Assess your coffee break routine: don't, for example, try to bring your energy level up with coffee and sweets. For more information on this, see the section on *Diet* in this chapter. Also assess whether your social contacts during coffee breaks are sapping your energy.

Concentrate on your work: lack of concentration usually drains energy. In general, when your concentration level goes down, you start running troubling thoughts through your head, and that takes a lot of energy. You can increase concentration by focusing your attention exactly on the senses involved with the task at hand: focus your eyes on colors and shapes of things related to your task; smell whatever there is to smell (unless it is noxious); listen to the sounds you make as you work; feel how your skin surfaces relate to the work.

You may want to use your imaginary doctor to help you examine your work environment for areas that can be improved.

WAYS TO HANDLE UNPLEASANT TASKS

There are many things that have to be done but which you may not enjoy doing. This is particularly addressed to short-term tasks like dishwashing, changing a tire, etc. The thing to remember is that the moments spent doing those tasks are not less important moments of your life than others. (In terms of your body, the commercials during the football game on t.v. are just as precious and real as the touchdowns).

In the case of necessary tasks, you can bring double pleasure and energy to your life during the times you are doing these tasks by finding ways to make your time with them enjoyable. Not that this is easy to do, nor is it always possible. But often it is possible, too. When faced with such situations, try these suggestions:

Stand outside yourself and watch yourself doing the task. Instead of saying or feeling, "I hate this job," say to yourself, "Now I am picking up a dirty dish, now I am putting it in the soapy water, now I am washing it off, now I am rinsing it, now I am putting it in the drying rack," or whatever is appropriate, and accurately describes what you are doing.

As you watch yourself in this way, look for potential sources of pleasure, however seemingly

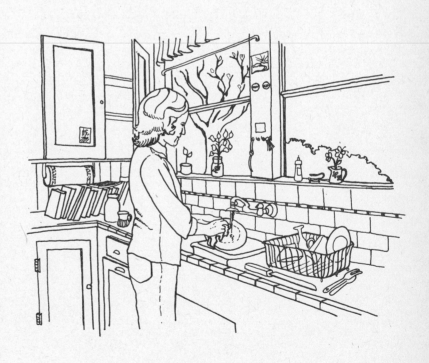

small, which are inherent in the work. Perhaps it is the sensation of dipping your hands into the water. Perhaps it is rinsing away the suds. Or maybe there is a pleasant view from a window to look at as you work.

Assess the work area to see if there are any ways to make your time there more enjoyable. Then go ahead and do whatever you can to improve it. It might involve adding color to the area, it might mean investing some money in tools which are nicer to handle, it might involve changing that work area to another place.

Turn your full attention to the parts of the task which feel good, look good, smell good, or which satisfy you mentally.

Sometimes, very small changes can turn necessary tasks into pleasure. Adding color to a work area, increasing the light, clearing away extraneous clutter, or making a more effective place to store your tools, are all small changes that can work in this way. Standing outside yourself as you work may bring attention to such details. Understand that in working out rest-work cycles in your life, you are in control of your energy levels; you can direct where your energy goes.

SLEEP

Everyone's sleep needs are different. Attempting to conform to the eight-hour sleep standard may very well prevent you from getting in touch with the sleep pattern that is normal for you.

Some people feel best going to bed early in the evening, getting a full night's sleep, and awakening early in the morning. Others feel best if they sleep during the day, and spend their waking hours at night. Some people use napping to supplement their sleep needs.

Many people's sleep patterns are determined by social patterns: their job, television schedules, family responsibilities, etc. We feel that it is healthy to get in touch with your own body's messages where sleep is concerned. When you sleep and for how long, is not in itself the important thing here; the important thing is that you can go to sleep easily and wake up feeling rested.

There is a sleep cycle which most people normally follow: you go from a light sleep to a deep sleep and back to a light sleep in 90 minutes. Some of this time is spent in a state of consciousness which sleep researchers call REM (rapid eye movement) sleep. This is the part of sleep where people dream. When people are deprived of sleep or if their REM sleep is constantly interrupted they become moody, irritable, depressed, have difficulty concentrating, and hallucinate. They may suffer a loss or gain in appetite and they are more susceptible to infection. Their muscular co-ordination becomes less efficient, their vision blurs, and their body rhythms may become erratic. It is known that "growth hormone," which is believed to be important in regeneration, is secreted only in deep sleep.

Sleep is also important when you are sick. If you are sick or injured, your body needs extra energy available for healing — for building up antibodies, for collecting and disposing of bacteria, and for creating new cells to replace cells destroyed or damaged by sickness. Your body's healing processes are activities that require energy, just as playing tennis requires energy. A good mental model to follow is that if your body gets a case of the flu, it will require about the same energy to heal itself as it would take you to walk about 150 miles over a three-day period with a 40-pound pack on your back. Additional sleep is one way to get the energy necessary for healing, since during sleep most of your body's energies will be reserved for healing activities.

GET IN TOUCH WITH YOUR OWN SLEEP PATTERNS

The message which your body sends out to you when it needs more sleep is one of the more obvious ways it has to tell you it wants something: you feel "sleepy." Upon arising each morning ask yourself how you feel: sleepy or well rested? If you wake up feeling sleepy, ask yourself why. The simplest answer will be that you went to bed too late. Another common complaint is that you got up several times during the night to urinate. This is usually remedied by not drinking fluids in the four hours before you go to bed. Other common causes of sleeplessness are an uncomfortable mattress, being too hot or too cold, or the light being too bright in the room. The remedy for each of these is obvious and very individualized.

If you have difficulty falling asleep, you will probably discover that you may be able to remedy the situation by cutting down on your intake of stimulants: coffee, tea, cola drinks, and pep pills. Similarly, if indigestion is the cause, don't go to bed directly after eating a large meal. Your stomach will not stop to rest until it has finished digesting your food.

The main thing to remember about sleep is that neither your body or your mind can rest and sleep until they are first relaxed. If you have difficulty going to sleep, try any of the relaxation exercises in this book. They will prepare your body and mind for sleep and will improve the quality of both sleeping and dreaming.

Sleeping medications affect your entire body and have many side effects. Furthermore they *fail* to help 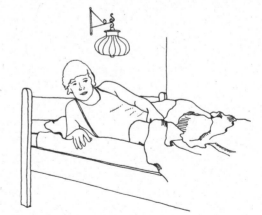 you deal with the causes of sleeplessness that we mention above. (See *Drugs Are Helpers* on *Barbiturates* for more information.)

Discovering why you can't sleep, doing things to improve your sleep, and getting in touch with your body's sleep needs are essential in maintaining maximum energy levels in each cell in your body and thus in maintaining good health.

DREAMING

Dreaming is a continuation of daily thought processes, but dreams tend to be more open and free than most people's waking thoughts usually are.

Dreams are sometimes gentle reminders to the dreamer about something that he or she has forgotten to do. For example, a woman may dream of having a baby and be reminded that she has forgotten to take her birth control pill that day.

Dreams often deal with problems and solutions to problems in everyday life.

Dreams reflect the emotional activity of the dreamer's personality.

Dreams have their own language. Each dreamer has his or her own language in dreams, a language of images and symbols which is seldom the same for any two people.

Depriving people of dreams by awakening them in the middle of the sleep period during which they are dreaming results in their becoming irritable, neurotic or psychotic, depending on the person and the degree of dream deprivation.

People can get in touch with their dreams. In this way, they can sometimes work out conscious solutions to conflicts and problems which they feel, instead of having to act out their dreams in their everyday lives.

Most people are taught that only waking experiences are *real* or valid. But we feel that dream experiences are as real to your mind as waking experiences.

Dreams are links with the *collective unconscious* and can provide you with pure information from it.

Dreams are connections with the *astral plane* — a totally different reality from that which you perceive in everyday life.

Many psychologists take the view that dreams are rooted in everyday reality, and are extensions of your daily experiences.

Doing the best you can to provide yourself with a healthy dream life would seem, then, to be important. Uninterrupted sleep, as discussed in the sleep section of *Preventive Medicine* is the key to good dreaming.

GETTING IN TOUCH WITH YOUR DREAMS

Everyone dreams. Some people remember their dreams easily, others with difficulty. The simplest way to get in touch with your dreams seems almost too simple. But it does work.

Before you go to sleep at night, and while you are very relaxed and ready to fall asleep, tell yourself that you will remember your dreams when you awake.

Keep a notebook and a pencil beside your bed. When you awake, and before you do anything else, remember your dreams and write them down. You may remember very little at first. By practicing this technique many people are able to remember as many as three or four dreams per night.

Keep your dreams in the notebook and refer to them from time to time, noting repetitions of whole dreams, parts of dreams, themes of dreams, and images. During the day, ask yourself what these dreams, themes, and images mean to you.

In this way, you will bring your dreams into your conscious life. They will become a more active part of your life. One dream researcher suggested that you learn to treat your dreams as though they were people, to look upon each one as an individual unlike any others. Like people, one gets to know their dreams by looking closely and by listening carefully to every movement and sound they make.

INTERPRETATION OF DREAMS

Sigmund Freud and other analysts have sought to create a sort of universal symbolism for interpreting the language and symbols of dreams. Although some people have found this method of interpreting dreams useful, others have found it less so. In more recent years, people studying dreams have come to the conclusion that each person creates his own "language of the unconscious" — a language of images, situations, words, and characterizations of people. In this respect dreams are like poems, songs, plays, and short stories or novels which you must listen to and read carefully before you fully grasp what the *author* is trying to say. The author, of course, is the dreamer.

One way to *make sense* of dreams is to act out the various roles and situations which occur in a dream. Here's how that can be done:

Recall the dream, particularly remembering people and objects.

Assume the character of each object or person in the dream. For example, let's say that I dreamed about a telephone call to a friend in another city. The characters and objects are myself, my friend and the telephone.

To act out the dream, I begin by taking on the character of the telephone, since it is apparently the least complex of the three. It is essential that I preface each statement I make about the character with "I am." You then express any *feelings* about each character or object — probably one of the most important parts of dealing with dreams in this way. Here's how my characterization of the phone might go:

"I am a telephone. I am an electronic device for communicating with people in faraway places. I am able to carry voices back and forth on a wire while the people talking neither see nor can touch each other."

As it happened, when I characterized the phone in this way I realized that I had chosen this form of communication with my friend for a specific reason — that being that I did not want to see or be able to touch my friend as I spoke to him. These revelations came to me naturally as I played the role of the phone describing the phone with the *feelings* that "being" the phone evoked for me. (It is very important to note that the phone will probably mean different things to different people and you would be doing yourself a diservice by using my interpretations of my dreams to interpret your own or someone else's dreams.)

Go on to the next character of the dream and assume its character, using your dream as the script.

Just as you have control of what you dream, you also have control of how you interpret a dream. You chose the thoughts and feelings. There are, for example, an infinite number of ways to describe a telephone. I might have said, "I am a telephone, an instrument for bringing people closer together when they are separated by long distances." Note the vast 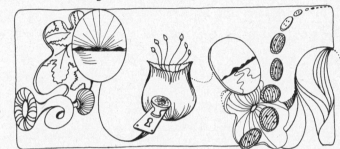 difference between that description and the previous one about the phone as a way of communicating without seeing or being able to touch the person you are talking to. Thus, your description can tell you as much about what you are thinking and feeling as will your interpretation of the dream itself.

Now put yourself in the situation of the dream. For example, with my dream I might sit down in a chair and dial an imaginary telephone, just as I had done in the dream. It is tremendously helpful to do the gestures with the words, moving and speaking just as though you were acting out the dream on a stage. So I dial the phone and speak to my friend just as I remembered speaking to him in the dream. As my friend answers and speaks to me I assume his voice, and his gestures, too, just as I remembered in the dream.

As you act out the dream in this conscious and deliberate way, you become increasingly more familiar with the dream. It is now taking place in your wakeful state of consciousness where you can study it, and act out its parts from the point of view of a person reading a book or seeing a play. You can even stop and repeat actions that you want to take a more careful look at.

More often than not, people leave their dreams in an unresolved state. Like a heated conversation with a friend or associate, you come away thinking of what you would have liked to have said but didn't. This represents a lot of *pent-up* emotion and energy. But the next step in this way of treating dreams is to *act out* what you wanted to say but didn't. This is accomplished by acting out the dream again, saying and doing whatever you wish, expressing the deepest things you feel.

In the privacy of your own room, as you work out your dreams, you can try out new ways of dealing with yourself, your friends and situations which have previously been difficult for you to deal with. You can, in essence, *try out* ideas that you feel timid about acting out in real life, using these exercises as rehearsals for something you will eventually do. In this way, you can avoid the pitfalls of acting out all your feelings in real life, which, if most of us were to do that would end up getting thrown in jail. For example, you might act out punching your boss in the nose, something you would not do in real life because it would result in your getting fired and perhaps even arrested for assault and battery. But acting it out in privacy allows you to test your feelings and to also let out anger that may be causing you to be irritable and distracted.

This method of interpreting dreams takes some time to learn, but it is well worth the effort. We recommend it because it allows the dreamer complete freedom in interpreting the language of their dreams.

INFLUENCING YOUR DREAMS

Just as your dreams can influence your conscious life, you can consciously influence your dreams. You can, for example, ask a question to yourself before you go to sleep and have the answer come to you in your dream. Here's how to do that:

Just before going to sleep do one of the relaxation exercises in this chapter. Then ask yourself the question you want answered. It can be any question that you have in your life. Tell yourself that you will get the answer in your dream and you will remember the answer when you awaken. The dream world seems to hold all the answers in the universe. When you wake up in the morning remember your dreams and write them down, if you wish. You may not get your answer on the first night you do this. It may take several nights of dreaming and doing this exercise before you are successful.

A famous example of getting answers through dreams, one cited in many medical books, involved a well-known chemist who was trying to determine the chemical structure of benzine. He saw the shape of the molecule in his dream, and later verified it in his laboratory!

It is possible to choose the characters in your dreams, what you dream about, and where the dreams take place. This will take more practice but you can do it using the simple exercise we describe above.

To increase your ability to more fully use your dream consciousness, to move in your dream consciousness as freely as you move in your waking consciousness, start with the following exercise:

Relax yourself using any relaxation exercise which you enjoy. Visualize in your mind's eye a simple image or shape. It can be any image which you yourself design: a geometric shape, a shape from nature, etc. Pick one that is easy for you to recall and toward which you feel positive. You may wish to draw a picture of this image on a piece of paper.

Before going to sleep at night, visualize this image in your mind's eye. Tell yourself that this image will appear in your dreams. You will be able to see it and recall it when you awaken.

When you awaken recall your dreams and try to remember if you saw your image there. This may take quite a bit of practice before you are successful.

This is a basic exercise for gaining the ability to consciously participate in your dream world. From here you can move on to more and more deliberate and conscious use of your dreams.

HELPERS IN DREAMS

Many people discover helpers such as imaginary doctors, spiritual advisors, alter egos or other personal consultants in their dreams. These characters or things often provide messages leading to positive changes in the dreamer's life.

You may want to seek these helpers in your own dreams, and you can do this by getting in touch with your dreams (page 129), putting emphasis on making contact with your helpers.

Once you have gotten in touch with your helpers you may find the exercise for influencing your dreams (page 132) useful in getting specific answers. You will also find it useful to bring your dream helpers into your waking life as you would do with your imaginary doctor (page 6).

LIFE RHYTHMS

Life rhythms are only beginning to be studied. Recent studies relate body rhythms to *cosmic* and *universal rhythms:* the human body interacting with sun, moon, earth, and other bodies in the universe. For example, studies have related unexplainable increases in aggressive behavior of certain groups of people to solar flare activity — magnetic storms on the sun.

Another study deals with cosmic rays and their effect on various forms of plant and animal life. A cosmic ray is basically a flow of energy from sources outside the earth's atmosphere. It is made up of protons, alpha particles, and atomic nuclei, including high energy electrons and protons. Since each cell of living tissue, both plant and animal, contains these same elements, it would not be really surprising to discover life rhythms varying with variations in cosmic ray activity. Ordinarily life on earth is protected from cosmic ray activity by the earth's ionosphere — electrically charged gaseous matter — which is held in place by the earth's magnetic field. This ionosphere acts as a shield to reflect back cosmic rays. But the density of the ionosphere expands and contracts by day and night cycles. At certain times within this cycle, cosmic rays can get through to interact with the cells of living things.

Researchers have related the color change of fiddler crabs to cosmic ray activity. They also found that the oxygen consumption of potatoes, carrots, shellfish, and rats went up and down on a scale directly relating to cosmic radiation and magnetic vibrations.

Since cosmic ray activity is so closely linked to magnetic energy (the ionosphere letting more or fewer cosmic rays through, according to the strength of the magnetic pull), people have begun to study the influence of magnetic fields on animal behavior. It has been found, for example, that worms and snails veer in given compass directions according to the times of the day, the month, and the year.

All living things may get information about their orientation in space and time from the interaction of their body cells with electromagnetic fields and cosmic ray activity in the external environment. These interactions of energy could be used by the central nervous system in ways that we have barely begun to understand. It is possible that heart beat is related to universal rhythms, perhaps even rhythms outside our solar system. The sensitive magnetic fields which man knows exist within each living cell certainly cannot help but be influenced by the energies of the universe.

The problem at this point seems to be to figure out what influences these energies really do have on our lives, and what, if anything, we want to do about it. Presumably we could improve our lives with such knowledge, varying our conscious activities to match what we know or suspect is happening with flows of energy outside ourselves which we have no way of influencing. Thus there may be times when the "powers of the universe" are truly working in our favor, within any given time and space that we choose to act.

BIO-RHYTHMS IN YOUR BODY

People have more colds in the winter than in the summer. This may be due to temperature changes, with the body putting out more energy to keep warm. However, other factors may be involved. In the winter the days are shorter, and plants as well as many animals are hibernating. Human beings seem to want to do the same amount of work the year around. This attitude may be ignoring signals coming in from universal orders: seasonal flux or daily changes of the earth in relation to other cosmic bodies. It may be that people need more rest in the winter than they do in the summer because there is simply less available energy during that time.

Indian tribes used to have harvest finished by the winter solstice. Then they'd go into their communal huts and mend their tools, and tell stories until spring. That fit in with their natural body rhythm. Now people are less in touch with their rhythms, and that's possibly one of the reasons they get sick in the winter more than in summer. All this gives us a new perspective on the Biblical saying, " . . . a time to live, and a time to die; a time to sow, and a time to reap."

Your body has minute rhythms, hour rhythms, daily rhythms, monthly rhythms, yearly rhythms. The adrenal gland releases a certain amount of hormone at a particular time of day: sexual hormones are secreted at a particular time of day, and so on. It is now known that the time of day that people are exposed to a bacteria or virus will determine how severely they get the disease, or if they get it at all. This may be due to the total body chemistry being different at different times of the day. Doctors don't know enough about this yet to suggest ways to use it to prevent illness.

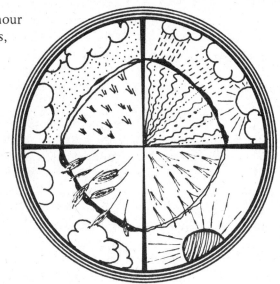

The menstrual cycle is a moon cycle, as opposed to a yearly or daily cycle. It is influenced — timed somehow — according to lunar time: 28 or 29 days, more or less. Most women have mood changes, hormonal changes, and blood changes, as well as changes in muscle tension, that correspond with these cycles. Once aware of this, they can plan activities to correspond with changes in their bodies.

Men have cycles similar to the woman's lunar cycle. But men don't have anything like a menstrual cycle to use as an easy reference point. One study made in England some years back showed that men who denied having cyclic life changes very predictably became moody and irritable, got into fights, and had marital difficulties every two or three months on regular cycles! The study also revealed changes in their blood chemistry and hormone secretions.

The body has various energy levels which correspond to the seasons: some people have more energy in summer, less in winter. Such a person might go to bed earlier in the winter as the days get shorter, work themself a little less, and relax more. It's a simple problem of conserving energy, *using your energy the best way you can in terms of your own body.*

The daily and seasonal rhythms of the earth probably affect the human body much more than we know. There's a hormone that doctors have recently named the "summer hormone," which is found in measurable amounts in the human body only during the summer, and which helps people keep their weight lower in the summer. This influences diet and the amount of fat on a person's body: less fat to hold in the body heat during summer months.

There's also the phenomenon of changing sides of your body: you breathe out of one nostril for several hours, then the other. And there's speculation that all the organs and glands that have *mates* — such as lungs, kidneys, and adrenal glands — may do this to some extent, letting one side rest while the other side works. Also, the skin temperature of the right side of the body is higher while you are sleeping than the left.

All of these things mean that the human body, and every living cell within it, is influenced by rhythms. If a person wants to use energy in the best way they can, they should try to get in touch with their own life rhythms.

A MODEST PROPOSAL

Your body, your own life, can become a laboratory for studying more about life rhythms. Keep records over a period of time, and you will begin to pick up on cyclic patterns in your life, and perhaps find that you are able to make adjustments in your conscious activities so that your energy is more in harmony with the energy of the universe. You will have to design your own system for doing this. Others have kept records relating mood shifts, energy levels, intellectual capacities and sexual drives to moon cycles, seasonal cycles. Book stores carry almanacs which tell about lunar cycles and the shifts of the seasons on a yearly basis. There are also astrological guides available in book stores if you want to go further.

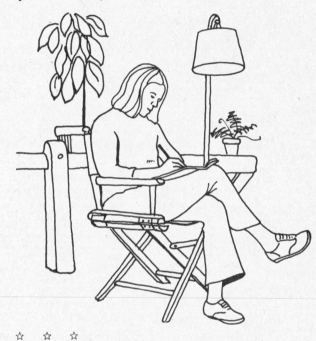

☆   ☆   ☆

Most medical research up to now has been done in large universities under big budgets. Lately most research has centered on highly specialized subjects. You have the greatest tool for research into healing and preventing disease: a human body. Your body contains all the answers it needs to keep itself healthy. By getting in touch with your inner self and by learning to read the messages of your body, you can learn things about healing which high-budget, highly-specialized medical research programs may never discover. If it works for you, your information will be just as valid as theirs.

WHERE YOU BE

Creating an external environment which expresses your own inner vision of what you would like your physical environment to be helps get you in harmony with your life and relieves tensions of alienation. When you are at home, at a job, or in a community situation which makes you ill at ease, angry, anticipatory, or in any other way upset, those tensions are expressed in the muscles of your body. The body's response to external *threats,* however seemingly mild those threats may appear, tends to be still based on the animal instincts of "fight or flight." This means that blood and energy move to the muscles of the arms, legs, and trunk, and that most of the vital organs get less blood and energy at such times. Probably everyone has had the experience of eating when angry or upset, and then getting a stomach ache. The reason for this is clear — your blood is not going to your stomach, but to your limbs.

When the muscles are in a constant state of tension, blood can't flow as freely, hormones can't get through to stimulate other body actions, healing foods can't get through. The result is that some cells within your body go un-nourished or under-nourished, and the cells cannot get rid of their excrements when the road is blocked by tension.

Any cell or organ of your body where blood flow is limited by tension or for any other reason, is more prone to disease and infection than an area that is receiving a good, strong, steady flow of blood. It will also take longer to repair itself following infection or injury because its supply of nutriment is limited and/or slow in coming. Nutriment is only part of what happens between the blood and the cells of organs and tissue: white blood cells also carry away bacteria, particles of damaged cells, and the waste products excreted by the cells in the usual course of their lives. A body free of tension and otherwise in fine shape means that these wastes are freely carried off and dumped out through your urine and feces, rather than lingering in your body where they can sap your energy.

CHECKING OUT THE SPACES

Living in spaces of maximum harmony with your inner self means less tension and more energy for every cell in your body. Evaluating the degree of harmony which you have, and figuring out what to do to increase that harmony begins with getting in touch with your inner self, wherein lies your vision of *the way things should be.* Here's a good way to do that:

Find yourself a quiet place where you will not be disturbed or distracted for twenty to thirty minutes. Late in the evening or early in the morning is usually a good time for this. Sit in a comfortable position with your arms and legs uncrossed. Do the relaxation exercise which you use to get your imaginary doctor. Close your eyes if it helps you to cut down on visual distractions.

Home Vision: Imagine a house in which you feel perfectly comfortable, where you feel absolutely at ease, and completely healthy, joyful and radiant. Imagine what the walls are made of. Since this house is completely in your mind, you can use any material that you can imagine. You can use materials that have not yet been discovered, or you can use materials from the past. There are no limits. Let yourself go. The house can be any size since money is no object. As you do this, bear in mind that some people will see the house, others will feel it, and still others will simply feel that they are *making it up* in their mind. Any of these ways of getting in touch with your inner vision is fine. Do not be disappointed if it is not as *real* as you would like it to be in your mind.

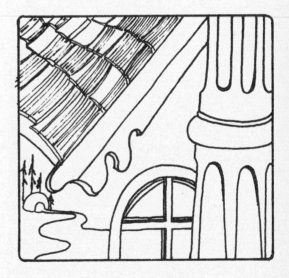

Come On In: If you are outside the house, imagine yourself walking up to the door, opening it, and going inside. If you are inside, look around you for a moment, picture the furniture, and then find a comfortable place to sit down. How does the thing you are sitting on feel to you? Is it hard or soft? How does it feel when you run your hands over it? Now picture the things on the walls of your imaginary house. Imagine the kinds of plants, aquariums, modern conveniences, artifacts, rugs, or whatever you want your home to have. What colors do you see around you? Furnish your imaginary home with whatever things make you joyful.

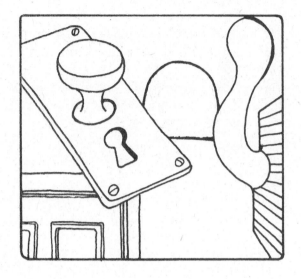

Tour The Grounds: Now imagine yourself getting up from your comfortable place in your imaginary house. Walk to the front or back door, open it, and walk outside. Look at the land around you. Is there water nearby? Are there hills? Is the land flat? Are there trees? What temperature is the air? Do you see concrete or earth? Breathe the air. How does it feel in your lungs? How does the sky look over your head? If it is nighttime, can you see the stars and the moon? Are there gardens, fences, flowers, lawns, open fields, or other things around you?

Community Organization: Go out into the community. Go on foot, by car, by helicoptor, by public transportation, or simply hover above the community in angel fashion. However you want to do it is up to you. Imagine how large the community is. Imagine what kinds of entertainments and stimulations you want there to be: schools, tools, libraries, civic buildings, general landscape, architecture, the kinds of transportation used. Imagine how the people work together and interact, and the kinds of community projects that they do together. Is it a community of high key activity, hustling and bustling, or is it low key, quiet, slow and easy?

Go To Your Work: Now imagine an ideal job. Imagine exactly what you would like to do. You have total choice. Present training and skills are no object in your imaginary job. You can have any training and any job you can imagine. Go as far as you want. If you can't pick a specific thing to do, just pick a mood and pick the kind of people you would like to have as co-workers. Decide whether you would like to be building something, designing things, engineering things, working with people, or what. Imagine a salary. Imagine what needs are being met economically by your job, and adjust your salary to this. Imagine little things around you, your office or working space, the sights outside your window, etc.

Going Home: Imagine yourself returning home from a day at work. Imagine the kind of vehicle that would convey you to your home: car, plane, walking, bus, train, etc. What kind of people are you with? Or are you alone? How long does it take you to commute? Finally you are back home. You open the door of your imaginary house. You enter the room where you are now sitting. Concentrate on how you feel right now. Many people who do this exercise feel warm, free, secure, and fully in control of their lives. It is a healthy feeling. It is the way it feels to get in touch with your inner self.

Once you have made these contacts, you can return to your imaginary home, job, or community any time that you wish, either by sitting down and actually going through the instructions again, or by voluntarily recalling them to mind. You may also find that, from time to time, your inner visions change.

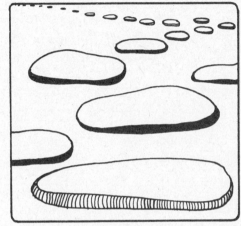

HARMONIES

Look for things in your external environment which closely resemble or perfectly conform to things which you saw when you went inside yourself. These can be the smallest things imaginable — a flower, the arrangement of objects on a table, the way light reflects from the surface of a window, wall, or a piece of furniture, or a way that you feel.

You can do things to work toward greater inner harmony immediately. To do this, go into your imaginary spaces: if you are now at home, go to your imaginary home; if at work, go to your imaginary job, etc. Look for things in your imaginary spaces which you can realistically buy, borrow, or make. Again, these may be small things: decorations, changing the color of a wall, rearranging objects on a table, rearranging furniture, etc. Or they can be large things: moving, building a house, changing jobs, etc. Even if they seem small, do not underestimate their importance. The effect is gradual and cummulative as you get things from your imaginary environment and put them into your real external environment. If you can change one thing in your external environment every couple of days to make it come closer into harmony with your inner self, that is more than 180 changes per year! People who do this exercise find that they can change their external environment radically in less than six months, even though they may be living in the same house, or going to the same job.

Remember how you felt either during or after doing this exercise. Understand that you have these feelings every day in your life but may not allow yourself to fully feel them. Now that you have made contact with these feelings allow yourself to bring them more and more into your everyday life.

RELAXATION SPACES

The main point is to provide space in your life where your body can relax, free of tensions created by your external environment. If you are unable to change your external environment, you can create relaxation spaces for your body throughout the day by learning to do one or more of the relaxation exercises in this chapter.

A psychiatrist friend of Mike's says that he makes a point of giving himself a minimum of four hours a day in the country, away from activity and people. Not everyone will be immediately able to do anything that radical, but everyone can plan their day to get a half-hour alone, probably in the evening, to completely relax their body and their mind. Try it.

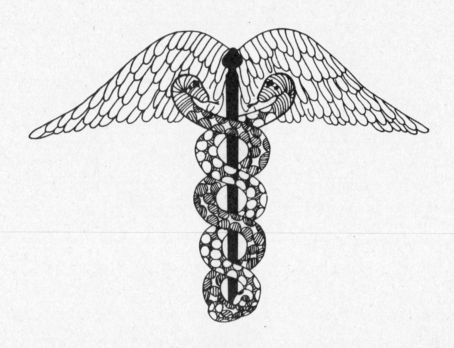

THE PHYSICAL EXAMINATION

THE PHYSICAL EXAMINATION

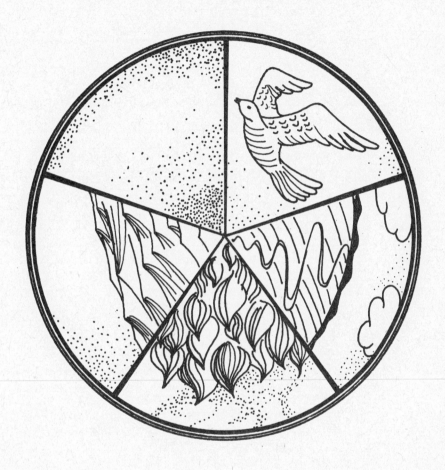

You can do a physical examination in a way that is warm and will make the person you are examining feel better. Calm your mind. Be gentle. Imagine that you are transferring healing energy from the universe, through your hands, into the body of the person you are examining. A psychic healer who we know suggests that you imagine yourself bathed in pure, white light before doing any kind of healing. That advice applies to the physical examination as well.

WHAT IT IS

In medical school a doctor learns the symptoms and "stories" of a large number of diseases. The physical examination helps doctors order their thoughts and feelings about a person's symptoms and the story of their illness. They then compare this information to "typical stories" of specific known diseases they have learned. Doctors are taught that most diseases progress through a series of changes as they run their course in your body. They apply this knowledge in diagnosing illness. Many diseases can have the same symptoms but the order in which those symptoms appear will help distinguish one disease from another.

Most doctors, after several years of medical practice, develop their own way of doing a physical exam, even though there is a more or less standard physical exam taught in medical school. We're going to show you how to do a physical exam in a way that covers the symptoms dealt with in this book. Sometimes we follow the standard physical exam, sometimes we depart from it. You may find our exam more detailed than some doctors', less detailed than others. But we do stay close enough to the standard so that you will know what your own doctor or clinic does when you are examined.

There are several reasons for learning to do a physical exam. You may want to learn in order **to evaluate your own present state of health,** or the present health of a family member or friend. Or you may want **to determine your own or a friend's present illness.** Or you may want to know how to do an exam in order **to understand what your own doctor is doing when you are examined.**

A LIST OF TOOLS

The most essential tools for doing a physical examination (called "P.E.") are your hands, your senses, your mind and intuition, and the sunlight. Most of the P.E. can be done with only these. But we recommend that you put together what we call the **Basic Tool Kit:**

The Well Body Book

A penlight flashlight: about $2.00. Get a two-cell type with a small bulb. With it you will be able to focus a very bright but narrow beam of light.

A thermometer: $1.50 and up. There are two types, those for taking temperature by mouth (oral), and those for taking temperature rectally (anal). If you have children up to the age of six you should take their temperatures rectally since the kids can't keep the thermometer under their tongues, and they sometimes bite off the glass tips. Oral and anal thermometers can be used interchangeably. If you intend to take adult temperatures only, just get an oral thermometer.

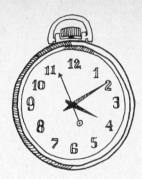

A clock, pocket watch, stop watch, or wristwatch with a second hand: $5.00 and up. You'll use this for timing pulse and respiration rates.

A butter knife: You'll use this as a tongue depresser.

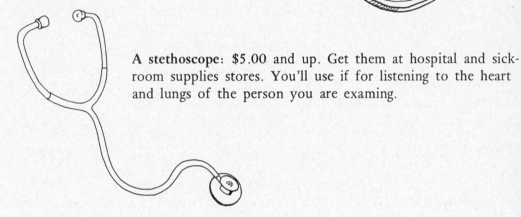

A stethoscope: $5.00 and up. Get them at hospital and sickroom supplies stores. You'll use if for listening to the heart and lungs of the person you are examing.

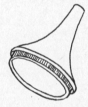

An otoscope cup (ear speculum): $0.50 and up. You'll use this, along with your flashlight, to look into ears. They can be purchased at hospital supplies stores. They come in different sizes: get medium for adults, small for children.

A couch, a bed, or the ground: Choose a place to lie down which will be well-lighted and where you will both be comfortable doing the physical exam.

You: . . . most important of all.

We've put together an *optional tool kit,* knowing that some people will want to have as complete a kit in their home as their family doctor has in their office. But bear in mind that these are *optional tools:*

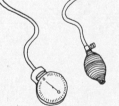

A blood pressure cuff: $25.00 and up. Most mail order houses, such as Sears, Wards and others, carry a blood pressure cuff at about this price. You can also buy one from a hospital supplies store. With this tool you will be able to measure your blood pressure exactly. If you or people you are examining regularly have family histories of high blood pressure you may wish to get one of these. But if you do the complete physical examination as we describe here you will not, in most cases, need the information that you would get with a blood pressure cuff.

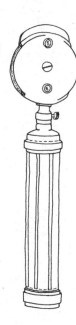

An Opthalmoscope: $30.00 and up. You can buy one at most hospital supplies stores. An opthalmoscope is one of those things the doctor uses to look inside your eye. They look through your lens and visually examine the retina. By looking at the blood vessels they find there, the doctor can sometimes tell the severity of diagnosed diabetes, high blood pressure, and eye diseases. We don't include it as a necessary tool here because of its specialized application.

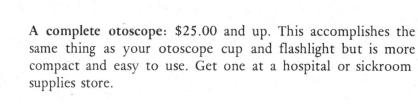

A complete otoscope: $25.00 and up. This accomplishes the same thing as your otoscope cup and flashlight but is more compact and easy to use. Get one at a hospital or sickroom supplies store.

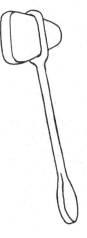

A neurological hammer: $3.00 and up. You can buy one of these at most hospital supplies stores. It is used to tap your knee to test reflexes. But we don't include it in our basic tool kit because you can accomplish the same thing with the edge of your hand.

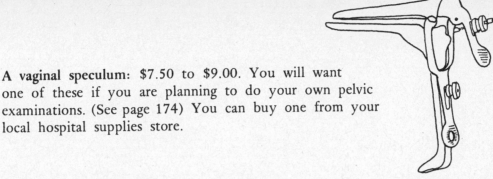

A vaginal speculum: $7.50 to $9.00. You will want one of these if you are planning to do your own pelvic examinations. (See page 174) You can buy one from your local hospital supplies store.

A bathroom scales and a ruler: $7.00 and up. You can buy these if you want to keep a record of the height and weight changes of people you are regularly examining. If you have young children in your family and you want to keep health records for them, the weight and height charts will provide you with a running record of their rate of growth.

Obviously there are other tools which you may have seen in doctors' offices, such as x-ray, E.K.G., and laboratory equipment, which we don't include here. We have included only those tools which you can use at home, and which are relevant to this book.

The first physical examination which you do will probably take about forty minutes. But after you learn the techniques we describe here you can do one in about a quarter of that time. You will find that the physical exam is easier to do than to read.

You can get photocopies made of the forms on pages 32 through 41 (*Systems Review*), as well as 184 through 190, (*Physical Examination Report*), for each person you want to examine.

STARTING THE PHYSICAL EXAM

For most doctors the **first part of the physical exam is the Present Illness,** or P.I. It is a story told by the person being examined, explaining why they have come to see the doctor.

Taking a P.I., and in general throughout this book, try to **reduce your ego overlay to zero.** Ego overlay is that mental state where you say to yourself, or feel "I'm better than they are, I'm worse than they are, I want to make them sexually, or I'm not as pretty as they are, etc," about the person you're examining. This overlay prevents you from receiving valuable information from the person. What you are doing is receiving messages from yourself instead. Minimizing ego overlay, we might add, is equally important if you are examining yourself.

The **best way to reduce your ego overlay** is to put yourself in the same relaxed and open state of mind you use to meet your imaginary doctor. Before you begin the physical examination go back to page 8 and do the exercise for getting in touch with your imaginary doctor. Do the entire exercise up to the place where you create your imaginary house, page 10. At that point your ego overlay will be very low. Stay with that consciousness to do the exam.

To do a Present Illness you ask the person you are examining: "What's wrong?" or "Why are you here?" or "Why do you feel that you need a checkup?" What you want, ideally, is a one sentence reply. This answer is called the *chief complaint* (C.C.). The chief complaint might be: "I have pains all over my body," or "My throat is sore," or "annual checkup" or even "My mother sent me." Probably the "chief complaint" of the first person you examine will be: "To learn how to do a physical examination." Record this one sentence answer under *Chief Complaint* in the *Physical Examination Report,* page 184.

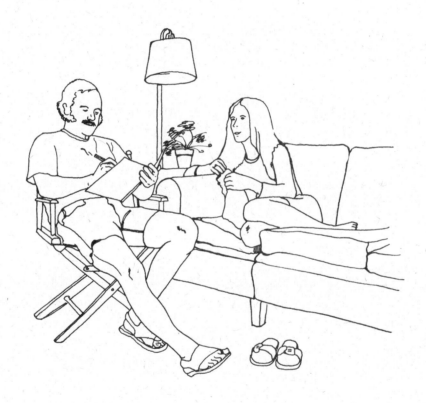

If the person you are examining has an actual illness, say to them, "Tell me the whole story of your illness." Then listen to them. Their story might go something like this:

"I was well until about five days ago, when I suddenly noticed that my throat was sore. I had a little difficulty swallowing and slowly I got even worse until I could hardly swallow at all. I also noticed that I had a fever. I started coughing about that time, too. Otherwise, everything is alright."

People who are not skilled in telling stories may tell rambling, disconnected stories, but they will usually come up with valuable information anyway. Listen to their whole story without interrupting them. Then, perhaps, you can ask them to elaborate on certain points by asking them more direct questions. For example, it is helpful to find out: *when they got sick, what symptoms they noticed, and whether these became, or are becoming, better or worse.*

If you are trying to get the story of a present illness, and you are not sure of what questions you should ask, it may be helpful for you to turn to the *Diagnosis and Treatment* section of this book (page 195), and read over everything we have written there about the target organ or system of their chief complaint.

To find out if the person you are examining has forgotten to mention any symptoms which may prove valuable in determining what they have, turn to the *Systems Review,* page 30. Ask them whether they have had the symptoms listed in the organ system that they are complaining about (or nearby systems that may be related). If you are in doubt about which symptoms are relevant to the illness, go through the entire *Systems Review.* As you gain experience in taking the *present illness,* you'll learn which symptoms are relevant and which aren't.

If you are examining someone who is not ill, the *Systems Review* will also be helpful because it will direct you to give more attention to examining his or her target organs or systems when you do the actual physical examination.

You may also ask the questions in the *General Information* section, page 19. Pay special attention to questions which seem to relate to the present illness. If you don't know which questions are relevant, ask all the questions.

If the person you are examining for a *present illness,* has **recently been to a doctor,** or **has previously been to a doctor with the same complaint,** ask them what the doctor diagnosed. Ask them what treatment was prescribed, if any, and what affect, if any, that treatment had on their getting better or worse. Also ask the person you are examining if they have been treating themself and what affect that treatment has had on them.

At this point, sit down and record your findings in the *Physical Examination Report,* in the *Present Illness* section. Be relaxed as you write. Record things spontaneously as they come to your mind, remembering that things which you feel are most important will probably come first, less important things next, and so on. You will not necessarily remember things in the same order they occured or were told to you. Be sure to note and record **when** the person became ill and **what symptoms** they have had.

In his own medical practice, Mike says he has found that taking **the present illness is the most important part of the physical examination.** In many cases this alone enables the doctor to make a correct diagnosis of the patient's disease. The doctor then uses the rest of the physical examination to confirm that diagnosis.

ADDITIONAL METHODS

At this point you have a complete story of the illness. You can go on to the actual physical examination. But we urge you to do something that most doctors may not do, which we call *Where The Person is At.* Try to find out what's happening in their life. Are they happy with their life? Are they unhappy with it? How do they like their job? What tensions do they feel? How is their family situation? What are the areas of deep satisfaction in their life? This information may help them and you to discover why they are sick or why they have chosen a particular organ or system in which to manifest a disease: why a musician has an ear infection, a singer a sore throat, a housewife migraine.

Look at the eyes of the person you are examining. Do they look happy, sad, about to cry, tense, in pain, overly concerned, defensive, or open and beautiful? Look at the way they hold their body. **Do a body reading:** are they holding themself erect and proud, holding themself hunched over, holding their hands to protect a certain part of their body, or are they relaxed and at ease with their body? One time Mike walked into an examination room in a hospital where he was working and found his patient lying in a fetal position in the corner, like a frightened infant. **How a person holds their body tells you a tremendous amount about how they feel toward themself.**

While doing the *present illness,* watch the person. Watch the way they move. Watch the way they hold their body. Watch the way they hold their head and their hands. Watch the brightness of their eyes. Then ask yourself how that person makes you feel: high, or low, or in between? If you wish, repeat the exercise to get to the relaxed state you use to meet your imaginary doctor (page 8). In this relaxed and open state of mind, ask, "How does this person feel?" **Be that person for a moment. Feel whatever they feel.** If they have an earache, try to feel that earache as your own earache. If they have a sore throat, feel that sore throat as you own.

Mentally define what you are doing as *working.* Say, "I am working now." When you are in this relaxed state and are working, all physical and mental feelings will come from the person you are reading. For example, if you are working and your ear suddenly hurts, the person you are reading — and not you — has an earache. (If you do this, be sure to finish the P.E. by doing the *Coming Out Healthy* exercise at the end of this chapter.)

☆   ☆   ☆

So, to determine where the person you are examining is at, you *watch them, you ask yourself how they make you feel, you ask why they hold their body as they do. You feel what they are feeling.* And with experience you will learn to trust this information. This is actually a whole other diagnosis system, different than the usual diagnosis system which most doctors are taught in medical school, but one which you will find to be just as valid. It is very similar to what good doctors do when they are using their *intuition.*

152

Record your observations in the *Where the Person Is At* section of the Physical Examination Report. Be sure to include a description of how the person looks and makes you feel, as well as areas of tension and satisfaction in their life.

You will now be turning your attention to specific things about the body of the person you are examining. You will find yourself focusing a great deal of your attention on one part or function of their body at a time.

DOING THE PHYSICAL EXAMINATION

The fewer clothes worn by the person you are examining the better, but you can examine quite a bit if they are clad as they might be to go to the beach. The first part of this section of the exam includes what is known as *"Vital Functions"*: Height, weight, temperature, pulse rate and respiration rate.

Height and Weight: If you wish to measure and record the weight and height of the person, do it now. Ask them if the recorded weight is different than their usual weight. If there is a large difference between usual and present weight ask them what the reason is for this change and record their reply in the physical examination report. The main reason for you to do weight and height is for the person you are examining to have a record of that information. With a child you might want the information to keep track of their growth rate.

Temperature: This will be most crucial if you are examining a person who is sick. But you may want to take and record temperature in order to have a record of the temperature which is "normal" for the person being examined. Although the average normal temperature for humans is 98.6°, many people have normal temperatures a degree or so above or below this. That's why it's nice to know what is normal for them.

To take a temperature, first clean the thermometer with cold, soapy water or rubbing alcohol. Shake down the thermometer until it reads 96° or less. Shake it briskly downward as though you were trying to shake droplets of water from the silver tip.

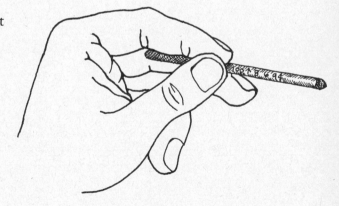

To read the thermometer, note that it is graduated from 94° to 108°. The scale of your thermometer will look something like this:

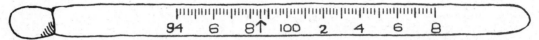

Each large mark indicates 1° of temperature. Between each large mark you will see five smaller marks. Read each smaller mark as 2/10ths of one degree. Thus 98.6° would be three small marks past the 98° mark. You only need to read the temperature within a half a degree.

You may find it difficult to read the thermometer since the color of the mercury inside is very close to the color of the reflection from the glass. Roll the thermometer back and forth until you see the thin line of mercury inside. The place where the mercury stops will be the temperature reading.

An oral thermometer should be held under the tongue. An anal thermometer used for infants should be dipped in vaseline and gently inserted in the rectum. In either case leave the thermometer in place for two minutes before trying to take a reading.

Record your reading in the physical examination report.

Pulse Rate: Taking the pulse will tell you how many times your friend's heart beats in a minute. There is considerable variation in normal pulse rate. Most healthy adults will be between 60 and 80 beats per minute, at rest. In young adults who are athletic, a pulse can be as low as 50 beats per minute. Young children range between 90 and 120 beats per minute. And 130 to 140 is not unusual in infants. If you have a fever, your normal pulse rate will rise 5 to 10 beats per minute for each degree of temperature.

In taking a pulse, you want to notice two things: the number of beats per minute, and the regularity of the beat.

To accurately read the pulse rate, first be sure the person you are examining is relaxed. Pulse rate goes up after physical exertion, and when the person is under stress. Take their hand, and place your fingers across their wrist like this:

Press your fingers lightly against the wrist until you feel the throbbing of the person's artery. Keep your eye on the second hand of your watch or clock and count the number of pulse beats you feel in 15 seconds. Multiply that number of pulse beats by four and record that sum in the physical examination report. If you wish you may count the number of beats for a full minute, but most doctors don't because they tend to lose count when counting to the larger number.

After you have counted the pulse rate, keep your fingers on the artery and feel for regularity: does the pulse speed up, slow down, or skip beats?

Note and record your findings in the physical examination report.

Respiration Rate: Respiration rate is how many breaths you take in a full minute. Most people breathe between 14 and 20 breaths per minute. With a fever this rate goes up about 4 breaths per minute for every degree of temperature above normal.

Measure respiration with the person at rest. Simply count the number of times their chest and/or stomach rises in a full minute. Most doctors count respiration while the person they are examining is unaware of them doing so. The reason for this is that many people become self-conscious and change their normal respiration rate when they know they are being watched. Another way to get an accurate count is to ask the person you are examining to visualize themselves doing something which they feel is both relaxing and thoroughly pleasurable: maybe basking in the sun on a seashore. This both relaxes them and takes their mind off their breathing.

Keep one eye on your watch and **count how many breaths they take in a full minute.** Record that number in the physical examination report.

Blood Pressure: Although some doctors take blood pressure in a complete physical examination we do not include it here. If you want to know more about blood pressure and how to take it, turn to page 180.

SKIN: There are great variations in the color and texture of skin. In spite of this it is possible to develop a sense of how healthy skin looks and feels. To do this, look for an area of skin on your own body toward which you feel absolutely positive.

Look at it, feel it, smell it; note its suppleness, warmth, moistness, or dryness. Ask the person you are examining to do the same with their skin. Compare your findings and discuss likeness and differences. Once you do this you will develop your own standards of healthy skin which you can use in future physical exams.

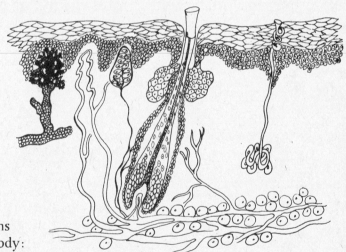

Examining the skin means examining all the skin of the body: the entire back from heels to head, under the arms, the folds inside elbows, stomach, between the toes, genital area, breasts, neck, behind the ears. You may wish to follow the *body tour,* page 57, which you learned to do in the section called *Mirror Mirror.* Make sure that you note on the report if the skin is pale, flushed, or yellow. Note pimples, rashes, moles, warts, boils, or any places that appear irritated. Write down their location and describe what you see. Record whatever comes to your attention.

HAIR: You will find that a healthy "unchemicalized" hair will be springy and elastic, and is slightly oily, though the oiliness is almost impossible to feel with your fingertips. Shininess or dullness of the hair is another variable quality. Note and record if the hair is elastic, dry, shiney, dull, oily, or covered with chemicals such as hairspray or lotions.

Examine the area around the roots of the hairs. Note any areas that seem red, obviously moist, or obviously dry and scaley. Note and record your findings in the physical examination report.

Few doctors pay much attention to hair, but a friend of ours who is a psychotherapist, says she uses a person's hair as one indicator of how they feel toward themselves. She says that as people progress in therapy their hair invariably becomes increasingly more attractive, shiney, and elastic. She points out that other animals, such as dogs and cats, reflect their well-being in the shininess or dullness of their coat.

HEAD: The examination of the head includes skull, eyes, ears, nose, mouth and lymph nodes. **The first thing to examine is the skull.** Do this by feeling it with your fingertips all over. Note any unusual bumps, or anything that your friend says is sore. Record your observations in the physical examination report.

Next **examine the eyes.** Have the person remove their contact lenses or glasses, if they have them. Look at the white parts of their eyes. If these look yellowish or pinkish, write down your findings in the physical examination report.

Now draw down the lower eyelids and note the color of the *mucosal lining* — the flesh inside. The best way to do this is shown here.

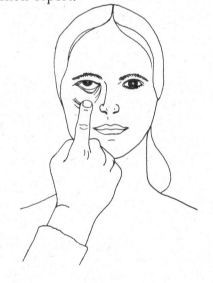

Healthy mucosa is moist and pink. If it looks reddish, grayish or swollen, note this and report it in the physical examination report.

Note if the person's eyes have puss in them, or have a discharge from them, or are irritated. Note any *crustiness* around the eyelashes. Record your findings in the Physical Examination Report.

To check for constriction of pupils, have your friend face you. The room should be dimly lighted. Have them stare at a dark area on the wall behind you. Their pupils will expand in size — dilate. Then, starting about a foot above their head, pass your lighted flashlight downward across the front of their left eye. As you move the flashlight, shine the beam of light directly into their pupil. As light strikes the center of their eye the pupil will constrict — become smaller. Do this for both eyes. Both should constrict at the same rate

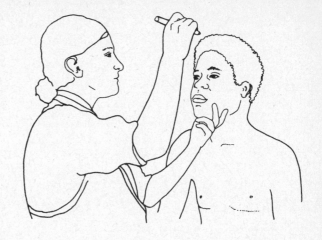

of speed, and should constrict about the same amount. Note and record any differences. Also note if one or the other pupil fails to constrict.

If you have difficulty seeing any constriction, go into a darker room and try again.

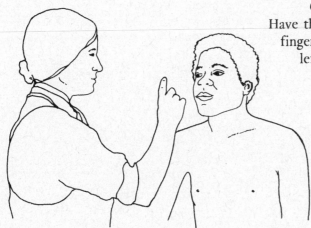

Check for co-ordination of eye muscles: Have the person you are examining follow your fingertip with their eyes. Move your hand left to right. Move it up and down. Then draw an imaginary "x" in the air in front of them.

Note jerkiness, inability to follow, one eye wandering off to the side as the other follows, or *crossing* instead of following. Write down your observations in the Physical Examination Report.

EARS: Examine the skin of the outer ear surfaces. Note and write down in the Physical Examination Report any redness, sores, moistness or scaliness. Then hold the person's ear like this:

Pull up and back. Pull gently. This helps to straighten out the ear canal. Use your flashlight to look down into the ear canal. A healthy ear canal will have a pale pink, slightly glossy surface, and you will also see some evidence of wax. Note any wax that actually blocks the canal,

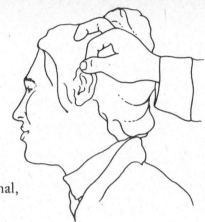

To examine the ear drum you will have to use the ear speculum — otoscope cup — and your flashlight. Make certain that the speculum you have is about the same size, or a little bit larger than the person's ear canal. Now pull the outer ear up and back and insert the ear speculum very gently.

Use the speculum both to straighten out the ear canal and to direct light from your flashlight toward the ear drum. You may have to manipulate the speculum in the ear to get the right angle.

When illuminated, the ear drum will look pearly gray and you'll get a shiney, bright mirror-like reflection, surprising the first time you see it because it has a definite *metallic* quality about it. However, keep in mind that the ear drum is extremely sensitive — a thin membrane sensitive enough to respond to the most subtle sounds. Some people have extremely curved canals which makes it very difficult to see the drum without an otoscope. Others have straight canals where you can see the drum without an ear speculum.

Note if the ear drum appears red, dull looking, or if it fails to reflect light. Record your observations in the Physical Examination Report.

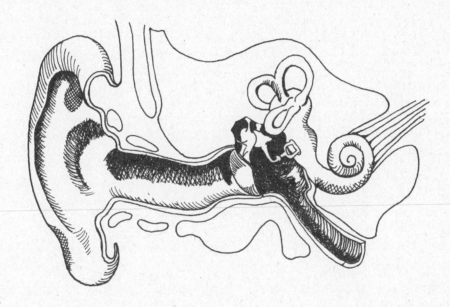

If you own a complete "otoscope" the examination of the ear will be the same as above, but the scope will make it much easier.

After completing the visual examination of both ears, you can go on to do a simple hearing test. Hold your hand about three inches away from the person's ear and rub your thumb and forefinger together very lightly. Experiment by doing this beside your own ear first. The sound that you want to make is more like an "airy rustling" 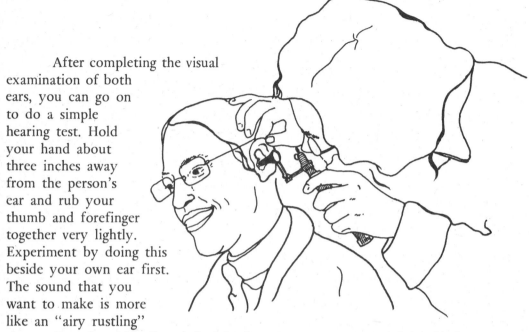 than a "rough rubbing" sound. Ask the person you are examining if they can hear the sound you are making, and if they hear it about equally in both ears. Another way to do this is with a ticking wristwatch.

Note and record your observations in the Physical Examination Report.

NOSE: First determine if the person breathes through their mouth or through their nose. The easiest way to do this is to simply ask the person which way they breathe.

To examine the inside of the nose, have the person tip their head back so that you can focus light into their nasal passages. You may wish to lift the outside of the nostril as the drawing shows.

Your main interest will be the *mucosa* which is the soft, moist tissue lining the nose. It is the same type of tissue as you find inside your mouth, under your eyelids, in the vagina, and lining the urethera. When completely healthy the mucosa is slightly pink and moist.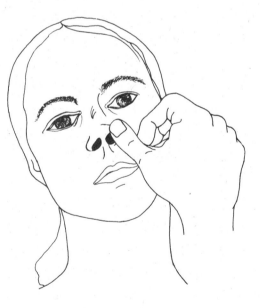

Note anything that looks swollen, red, bluish, or which gives evidence of bleeding. Record your findings.

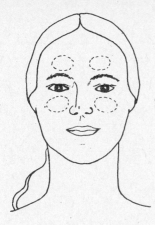

Sinuses: This is the last part of the nose exam. Place your fingers on the sinuses as located for you in this drawing, and press firmly on them.

Try it on yourself first to establish how much pressure to apply. Then do it on your friend and ask them to tell you whether or not they feel any pressure or tenderness. Record your observations.

MOUTH: Have the person you are examining open their mouth as wide as possible. If they have dentures, ask them to remove them, both top and bottom. **Examine the gums.**

In their most healthy condition, gums are pink, sometimes with a slight gray cast to them. They are also firm and strong, and they grow tightly around each tooth forming a seal against liquid, bacteria, and air that might otherwise work down around the base of the teeth. Note if the gums appear to be pulling away from the teeth, or if they appear to form an imperfect seal around the teeth. Note if they appear red, puffy, bleeding, swollen, or sore. Record your observations.

Now **examine the teeth.** Check between the teeth; where the flesh of the gums meets the teeth; and in the grooves on top of the teeth. You will be looking for any signs of cavities. They will show up as small or large dots or holes which are brown or black in color. Grayish, yellowish, or light brownish stains may indicate *plaque* which leads to decay and should be cleaned off by a dentist. Record your observations in the Physical Examination Report.

If you want to find out how to do a complete dental exam, and also how to take care of your gums and teeth, see *The Tooth Trip*, by Thomas McGuire, DDS. It's a Random House — Bookworks book.

While their mouth is open, **examine the person's tongue.** Usually it will look pink and moist. You may find the tongue stained nearly any color you can imagine. These stains are caused by food or drink, and you should not consider them a symptom of a disease. The *texture* of the tongue is normally smooth to hairy, according to what the person has eaten, drunk, or smoked.

Note and write down in the Physical Examination Report any parts of the tongue or mucosa that are bright red, or have curd-white patches.

Ask the person to move their tongue around, up and down, from side to side, in and out of their mouth. If they have any difficulty with any of these movements, note them and record them.

Now examine **the throat**. Have the person open their mouth wide and say "ahhh!" If necessary, take your butter knife and use the flat side of the blade as a tongue depresser to press down the back of the tongue so that you can see into the throat.

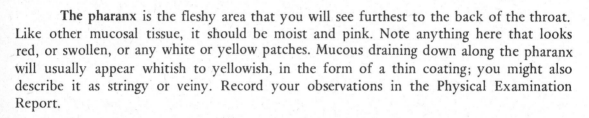

Tonsils are masses of lymphoid tissue which in childhood probably help protect the body from infection. Their size varies, but the color is pink like other healthy mucosa. If a person has had their tonsils removed, you won't, of course, see the tonsils. Also, in adults, tonsils may be normally shrunken and difficult to see.

Note red, swollen, or white to yellow patches on the tonsils. Record in the Physical Examination Report.

The pharanx is the fleshy area that you will see furthest to the back of the throat. Like other mucosal tissue, it should be moist and pink. Note anything here that looks red, or swollen, or any white or yellow patches. Mucous draining down along the pharanx will usually appear whitish to yellowish, in the form of a thin coating; you might also describe it as stringy or veiny. Record your observations in the Physical Examination Report.

Examine the person's lips. Healthy lips are slightly moist looking and pink. Note and record any sores or white spots or areas that you find on the lips.

Examine the mucosal lining of the mouth and record anything that you notice in the way of sores or white spots on the insides of the cheeks, inside the lips, or anywhere else in the mouth. Then you will have completed the mouth examination.

Lymph Nodes: (For an explanation of what lymph nodes do, where they are located throughout the body, and how they work, see page 341.) To examine the

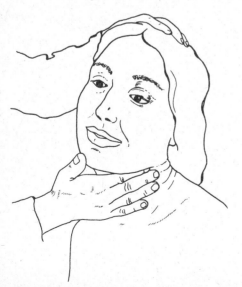

lymph nodes, stand in front of the person being examined, as they sit in a chair. Have them relax their jaw and neck muscles. Place your hand directly under their jaw on one side or the other. Now tell them to tilt their head slightly toward the side where your hand is. Starting under the chin, feel gently with your fingertips for little lumps — the lymph nodes. Work from the soft area under the chin, all the way around to the last node under the ear. The drawing on the next page shows you the locations of the lymph nodes.

When a person is healthy, their
lymph nodes are so small that you won't
be able to feel them. With a minor infection
the nodes may feel firm and may be as large
as a lima bean. Examine both sides of the jaw
the same way. Note and record what you find in
the Physical Examination Report.

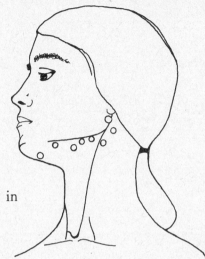

NECK MOVEMENTS: Have the person tip their head back as far as possible without straining. Ask them to swing their head to the extreme right, tipping their head toward their shoulder. Now ask them to drop their chin to their chest. Then ask them to swing their head to their left, tipping it toward their shoulder. Ask them if they felt any pain, discomfort, or had difficulty doing these movements. If they did, record their reply in the Physical Examination Report.

BREASTS: The first part of this exam is visual. Have the person sit facing you with her arms hanging loosely at her sides, breasts uncovered. Study her breasts for a moment, comparing one to the other. Note symmetry and asymmetry. Most women have one breast slightly larger than the other — which may or may not be immediately perceptible. In spite of the size differences they will be shaped about the same, one side matching the other even though different in size. That's the symmetry you want to look for. Lack of symmetry means dimples or bulges which appear in one breast but not in the other. Note these and write them down in the Physical Examination Report.

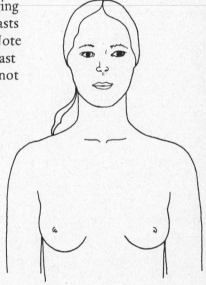

While the person is sitting up, examine her nipples close up. Nipples vary in shape, size, and coloration from person to person. The color of the nipples, as well as the size of the breasts, may change during menstruation. Tenderness of the breasts may also occur. Note and record any redness, discharge, or sores.

With your fingers spread slightly apart and extended, press gently against the person's breast. Start at the top of each breast and move down. Use a slight, circular, gentle massage-like motion to feel the breast tissue. The breast is a complex arrangement of ducts, muscles, and connective tissue, and unlike muscle or fat it will be highly textural in quality. If you find any irregularities, or lumps, place one hand on the irregular place and the other hand on the other breast in the matching place. Sometimes irregularities are simply the way the person is made, so if you find what you believe to be matching irregularities in both breasts the chances are that these irregularities are normal for that person.

Note any irregularities or lumps which you find and describe them as to location, shape, size, moveability, firmness, and tenderness. Write them down in the P.E. report.

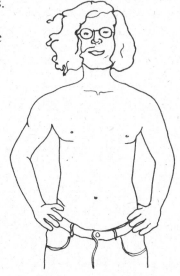

Now have the person lie down. Repeat the same examination of the breasts in this position. This new position will allow you to do a more complete exam of the person's breasts because the position of the breast tissue changes considerably from sitting up to lying down.

Most doctors examine only the skin surfaces of the man's breasts, but there is no reason to leave the man out of this part of the P.E.

CHEST: This exam includes the person's heart and lungs. Begin with the lungs.

Lungs: The first part of the lung exam is visual. The person you are examining should be sitting in a comfortable position with their shirt off. You should stand in front of them, facing them. Watch their chest as they breathe.

Normal breathing is smooth, quiet, relaxed, and rhythmic. Note and record breathing that appears forced, noisey, uneven, panting, or in any way difficult.

Watch to see if both sides of the chest expand approximately equal. Note and record anything unequal.

Watch their chest and stomach as they breath. Note and record in the Physical Examination Report whether they breathe predominantly from their stomach or from their chest.

This completes the visual exam. The second part of the lung examination is done by percussing.

Directions For Percussing:

Percussing is when the doctor thumps on your back, chest, or abdomen, with their fingers. By listening to the sounds made in percussing you can tell certain things about parts of the body that you can't see.

To percuss, use your two middle fingers. If you are right-handed, use your right middle finger to strike your left middle finger. (Reverse these directions if you are left-handed.) We suggest that you practice percussing, using the following directions, on yourself or on a table top, before you try it on a friend.

When percussing, your hands should be in a position something like this:

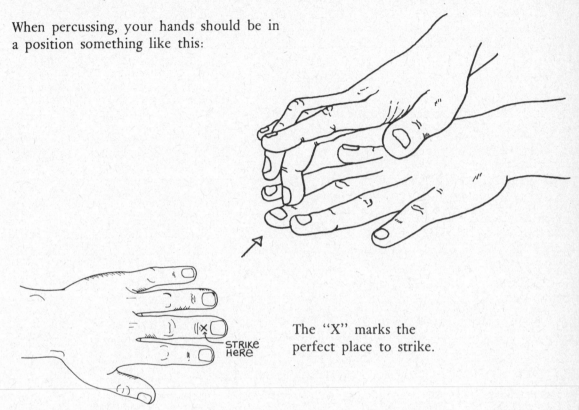

STRIKE HERE

The "X" marks the perfect place to strike.

Place your left hand on the area to be percussed. Press firmly with your middle finger only, letting the other fingers relax.

Now bend the middle finger of your right hand slightly, and strike the left middle finger a sharp, quick blow. To do this, be sure the fingernail or your right middle finger is short, or you will injure the finger you strike. The action of the strike must be in the wrist, and the striking finger should be withdrawn quickly after the strike. Strike the left finger exactly between the cuticle and the first joint.

First become accustomed to the mechanics of percussing. Then go on to learn to distinguish between the **three basic sounds: RESONANT, HOLLOW,** and **DULL**.

To produce a resonant sound: Percuss anywhere in the ribcage on a person's back. A resonant sound is heard over parts of the body that have both air and mass: for example, the lungs.

To produce a hollow sound: Percuss the middle of a relaxed abdomen, near the naval. A hollow sound is heard over parts of the body that have air in them: for example, the stomach.

To produce a dull sound: Percuss the top of your thigh muscle. A dull sound is heard over parts of the body that have mostly solid mass, such as muscles.

Practice percussing until you feel familiar with these three sounds and can recognize them. If you are doing the physical examination with a friend, go over their body to see what different sounds you get. In a healthy person you will get a **resonant sound directly above the lungs.** You will get a **dull sound in the body areas above solid organs such as the liver or thigh.** And you'll get a **hollow sound in the abdomen.** With practice you may "feel" these sounds with your fingertips in addition to hearing them with your ears.

Now you can percuss the lungs: Ask the person to slump slightly forward. This will make it easier for you to percuss their back. Use the drawing below to give you an idea of where to percuss.

    The back is the most important part of the lung exam because it is easy to detect problems there. So we suggest that you spend most of your time on the back for both percussing and stethoscopic exams.

    Thump, listen, thump, listen — *do not* thump, thump, thump like a woodpecker.

    In a healthy person, you will hear resonant sounds in the places noted in the illustration. Compare the sounds on the left side of the spine with those on the right. Note and record any areas that percuss dull, and describe their location.

    After you have percussed the person's back, continue percussing the sides of their ribcage. Start under the ribcage and work down. You may find it helpful to ask the person to raise their arms and place their hands behind their head as you do this part. Note and record any dull sounds that you hear. Describe their location in the P.E. report.

NOTE: As you percuss the person's back and sides, you may come upon flat sounds as you approach the bottom of the ribcage. Don't let this worry you. You are hearing where the diaphragm begins, and it will normally produce this dull sound. So don't record it in the Physical Examination Report.

    When you first try percussing, you may feel a little lost. Don't panic. Just take your time with it and have fun.

The next part of the chest exam is listening to the sound of the person's breathing: You can listen by putting your ear directly on a person's back, but a stethoscope makes it easier. The first thing to note about the stethoscope is that in most models the ear pieces are set at a slight angle. Put them in your ears so that the ends are pointed forward, rather than back. Note drawing.

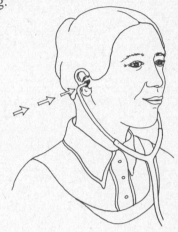

The forward pointing position directs sound against your ear drum. The backward pointing position will bounce the sound off your ear canal.

Start the exam on your friend's back. Try various pressures with the end of your stethoscope until you find the pressure that gives you the best volume.

In doing the stethoscopic exam, the following drawings show you where to listen.

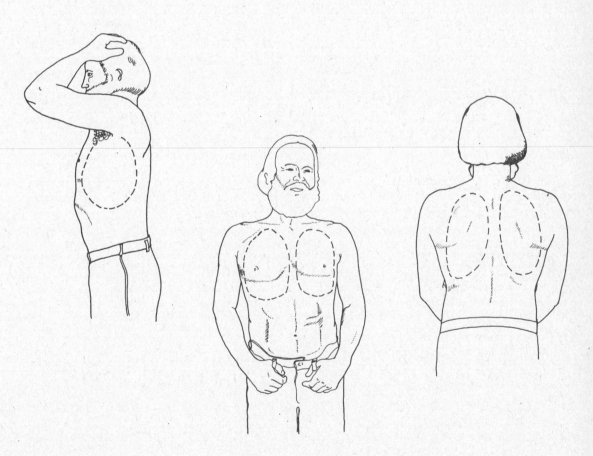

At each point, ask the person to take a deep breath through their mouth and exhale slowly. Healthy breathing sounds like air rushing through a clear tube. Listen to your own and other people's chests in lung areas to learn how a normal breath sounds. There are other breath sounds that you may hear if a person has an illness involving their lungs. They are:

Rales: (prounounced "ralz" — rhyming with "pals") You can approximate this sound by removing your stethoscope from your ears and rubbing a bunch of hairs from your head lightly between your thumb and forefinger next to your ear. You'll hear a sort of dry, crackling sound. Rales are thought to be caused as tiny, abnormally blocked air passages (alveoli) in the lungs pop open.

Rhonchi: (prounounced "Ron-Kie") This sound is best described by the words "bubbles popping." It is thought to be caused by the abnormal presence of vibrating, thick, wet mucous in the large air passages (bronchi) of the lungs.

Wheezing: This is a hoarse, "musical," whistling sound, caused by air being pushed through a constricted passage.

Absent or greatly decreased breath sounds: Breath sounds are sometimes difficult or impossible to hear in very fleshy or heavily muscled people. If you can't hear a person's breath sounds for this reason, record that fact in the Physical Examination Report.

In doing the stethoscope examination, note and record any rales, rhonchi, or wheezing that you hear, and describe their location.

While doing the stethoscopic examination you may pick up sounds caused by congestion in the nasal passages. Sometimes this sounds exactly like rales or rhonchi. So when you think you hear the latter two, have the person hold their nose and breath through their mouth as you listen once more. In some people you will still get a bubbling sound in the back of their throat, caused by congestion, but sounding much like rhonchi. Check this out simply by listening with your naked ear to the sounds coming out of their mouth. With practice you will be able to distinguish easily between sounds coming from the lungs and sounds from the mouth and nose.

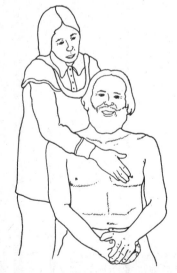

Now do the heart examination: The first part is to locate the **point of maximum impulse** (called P.M.I.). The P.M.I. is where you feel the heart beat the strongest. Place your hand against the left side of the person's chest in approximately the position noted at the right:

Press your fingertips lightly against the rib cage and you can feel where the heart beats the strongest against your hand. If the P.M.I. is way off to the side of the person's ribcage note its location and record your findings in the Physical Examination Report.

Do the second part of the heart exam with your stethoscope: Place the end of your stethoscope on the P.M.I. and listen to the heart beat. You will hear something that sounds like:

"lubb, DUP, lubb, DUP, lubb, DUP"

The "lubb" is low pitched and dull and is called "the first heart sound." It is thought to be due to the sudden tensing of the heart muscle during normal heart beat. The "DUP" is shorter, sharper, and higher in pitch. Doctors call it "the second heart sound." It is due to the closure of the heart valves during normal heart beat.

Normally during a physical examination, the doctor hears only this lubb, DUP sound. He routinely includes this part of the exam for the purpose of detecting an uncommon heart murmur. A murmur is a "shhh" sound, or a "rumbling" sound heard between heart beats if the valves are not functioning normally, and are disrupting normal blood flow. If a murmur was present, you would hear something that sounded like: "lubb, shh, DUP" or "lubb, DUP, rumble." Murmurs are not common. So in doing a P.E. just listen to the sounds of the heart, and enjoy them. Describe the sound that you hear in the P.E. report. ("Hear normal lubb, DUP" or "Hear lubb, shhh, DUP, etc.")

THE ABDOMEN: Have the person lie on their back on a firm surface, naked at least from their chest to the hair line of their pelvis. Have them place their hands on their chest since this will be more relaxing for them than placing them at their sides or under the back of their head. Make them as comfortable as possible. A pillow under their head and a comfortable temperature in the room will aid in this. Have them bend their knees slightly so that their legs are a couple of inches above the bed. This helps the abdominal muscles to relax.

For the purpose of getting your bearings on the abdomen, the usual thing to do is to divide it into four quadrants, as follows:

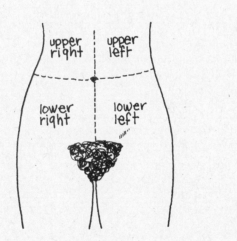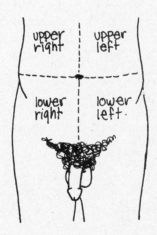

Use your hands as shown:

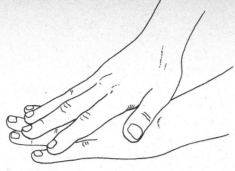

Use your top hand to provide pressure, leaving your bottom hand to feel the abdomen.

Go over the entire abdomen, covering each quadrant, pressing very lightly, in whatever order you wish. Obviously, if you press very hard anyone will complain of tenderness. So work lightly in such a way as to put the person at ease. As they relax and become more accustomed to your hand, press more firmly, going from quadrant to quadrant at a comfortable pace. Ask the person you are examing if they feel any tenderness as you do this.

You may feel the person tense up as you press an area. This is called "guarding." When a person guards ask them if they feel any pain. They may reply that you are tickling them. If this is the case, try to press in such a way as to not tickle them. Try to determine if they are perhaps feeling some pain after all. If they complain of pain in any area, do not press that area further. Note and record any areas of tenderness that you find in the P.E. report. Also note any areas that are rigid to the touch.

If a person complains of pain in one quadrant before you start you will want to begin your exam in the quadrant furthest from that point, and work gradually up to the uncomfortable area, in order to put the person being examined at ease.

A healthy abdomen will be soft and you will feel no organs or other masses. Sometimes it is possible to feel an edge of the liver, but most of it lies under the ribs in the right upper quadrant.

To check the liver press in the right upper quadrant with your fingers very close to the ribcage.

If the liver is healthy you probably won't feel anything. If it's enlarged — such as it might be with Hepatitis (see page 260) — you may be able to feel a firm, flat mass with your fingertips. If you are able to feel such a mass, note and record your observations in the P.E. report. Also note any tenderness in this area.

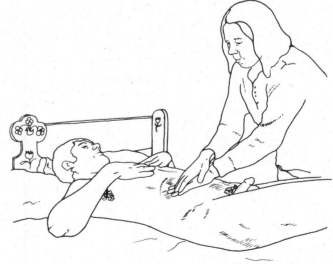

To check the spleen press in the left upper quadrant. Feel for it the same way you did for the liver. Normally you will not feel the spleen. If it is very enlarged — such as with Mononucleosis (see page 281) — you may be able to feel it as a firm mass. Note and record such findings in the P.E. report. Also note any tenderness.

To check the lower left and right quadrants: In a healthy body no organs can easily be felt in either of these quadrants. If any masses or tenderness is noted here, record your findings in the P.E. report.

Now percuss the abdomen. Start about the width of four fingers below the person's ribcage, only on the person's right side. Percuss upwards toward the liver.

Normally the abdomen will percuss hollow. If the liver is enlarged it will sound dull, because you are percussing against a solid mass. Percuss only to the edge of the person's ribs. This completes your percussion of the abdomen. You will not need to percuss other quadrants. Note and record any dullness you hear in the P.E. report.

To finish up the examination of the abdomen *listen for bowel sounds with your stethoscope*. Place the end of your stethoscope in the center of the person's abdomen. Press lightly. You will intermittently hear quiet and slow bubbling and gurgling sounds — the normal sounds of digestion. Listen for about one minute. Note and record in the P.E. report if the sounds are either absent, or are loud and constantly gurgling.

GENITALS (MALE): Since the examination of the male genitals is easier than that of the female, we start with that. The male genital exam is largely visual.

Look closely at the shaft of the penis and note any sores, red spots or "pimples" that you see. Look at the uretheral opening at the tip of the penis and note any liquid discharge or redness of the mucosa. The mucosa is that soft moist flesh that lines the urethera, so you may have to ask the person to hold his penis in such a way as to make it possible to see the edge of the opening. Record your observations in the P.E. report.

If the penis is uncircumsized ask your friend to draw back his foreskin. You will now be able to see the head of the penis and the surrounding area. You may also note a waxey substance along the inside of the foreskin which acts as a natural lubricant for the folds of flesh. Note and record any sores, red spots, or pimples that you find under the foreskin.

Be sure to examine the underside of the person's penis as well as the top.

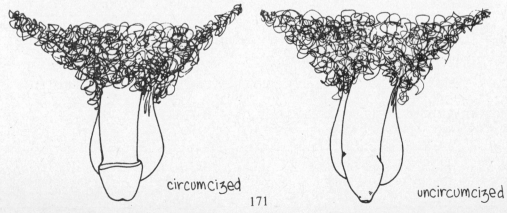

circumcized

uncircumcized

Now examine the person's scrotum — the sac holding their testicles. Note any sores, red areas, or pimples, and record them in the P.E. report.

Examine the insides of both thighs for sores, red areas, or pimples, and record any that you find in the P.E. report.

The next part of the male genital exam is done by touch. Have your friend stand up. Feel his testicles very lightly. Note if there is extreme variation in size, and note if there is extreme sensitivity to the touch. Normally one testicle hangs lower than the other. Most men's testicles are extremely sensitive if any pressure is applied, but touching them lightly will not cause discomfort.

Now reach up halfway between the testicles and the place where the scrotum joins his body. You will feel a cord going from the body to the testicle — one for each side. Gently feel this cord, rolling it lightly between your thumb and forefinger. This is the tube through which sperm and semen pass as part of the reproductive process. Remember, it is a delicate part of the person's body, and should be treated with care and gentleness. Note and record any extreme sensitivity in the cords.

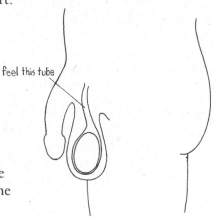

feel this tube

To finish the male genital exam, check for hernia. Have the person cough hard and strain. As they do this, watch the area just above their scrotum and **note any bulge** that did not appear there before. The area to watch is that circled by the dotted line in the drawing below.

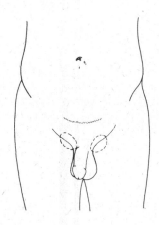

Note and record your findings in the P.E. report.

GENITALS (FEMALE): The first part is visual. Examine the *mound of venus* and other hair-covered flesh above and around her vagina. Note any sores, red areas, or pimples that you find here, and record them in the P.E. report.

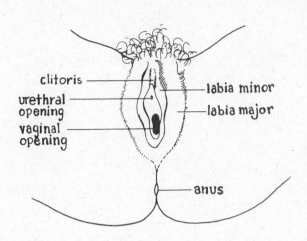

Now examine the *labia,* or lips of the person's vagina. Ask them to lie down, draw their knees up, then spread their knees apart. This will tend to stretch the flesh around the vagina slightly, making the exam easier and more complete. Medical people speak of two sets of labia, the *minora* and the *majora.* (Note picture above.) Examine the flesh of each labia carefully, and record any sores, discharge or red mucosa that you see.

If you are doing the examination during menstruation, you should understand that the menstrual discharge will mask sores, discharge, or mucosa. Because of this, it is best to postpone this part of the exam until after menstruation.

The next part of the exam is done by touch. Since you will be using your fingers to examine the person's vagina, they may prefer that you lubricate your fingers very lightly with vaseline before proceding. Often, however, the natural lubrication of the vagina will be enough. Ask the person you are examining which they prefer.

Now ask them to lie down with their knees drawn up and slightly spread apart. Go over each fold of skin that you find, using your fingers to spread the space between the *labia majora* and *minora.* Do first one side and then the other. Note any sores, discharge, or red areas and write down what you find in the P.E. report.

Now spread the labia at the top of the vagina, and where the labia come together you'll find a slightly moist, glistening node of flesh which projects down toward the vaginal opening. This is the *clitoris.* It will be pink in color just as other mucosa is pink. Note any sores, redness, or discharge in this area and record it in the P.E. report.

Look below the clitoris. You will find a slight indentation or opening: the uretheral opening — where the urine comes out. It may appear as a slight indentation or a definite opening, and will vary in size and shape from person to person. The uretheral opening, being mucosal tissue, will be pink in color and moist. Note any redness or swelling that you find here and record it in the P.E. report.

Bartholin's gland. This is a small gland which lies within the lower labia majora. (See drawing of vagina for location.) With one finger or your thumb inside the labia, and the other outside, press this area lightly. Ordinarily you will feel only the flesh of the labia in this area, not the gland itself. If it is swollen or tender, note that in the P.E. report.

Now have the person relax all the muscles in their pelvic area.

Gently put two fingers into the person's vagina as far as it is comfortable to go. Feel the insides of the vaginal walls, on both the right and the left sides. They will feel moist and smooth. Note any tenderness or soreness and record it in the P.E. report.

Feel for the *cervix*. This drawing will show you where to find it.

When you touch the end of the cervix with your finger, you will feel a small, firm protrusion. Once you find the cervix move your finger around the sides to establish its approximate size and position. It may be straight on, it may be tipped to one side. It will be fairly mobile, easily moved from one side to the other, and up and down. Next feel for the opening into the cervix. It is called the *os*. It will usually

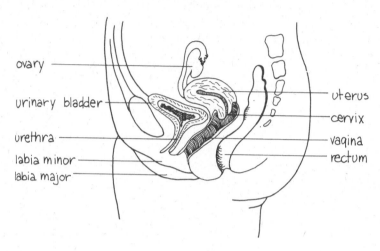

feel like a slight indentation, or dimple, in the tip of the cervix. If the person being examined has an *intra uterine device* (I.U.D.) for birth control, you may feel a small string coming out of the os. Ask the person if they do have an I.U.D. If they do, but you cannot feel the string, note this in the P.E. report.

The visual internal examination of the vagina: Some women will want to do this part of the genital exam, others may prefer not to. Here's what you will need to get started:

A vaginal speculum. (See page 149 for details on what to get.)

A pan of warm water, such as a medium-sized saucepan, to warm the speculum.

A small amount of vaseline, if you want it.

A good light source, and/or your penlight.

A hand mirror if the person being examined wants to see her own vagina.

Doctors usually wear surgical gloves when doing pelvics. One reason for this is that the gloves provide a smooth, even surface, and thus protect mucosa from irritation by rough hands or fingernails. If you wish to use gloves, you can get inexpensive, disposable surgical gloves from most sick room supplies dealers. If If you have long fingernails, either trim them or use gloves.

Before getting started with this part of the exam, you may wish to read over and discuss it with the person you will examine. It is easier to do when both people doing the exam know what is happening.

Make certain that you feel fully at ease with the way the speculum operates. Make it go from closed to open. Try the thumb nut or lever which locks it in open position. DON'T TRY TO USE THE SPECULUM UNTIL YOU ARE COMFORTABLE AND ADEPT IN THE WAY IT WORKS.

Fill the sauce pan with water which is warm but not hot to the touch. Clean your speculum with soap and water, rinse it, and place it in the pan of water to warm up. This will bring the speculum up to body temperature, and the water will also act as a lubricant, making the insertion of the speculum much more comfortable.

Set up a light which will provide plenty of illumination wherever you will be working.

The person being examined should be lying comfortably on their back, preferably with a pillow under their head. Ask them to raise their knees and spread them as fully as possible to allow easy insertion of the speculum into the vagina. Have them relax all the muscles in their pelvis area. The speculum cannot be inserted when these muscles are tense.

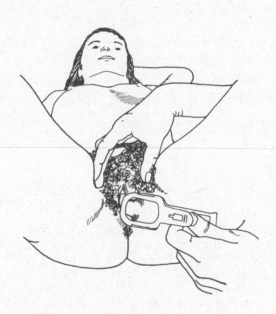

To insert the speculum, hold it closed with one hand as you place two fingers just inside the person's vagina toward the bottom. Spread the labia slightly. With the other hand insert the closed speculum so that the handle is pointed off to the side. This drawing shows you how it will look after you have inserted the speculum.

Push the speculum gently and slowly, straight into the person's vagina, allowing the sides of her vagina to guide it in. Now turn the speculum so that the handle points downward, as in this drawing.

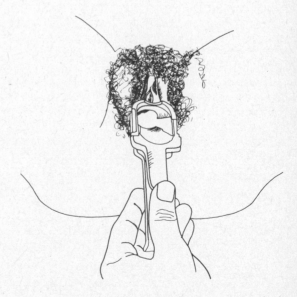

175

Open the speculum slowly until the person you are examining feels a slight pressure against the top and bottom of their vagina. Ask them to help you guide the speculum in and open it if you feel in doubt. Then lock the speculum in its open position.

When the speculum is properly inserted it can be moved slightly to one side or the other, up or down, to inspect the walls of the vagina or to look at the cervix.

The walls of the vagina will be pink and moist, much like other mucosa tissue you have seen in other parts of your body. You will see, also, a slight discharge secreted from the walls of the vagina, which will vary from being clear and watery to being slightly milky in color. Every woman has her own *normal* discharge, which varies from woman to woman. This normal discharge will also change according to ovulation and menstration, emotions, exercise, sexual relations, childbirth, and even diet. Note in the P.E. report any discharge that is different than the above description of a normal discharge. Also note any sores or irritated areas that you see in the deep walls of the vagina.

Move the speculum gently until the cervix becomes visible in the center of the speculum. Since every woman's vagina is different, it is difficult to give exacting directions for doing this. But once you are doing the pelvic exam with the speculum you will find it easier to do than it may look on paper.

You will find that the cervix is about one inch (2 centimeters) in diameter, and is ¾ to 1½ inches (2-4 centimeters) long. It will be slightly glossy, and probably pink in color, but this description will vary somewhat from one woman to another. For example, if your friend is taking birth control pills the cervix may be at least slightly on the red side due to the stimulus of the hormones contained in the pills.

The last thing to check out is the *os* — or opening of the cervix. The size and shape of the *os* varies from being very small and round, hardly more than an indentation, to being a noticable slit in women who have given birth to children.

If the person being examined uses an intra uterine device (I.U.D.), you may see a string coming out of the os. Note and record any redness or discharge around the cervix and os, and note whether or not you can see the I.U.D. string if the person has one.

This completes the pelvic exam. Now unlock the speculum, and slide it gently out of the vagina.

ANAL EXAM: (for male and female) This is a visual exam. The doctor usually does it with the person lying on their side. Lift the top buttock with your hand. The anus is a *sphincter* muscle — a donut-shaped muscle which expands and contracts. The skin here is smooth and variably pigmented. It becomes mucosal tissue as it enters the body. Note any sores, bulges, or small tabs of skin anywhere on the anus. Record your findings in the P.E. report.

NEUROLOGICAL EXAMINATION: Abnormal findings in the neurological exam, not due to injuries, are uncommon. But we include it here because it is fun to do and provides you with information about what the doctor is doing when you get a P.E. at a clinic or doctor's office.

Checking out eye movements and hearing are parts of the usual neurological exam. You have already done these in the ear and eye sections of the P.E. and there is no need to repeat them here.

Ask the person to face you, either seated or standing. Ask them to raise their eyebrows together, and watch their eyebrows as they do so. Note whether or not they can raise them together. If not, describe how they do it in the Physical Exam Report.

Take a small ball of cotton or a softly wadded tissue. Brush their right cheek lightly and ask them if they can feel this. Do the same with the left cheek. Ask them if the right and the left feel about the same. Now brush the right forehead, just above the eyebrow and ask them if they can feel that. Do the same on the left forehead. Ask them if right and left feel about the same. This test checks the sensory nerves in the upper and lower face. If your friend doesn't feel one of the spots checked, or if they feel them unequally, note your findings as well as your friend's comments about the findings, in the Physical Examination Report.

You can extend the cotton ball test to all other areas of the body, such as arms, trunk, and legs. Touch one side first, then the other, and compare the two sides as above. Record your findings in the Physical Examination Report.

Have the person swallow. Their throat will move in a *bobbing* motion. Note any problems they have swallowing; ask them if they know why they are having trouble, then write down their comments as well as your own observations in the Physical Examination Report.

Place your hands on their shoulders and press down slightly. Tell them, "Raise your shoulders." As they do so, note the strength in their shoulders. Describe how they do this, and write it down in the Physical Examination Report. This tests co-ordination of the upper back muscles.

Hold out your index and middle fingers, and ask the person to grasp them tightly, as shown in this drawing.

YOUR FRIEND'S HAND

YOUR HAND ↑

This is a test for muscle strength and co-ordination of the fingers, wrist, and so on. As the person grasps your fingers, try to pull your fingers away. If you can, tell your friend, "No, grasp them tightly." If you can still pull them out, write down your findings in the Physical Examination Report. Do this test for both hands.

Tell the person to push against your hand as the drawing shows, *using their wrist muscles only.*

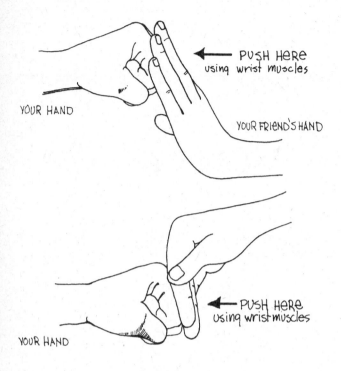

PUSH HERE
using wrist muscles

YOUR HAND

YOUR FRIEND'S HAND

PUSH HERE
using wrist muscles

YOUR HAND

This test checks the strength in the lower arm muscles, the wrist muscles, and their co-ordination. Do both arms. If you note any significant differences between one side and the other, note these differences in the Physical Examination Report.

Tell the person to hold their arm out straight with their palm down. Then tell them to push *up* on your hand, then push *down* on your hand, as the drawing shows.

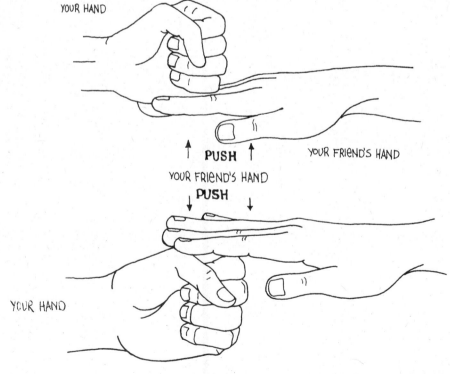

YOUR HAND

↑ PUSH ↑

YOUR FRIEND'S HAND

YOUR FRIEND'S HAND

PUSH

YOUR HAND

Have them do this with both arms. This tests for strength and co-ordination of the upper arm muscles. Again, note whether the strength is equal in both arms. If it isn't, repeat the test, and make certain that your friend has fully understood the instructions. If still unequal, note the differences and write them down in the Physical Examination Report.

With the person seated, place your hand on top of their knee and tell them to push up. Feel the pressure they exert, first on one side and then on the other side. This tests for strength and co-ordination of the thigh muscles. Again, report any differences that you feel between the right and left sides.

With the person seated, kneel down and hold their ankle, as shown in the drawing.

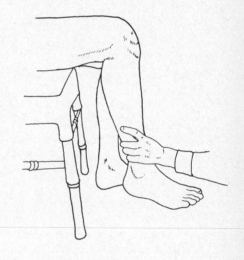

Ask them to push their leg out. Then ask them to pull in. As they push out or in, draw back or push against the force of their muscles with your hand. Do this with both left and right legs, and make notes of any differences in strength between the two. This tests lower leg muscles for strength and co-ordination. Write down your findings in the Physical Examination Report.

Check the knee reflexes now. To do this, support the person's leg so that their foot is off the floor an inch or more, as shown in the drawing below.

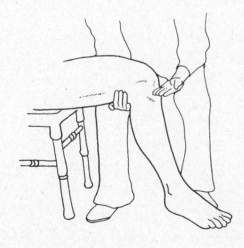

Feel their knee for the first soft area below the kneecap. Strike this point with the heel of your palm as the illustration shows. Strike it firmly but not any harder than you would want them to hit your knee. Sometimes, the exact reflex spot is difficult to find. So try again if you miss the first time. When you hit it right, the knee will jerk perceptibly. If you really can't get a good knee jerk after a couple of tries, try the other leg, then come back to the first. If you still can't get it, note this in the Physical Examination Report.

This completes the neurological examination.

BLOOD PRESSURE: This part of the exam is optional. If you do it, you will be recording your findings in the *Vital Functions* section of the P.E. report.

To take a blood pressure, you will need a stethoscope and a blood pressure cuff. The following drawing shows you the working parts of a common cuff:

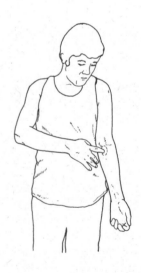

Blood pressure cuffs vary somewhat in design. So get accustomed to the way yours operates before you do this part of the exam. Practice inflating and deflating it, particularly.

The person whose blood pressure you are measuring should be seated and relaxed. Nervous tension, physical exertion and fatigue all effect blood pressure, so be sure that the person is at rest if you want to get a meaningful reading. Also, their arm should be bare from the shoulder down. In taking blood pressure you will be listening to a pulse from an artery in the person's arm.

Deflate the cuff completely and wrap it snugly around the person's arm as indicated in the drawing below left.

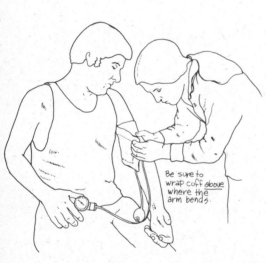

Be sure to wrap cuff above where the arm bends.

Put your stethoscope in your ears, and place the bell at the end of it on the following place on the person's arm:

Be sure the stethoscope bell is not touching the cuff itself or any part of the tubes coming from it. Make certain that the gauge of the cuff is situated so that you can easily read the dial.

Now close the valve of the blood pressure pump and inflate the cuff rapidly until the gauge reads 200. *Immediately open the valve and release the pressure fairly rapidly.* Watch the dial and listen for the approximate places where the pulse sounds — heard in the stethoscope — appear and then disappear.

As you deflate the cuff, you will probably first hear the pulse sounds at between 150 and 110 on the gauge, and you will probably continue to hear them until the gauge reads between 90 and 60, where the sounds disappear. (If the person you are examining is over 45 years of age, these figures may be higher.)

Inflate the cuff again until the pressure is 10 to 20 points above the point where you first heard the pulse sounds on your previous try. Deflate the cuff slowly until you hear the sounds again. This will be the *systolic* (heart pumping pressure) blood pressure reading. Make a clear mental note of it.

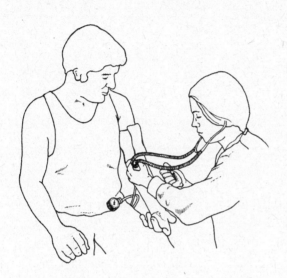

Deflate the cuff more rapidly until your guage reads 10 to 20 points above where the sounds first disappeared on the lower end of the reading. Then slowly deflate the cuff until you no longer hear the sounds at all. At the place where the sounds disappear, make a mental note of the number on your guage. This is the *diastolic* (heart resting) blood pressure reading. Note it mentally.

Open the valve of the blood pressure pump completely. Remove the cuff.

Now record the *systolic* and *diastolic* blood pressure readings on the P.E. report.

Normal blood pressure: For adults under 40, a normal systolic pressure is considered to be between 110 and 150; normal diastolic varies between 60 and 90. In people over 45, these figures are often higher: 185 systolic, and 100 diastolic not, in themselves, considered abnormal.

This completes the physical examination.

COMING OUT HEALTHY

Many healers, from both primitive and modern cultures, do things to prevent a sick person's disease energy from entering their own body, and the bodies of others in the same room, after a healing session. This usually consists of a ritual to strengthen and increase the healer's own healthy energy. The ritual itself is a form of preventive medicine which works through the mind. Some American Indian healers paint a dot of herb powders on the foreheads of people present at healings to protect them from disease. Western medical people wear masks and gowns for protection, which they later shed — even though it has been proven that masks and gowns work poorly, if at all, to prevent the spread of germs.

Our ritual for **The Well Body Book** is called **Coming Out Healthy**. When you finish doing a P.E., or any other healing process, sit down in a quiet place and close your eyes. Relax and rest. Take a few deep breaths, exhaling each breath slowly.

Now imagine, as you inhale, that you are taking positive healing energy from the universe and drawing it into your own body. As you exhale, imagine disease energy is leaving your body. Do this exercise until you feel strong and healthy. Say to yourself, "I am stronger and healthier than before."

You may wish to go further with this. As you inhale imagine that your breath is drawing positive healing energy from the universe. It is coming into your body through your third eye (the pineal gland between your eyes). Imagine that this healing energy radiates with pure, white light. Exhale strongly through your nose. Imagine disease energy leaving whatever part of your body that you feel might be prone to disease at that moment. Imagine that the disease energy leaving your body is brownish in color. Continue doing this exercise until you imagine that the energy leaving your body is as clear and pure as the pure white light entering it. To finish the ritual, say to yourself "I am stronger and healthier than before."

Some people may wish to do the exercise for getting in touch with their imaginary doctor as a **Coming Out Healthy** ritual. Then you can have your imaginary doctor do either of the above exercises with you, or you and they can work out your own rituals for accomplishing the same things. If you do use your imaginary doctor to get a new ritual, we recommend that the ritual include two elements: the taking in of healthy energy in some form, and the catharting of disease energy from your body.

HOW TO USE THE PHYSICAL EXAMINATION REPORT

First make notations as instructed in the chapter on how to do a *Physical Examination*. You can either make photo copies of the P.E. Report Form or you can use the P.E. Report Form as a guide and make your own notations on a separate sheet of paper.

After you have completed the physical exam and have written down your findings, read over any notes which you have made. Sometimes we give you page numbers where you can read about the probable cause or causes of whatever you found to report. Usually we refer you to the *Diagnosis and Treatment* chapter. (If you have any questions about how to use that chapter, read pages 195 — 197 first.)

If in doing the P.E. you find symptoms which we do not ask you to note, first write them down in the P.E. report, then turn to the *Index,* page 347 — 349. This index lists more specific symptoms and refers you to pages where you will find more information about their probable cause.

On pages 191 — 192 we give you specific instructions for each portion of the physical exam report, whenever such instructions are relevant. We suggest that you read these after completing the P.E. report if you have any questions.

Although these instructions may seem complicated at first, once or twice through the exam will make it obvious and familiar to you. The P.E. report form can become your abbreviated guide for doing a physical exam, after you have done it a few times following the more complete instructions.

If for one reason or another you are unable to find the cause or causes of a present illness, go to your doctor for further help. Our chapter on *Your Doctor As A Resource* will help you do this.

PHYSICAL EXAMINATION REPORT FORM

Name _____ Date _____

PRESENT ILLNESS

CHIEF COMPLAINT: (What's wrong?)

Present Illness: (The story of the illness, including when they got sick, what symptoms they noticed, and whether the symptoms are becoming better or worse. Ask about any previous diagnosis by a doctor, or any self treatment.)

Where The Person Is At: (Areas of satisfaction and/or tension in their life; how the person makes you feel and how the person looks.)

VITAL FUNCTIONS

Height   Weight   (Note any gain or loss)

Temperature   Pulse rate   (note if irregular)

Respiration rate   Blood pressure (Optional)

SKIN AND HAIR

Skin: Note any pimples, rashes, moles, warts, boils, irritated areas, page 201 – 217; yellow skin, page 260; paleness, page 283.

Hair: Note shiney, dull, dry, oily, or chemicals, page 87.

Scalp: Note any red, or moist areas, page 201 – 217.

HEAD

Skull: Note bumps, soreness, page 291.

Eyes: Note whether the white part is yellowish, page 260; pinkish, or the mucosa is reddish, page 220 – 223; mucosa looks grayish, page 283; swollen or has discharge with pus, page 220 – 223. Note differences in the constriction of pupils, page 291. Note inability to follow finger, page 192, Neurological exam.

Ears: Note if the skin of the outer ear is red, moist, or scaley, page 201 — 217. Note wax blocking ear canal, page 223; redness in canal, or discharge, page 224 — 226; note if the eardrum is red, dull, or fails to reflect light, page 225. Note inequality of hearing, page 225.

Nose: Note if the mucosa looks swollen, red, or bluish. Note any discharge, page 227, 233 — 239, and 243.

Sinus: Note tenderness, page 227.

Mouth: Note if the gums appear red, puffy, bleeding or sore. Note brown areas on teeth. Note areas of the tongue or mucosa that look red, or have curd-white patches, page 228.

Throat: Note if the tonsils are swollen, red, or have white patches, or if the pharanx looks red, swollen, or has mucous, page 233 — 239.

Lips: Note sores, page 208, and 210; or white spots, page 228.

Mucosal linings: Note sores, page 208 and 228; or white spots, page 228.

Lymph nodes: Note any swollen lymph nodes and their location, page 163 and 341.

NECK MOVEMENTS

Note any paid or difficulty with neck movements, page 233 — 239, 191, and 292.

BREASTS

Note asymmetry, redness, sores, or discharge from nipples, any irregularities or lumps, page 230 — 231.

CHEST

Lungs: Note forced, noisy, uneven or difficult breathing, page 239 — 247; unequal expansion of chest, page 241; areas that percuss dull, page 241; note rales, page 241; rhonchi, page 239; or wheezing, page 245.

Heart: Note if the PMI is way off to the side. Note murmurs or any other irregularities, page 191.

ABDOMEN

Note tenderness or rigidity, page 255 — 262, 191; note if the liver is enlarged, page 260; note if spleen is enlarged, page 281; note dullness on percussion, page 260; note absent, loud, or constant bowel sounds, page 249. Note any masses felt.

MALE GENITALS

Penis shaft: note sores or rash, page 201 — 217, and 271.

Urethral opening: note liquid discharge or redness, page 267, and 273.

Scrotum: note sores, page 201 — 217, and 271; tenderness in testicles or tubes, page 192.

Hernia: note any bulge when the person coughs.

FEMALE GENITALS

Area around vagina and labia: note sores, page 201 — 217 and 271; discharge or red mucosa, page 265 — 269.

Urethra: note swelling, redness, page 265 — 269.

Bartholin's gland: note if swollen or tender, page 271.

Vaginal walls: note tenderness or soreness, page 265 — 270.

Cervix: Note if I.U.D. string is present.

Speculum exam: (OPTIONAL) note discharge, page 265 — 270; sores, page 201 — 217, 271, and 192. Check I.U.D.

ANUS

Note sores, or small tabs of skin, page 201 — 217, 271, and 262.

NERVOUS SYSTEM

Eyebrows: note if person raises them unequally.

Cotton ball test: note if person feels cotton touch unequally.

Swallow: note if person has trouble swallowing.

Shoulder raising: note if person is unable to raise shoulders.

Hand: note if the strength is unequal in the hands.

Arm: note if the strength is unequal in arms.

Thigh: note if strength is unequal in thighs.

Leg: note if strength is unequal in legs.

Knee reflexes: note if knee reflexes are absent.

End of the P.E. Report Form.

SPECIFIC INSTRUCTIONS

VITAL FUNCTIONS: Your findings in this section will help you in diagnosing diseases involving specific organ systems. For example, in the *Diagnosis and Treatment* chapter you may find increased respiration or fever listed as a symptom of many different diseases. You will thus use all your findings in the physical exam to help you determine the cause or causes of a present illness.

SKIN AND HAIR: Some skin symptoms are also listed under other organ systems, and these will become clear to you as you continue with the exam. For example, you will be asked in the Genital exam to make note of pimples, and will also be told where to turn for further information.

If the person you are examining looks flushed, check for fever.

HEAD: No specific instructions.

NECK MOVEMENTS: People often complain of neck pain when they have muscular aches accompanying upper respiratory infections. Severe discomfort or inability to move the neck may have other causes; use your doctor to help you diagnose probable causes.

BREASTS: No specific instructions.

CHEST: Lungs: No specific instructions.
PMI: We don't deal in detail with heart problems, so if you discover an irregular PMI, a murmur, or other heart irregularity, have your doctor help you diagnose the cause.

ABDOMEN: Masses in the abdominal area may have many causes which we do not deal with in this book. In very thin people you may normally be able to feel some internal organs, such as ovaries, bladder, etc. Since it takes some practice to feel an abdomen, we suggest that you have your doctor help you if you feel any masses.

MALE GENITALS: Pain in the testicles or tubes can be due to many causes besides Gonorrhea. In any case, your doctor will be your best resource in diagnosing and treating the cause or causes of these symptoms.

Because hernia often requires surgical correction, see your doctor for help with this.

FEMALE GENITALS: The I.U.D. should occasionally be checked by a doctor. Have your doctor help if you find any irregularities here.

ANUS: No specific instructions.

NEUROLOGICAL EXAM: We do not deal with neurological troubles in this book. If you do discover irregularitites which you do not already know about, have your doctor help you diagnose the cause.

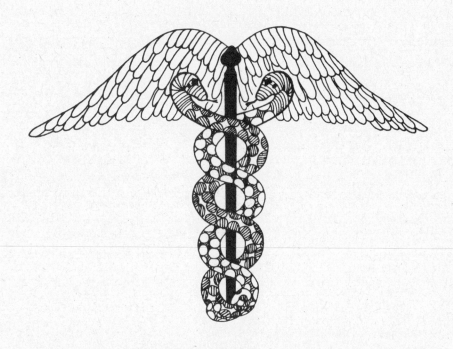

DIAGNOSIS AND TREATMENT

DIAGNOSIS AND TREATMENT INDEX

ORGAN SYSTEMS

DISEASES

DIAGNOSIS AND TREATMENT

In this chapter we tell you how to diagnose and treat a number of common diseases. By common diseases, we mean diseases for which people actually go to a doctor to receive treatment. The diseases in this chapter are not *fantasy* diseases, are not rare and exotic diseases which you have seen on television, or which you worry about having but which are, in reality, very uncommon. They are real diseases that real people get. They are the diseases that general practioners spend most of their time treating, and which are common to people between the ages of fifteen and fifty. We do not deal with the so-called "childhood diseases," such as measles, since this information is readily available from many other home medical encyclopedias.

We have chosen diseases in which the person being healed can easily take an active role in the healing process. In some of these we tell you how to diagnose and treat the disease yourself. In others we tell you how to use a doctor or a clinic to help your body heal itself.

You do not have to be ill or have one of the diseases we list here to benefit from reading this section. You will find, as you read through this chapter, that each disease presents and explains something about how your body interacts with Nature: what makes it get sick and what makes it heal. The stories and the principles of these illnesses will apply to many illnesses besides the ones we list, and will help you develop skills for staying well. The total chapter is a model for you to begin developing your own philosophy of disease and healing.

The models of disease which we describe in this chapter are taken from what Western medicine (as opposed to Psychic Healing, Acupuncture, etc.) has learned about the nature of disease. There are large numbers of "facts" which we present, but don't feel that you must memorize or completely understand them in order for this information to work for you. Understand that medical researchers change these "facts" periodically, often without apparently changing their effectiveness as diagnostic or healing tools. This is probably not the view of medicine that you have been taught; you have probably been taught that medicine is an exacting science and that the "facts" of medicine are *real* and never-changing. The truth is that medicine is a dynamic, ever-changing art — a system of looking at the world of disease and healing that will no doubt be completely different in another hundred years. Does this mean that these facts are of no value to you now? On the contrary . . .

The "facts" and the stories of diseases which we present in this chapter are useful to you in that they help you organize your thoughts, your feelings, and your energy in order to heal yourself. They allow you to visualize what is going on in your body when it is sick, when it is healing, and when it is well, allowing you to reduce swelling, increase blood flow, and direct healing energy for positive change in your life.

HOW EACH DISEASE IS ARRANGED

You will find each disease (or model) organized under the following headings:

Symptoms: Messages from your body which tell you that you're sick.

Physical Exam: Specific abnormal findings which apply to diagnosing a particular disease.

What's Going On?: A description of what is happening in your body as it reacts to the disease.

Treatment: How to help your body heal itself.

Your Doctor As a Resource: How you can use your doctor or clinic to help your body heal itself.

Preventive Medicine: How to keep yourself well.

The diseases are organized, also, according to *organ systems,* just as the *Systems Review,* page 30, was arranged according to organ systems. Thus, if you have symptoms on the skin, perhaps a rash, look under *Skin,* the organ system involved, and then skim the symptoms of all the diseases in that section until you find the symptoms, and thus the disease, that most closely corresponds to what you have.

LEARNING BASIC PRINCIPLES

A selection of diseases in this chapter demonstrates basic principles of disease and healing. You may want to spend your time studying those, since they are the ones that will most help you develop your own system of diagnosis and treatment. Look upon these as basic models: Fever, Pain, and Symptoms of Healing; Contact Dermatitis; Tension Headache; Infections of the Middle Ear; Common Cold; Strep Throat; Bronchitis; Hay Fever; Diarrhea; Hepatitis; Gonorrhea; and Lower Back Pain.

Principles which you'll discover will include:

Tension — When you tense up muscles in an area of your body, blood flow slows or stops, affecting the supply of nutrients to that area, as well as slowing down the rate at which waste products are carried away, and causing nerve ends to send messages of pain to your brain.

Stasis — When body fluids are not moving in an area of your body that area becomes a good place for bacteria to grow.

Communication of Disease — How disease is transmitted from one person to another.

Use of Energy — How harmony or disharmony in the way you direct your energy between muscle and bone can affect your health.

Other principles of disease and healing are discussed in this chapter but these are among the most basic ones.

YOUR SYMPTOMS MAY BE DIFFERENT

Bear in mind that these medical models describe *average* diseases. But each person's body reacts *differently* to disease. This means that the *symptoms you feel, what you find on the physical exam, and the description of what's happening in your body will probably differ from the model we describe.* You may have *only one* of the symptoms when we describe several, you may have *ones that we don't describe.* But from the information we give you will be able to find the disease that most closely corresponds to your feelings.

You will find this section of the book most helpful if you use the information which we present here to guide you in dispelling fears about disease. Your understanding of how your body reacts with Nature, in times of both sickness and health, will allow you to use your energy to heal your body and keep it well.

We suggest that after you read parts of this chapter, either now for general information, or later if you are ill, that you finish your reading by doing the exercise, *Coming Out Healthy* which we describe at the end of this chapter.

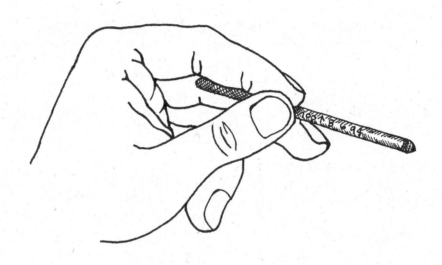

GENERAL SYMPTOMS

Most diseases involve very common symptoms which are signals of a disease. The two which most doctors recognize as "general symptoms" are *pain* and *fever*. In most diseases either one or the other of these symptoms is present to some extent. The pain may be little more than the mild discomfort of a cold or it may be more pervasive, as with a broken bone. Likewise, fever may be slight, sub-normal, or several degrees higher than normal. In any case, fever and pain are valuable signals, messages from the body to tell you to direct your energy toward healing.

FEVER

The next time you have a fever, be thankful that you have it since the fever may very well be helping your body to heal itself.

The body's normal temperature is 98.6°. This is the average normal temperature. Yours may normally be higher or lower than this. The temperature of your body also varies normally with exercise, with the temperature of your surroundings, during digestion, during the menstrual period and at other times.

Fever affects different people in different ways. Some people feel hot and sweaty, others feel chilled, and others feel nothing at all. When you suspect a fever, and you want to make sure whether or not you really have one, use a thermometer to check it out. (See the *Physical Examination* chapter for instructions.)

The treatment of fever varies with the treatment of the specific disease causing the rise in your body temperature. In this country most people treat fever as soon as it appears by taking aspirin. (See *Drugs Are Helpers* for information on aspirin.) But it is important to understand that, in most cases, *fever is okay*. The only reason to bring it down is if it is making you uncomfortable. The only exception to this is with infants having a rapid rise of fever. In this case, do what you can to reduce the fever or keep it from rising.

If you have a fever and it is making you very uncomfortable, there are some ways to get relief: increase your fluid intake; sponge your body off with cold water; rub your body with rubbing alcohol. A warm bath causes opening of the skin blood vessels, which brings your blood closer to the surface and helps to bring the fever down. Ice bags are sometimes used to reduce body fever, too.

PAIN

Pain, like fever, is not a disease; it is a symptom. Look upon pain as a signal from a part of your body that is injured or sick, to your mind, to tell you that something is wrong and needs to be fixed.

No one can ignore pain. When your mind registers pain it stops everything else and turns your attention and energy to relieving the cause of it. Everyone has a different pain threshold — the amount of pain that you can tolerate. This threshold varies with fatigue, tension and fear. The more relaxed you are the less the pain will bother you. The less it will make you afraid.

Once the signal is received and a move has been made to alleviate the cause of the pain, total body relaxation and mind relaxation can usually serve to diminish its affects on you. If you use a drug to reduce pain without treating the problem that caused it, you may be doing yourself more harm than good. Unless you correct the cause the pain will only return when the drug has worn off.

To be told to relax when you are actually suffering pain may prove futile, and may be insulting to the person suffering it. It's a good idea, then, to practice the relaxation exercises in this book when you feel well so that you will have developed skills for dealing with pain the next time you experience it.

Several years ago a friend of ours was injured in a motorcycle accident. He broke his pelvis, hip, and several ribs, so naturally a great deal of pain was involved. On the way to the hospital he was fortunate in having an ambulance attendent who was both wise and sympathetic about pain. The following is an exercise derived from his experiences with that attendant:

Look upon your pain as a signal that something is wrong and needs to be fixed. Your injury is now receiving care. In a short time it will be fixed. Now close your eyes and imagine that the pain you feel is outside you. Imagine that it is a telephone ringing. But you already know who is calling. You have already done something about it. You do not have to answer the phone. Let it ring. Do not pick up the receiver.

Few people will ever have the good fortune to have such help when they need it, so we pass this exercise on to you now.

Fear and pain work together in an endless circle. Pain makes you afraid; your fear lowers your pain threshold; your pain feels worse; your fear increases, etc. The trick is to break the circle, and to interrupt the cycle. When you are in pain, focus your attention on whichever part — pain or fear — you feel most able to master. Thus you will be able to break the circle and reduce both your pain and your fear. The next step is relaxation, which brings healing energy to the injured parts. Focus singlemindedly on doing whatever is necessary to bring healing energy to your body. Relinquish fear, put the pain outside you, and relax to bring healing energy to your body.

RECOGNIZE SYMPTOMS OF HEALING

In some diseases we recommend getting *cultures* to determine when your body has fully recovered from an infection. We tell you more about these in the specific diseases for which they are relevant. But in general, focus your attention on symptoms of healing when you are sick. These symptoms are usually manifest in your fever balancing back to the temperature that is normal for you, and, if you are not taking pain drugs, a slow return of comfort. A return of energy and a feeling of well-being are messages from your body telling you that it is healing itself.

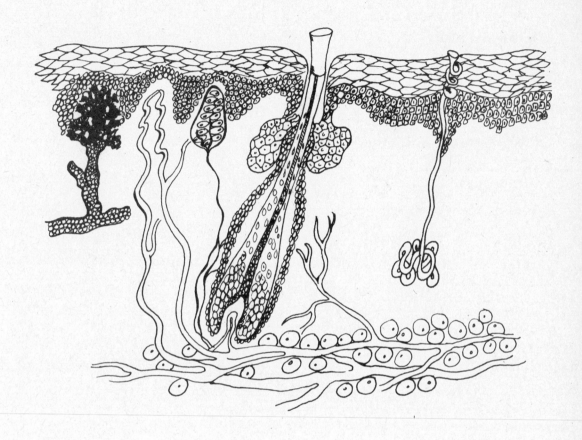

SKIN

Unlike many other organ systems, your skin shows. You can see it and you can touch it. It can reflect what is going on inside your body and how you are taking care of yourself. It is affected by things in the external environment, like heat, chemicals, the sun, and plants like poison oak and ivy. A general rule about treating skin disease is, "If it's dry wet it, and if it's wet dry it."

As you read through these skin diseases for the first time it may seem to you that one skin disease looks pretty much like another. But when the time comes that you find yourself diagnosing and treating an actual skin problem, you will discover that you'll be able to distinguish between one and another quite easily.

CONTACT DERMATITIS
(Poison oak, poison ivy, detergent reactions, etc.)

Symptoms: Itching
Burning
Stinging
The skin area may be hot and swollen
The person's chief complaint may be that they have a "rash"

Physical Exam: Upon examination you will find a red area, slightly swollen, with small red dots, some of these with water in them, some looking like pimples, some weeping (dripping or oozing water). You may also find crusting or infected areas or areas that appear to be filled with pus.

What's Going On?: Contact Dermatitis is caused by various substances that irritate the skin: chemicals, hair tints, shampoos, skin creams, detergents, plants (poison ivy, oak, and nettles, etc.) It is an extremely common skin disorder. The body reacts to irritants by releasing its own chemicals. Increased blood flow produces characteristic redness. The weeping is produced as histamines are released. The pus is made up of white blood cells carrying away dead body cells injured by the infection. All these "symptoms" are evidence that your body is defending itself from chemicals it feels are a threat to its well being and is going about the business of healing itself.

Sometimes the body's reaction to these substances appears to be an exaggerated one. The same substances which can cause one person to react violently will not affect others at all. Each person's body has its own idiosyncracies.

If you find it difficult to tell the difference between Contact Dermatitis and other skin diseases, ask the person about their exposure to plants or chemicals, and about any new clothing they may be wearing. Clothes sometimes contain substances, such as detergents and other chemicals, that can cause skin reactions. From this information you will be able to make a more accurate diagnosis.

Distribution of the rash will often give you a clue to its cause. If the person has a rash which is just on their hands, and they work with a strong dishwashing detergent, that detergent itself should be considered as a cause. If the rash is only in the underwear area and the person has either recently bought new garments or is using a new detergent to wash their clothes, explore the possibilities that the dermatitis may be caused by substances in the underwear or in the detergent used to wash the underwear. If the rash appears on the scalp it could be caused by a hair tint, shampoo, or other preparation used in the hair. If a combination of chemicals are being used in the hair, such as tints, shampoos, and hair sprays (not unusual) these chemicals reacting with each other may be the cause. If the rash appears under a ring, it could be caused by a reaction to the metal in the ring. Suspect cosmetics as the cause of the dermatitis if it appears in a body area where cosmetics are frequently used.

Plants such as poison oak or ivy will cause skin reactions in those areas which have been exposed to the oils from the plant. The hands, face, neck, and ankles are typical areas of poison ivy or oak exposure. But since a person can spread poison oak or ivy oils to other areas of their body by scratching or simply touching those other areas with hands carrying the toxic substances of the plant, don't rule out these plants as causing the reaction if the rash appears elsewhere.

Sometimes it is very difficult to diagnose the specific cause of Contact Dermatitis, and doing so will take a great deal of thinking on your part and on the part of the person with the dermatitis. Consult your imaginary doctor in diagnosing the cause if you feel you need this extra help.

Treatment: Keep the affected areas clean so that they don't become secondarily infected. (Secondary infection is where bacteria that normally live on your skin or which are in the environment, get into a body area at a weakened point such as that made by a cut or a rash. See *Impetigo* section of this chapter for more on this.) A secondary infection can be more severe than the Contact Dermatitis itself. So keeping the affected area clean is the first thing you should do.

To relieve the itching cool down the area that itches. This can be done by: cool baths; cool washcloths placed on the part that itches; cool baths with baking soda. Heat will make the itching worse. Some over-the-counter drugs to relieve the symptoms of poison oak help some people and do nothing for others. Understand that the lotions, creams, etc., do not *heal* the poison oak. They only treat symptoms. The present attitude of many doctors is "keep it clean, keep it cool, and the skin will heal itself."

Sometimes a doctor will prescribe steroids for severe cases. (See the chapter called *Drugs Are Helpers* for an explanation of steroids.) Steroids are the same substances that you normally release from your adrenal glands. Most milder cases of dermatitis are cured by your body responding to the illness and sending these steroid substances to heal it. By conscious control you can learn to increase the amounts of steroids that your adrenal glands normally secrete. The ability to control the various functions of your body improves with practice. Likewise relaxation exercises can increase the flow of blood to and from the affected area, and this enhances the healing process by bringing in nutrients and healing substances, and carrying away toxics and wastes.

Turning your attention to other things plays a dramatic part in the healing of Contact Dermatitis. "Poison ivy consciousness" is what I call it when a person thinks of nothing but his dermatitis, and this always makes the condition worse. However, if you relax and think about skin areas that are healthy, you can concentrate positive healing energy on your skin and this helps your body to heal itself. Positive mental and emotional energies have a tremendous affect on healing Contact Dermatitis.

Your Doctor As Resource: If contact dermatitis develops into swelling of large areas of your body, or leads to your eyes swelling closed, a doctor can prescribe steroids to reduce the swelling. Or if the affected area becomes secondarily infected, seen as hot, red, swollen areas that are painful and contain pus, the doctor can prescribe antibiotics to help your body heal the infection.

Prevention: To prevent contact dermatitis, diagnose the specific cause and then avoid contact with the irritants. Avoid chemicals on your skin.

Dermatitis caused by poison oak in our community, which is a small rural community, is most often suffered by new people moving in from the city or by people who can't recognize the plant or don't know how it can affect them. After people have lived here for awhile they get it less. This is possibly due to de-sensitization, or to the fact that you learn to wear gloves when you're working around the plant, or you remove it from areas that you frequent.

It may help you to avoid getting poison oak or ivy if you wash with brown soap (Naptha) shortly (15 minutes) after contact. It is especially important to wash under your fingernails because oils collect there and spread to other areas of your body when you scratch. Scratching also causes secondary infection.

HIVES

Symptoms:
Large, red, raised areas on the skin, called "wheals" which vary greatly in shape and degrees of swelling
Intolerable itching
Some tiredness and fever may be present
Person may complain of nausea

Physical Exam: The main things you will find on examination are the "wheals" as described in the symptoms section above. In some cases, there may be total body symptoms such as tiredness, fever, and nausea. The person who has hives will complain of intolerable itching.

What's Going On?: A person with hives may be red over large areas of their body, and may be swollen around their eyes. Hives is the body's reaction to substances which for one reason or another it recognizes as threatening, and the symptoms are the result of that phenomenon taking place. Each person who gets hives will find that their body has its own things that it reacts to. It is seldom the same for any two people, but there are some substances which seem more prone to causing this reaction than others. They are foods such as: shellfish, strawberries, eggs, milk, or chocolate; drugs such as penicillin and other antibiotics, aspirin, and bromides; and any number of kinds of insect bites. Some people never get hives. But if you were a person who was sensitive to mosquito bites one small bite could make your whole face, arm, or hand swell up.

Sometimes hives are brought about by emotional disturbances. There's a disease called *angioneurotic edema.* In this disease, when a person experiences emotional shock, fright, or stress they get hives just as severe as hives caused by food or drug reactions. This demonstrates how your conscious mind, and your feelings which may be less conscious, can bring about hives. If you have the power to bring it about, you also have the potential power to prevent the hives from occuring in your body.

Treatment: Just as hives can be brought on by stress, you can heal them by mellowing your body out, relaxing, and allowing your blood to flow more freely into and out of the affected area to heal you.

Your Doctor As A Resource: The only threat in hives is swelling of the mucosal tissue in the throat which then becomes a breathing problem. If this even begins to occur it is essential to get help from a doctor to help open the air passages. If breathing problems develop, or when very severe swelling of the whole body with intense itching occurs, your doctor can give you *epinephrine* (a hormone) injections which bring prompt and spectacular relief.

Doctors may also prescribe antihistamine drugs to block the body's histamine release which produces the symptoms of hives. These drugs may be given in cases of severe facial swelling if the person has difficulty seeing.

Prevention: Hives usually last only a few days, and always goes away by itself soon after the food or other cause of the reaction is removed. For these reasons, it is known as a "self-limiting" condition. To prevent hives, learn which substances in your life cause the reaction and then avoid them.

HEAT RASH

Symptoms: Burning
Itching areas on the skin
Fever and extreme tiredness may sometimes occur

Physical Exam: On examining the person's skin, you will see small vesicles, which are water-filled blisters, and general red areas. The person with heat rash may also have a fever and complain of extreme tiredness.

Affected areas will usually be around areas where tight-fitting clothes are worn or in body folds where the affected area can't breathe. (Also read the *What's Going On?* section for *Contact Dermatitis.*)

What's Going On?: Heat rash takes place in hot, moist climates. The sweat ducts in the skin become plugged. When they balloon and rupture, an irritating stinging reaction occurs and blisters and redness develop. Heat rash is usually a very mild disorder.

Treatment: Treat the symptoms with towels soaked in cool water. Your body knows how to heal itself of this complaint with relative ease. Prevention is the main "treatment."

Your Doctor As Resource: If you have questions in your mind as to what is actually causing your "rash," a doctor can help you diagnose it.

Prevention: Avoiding very hot conditions, and avoiding clothing which causes you to sweat (leading to blockage of your sweat ducts) are important things to keep in mind. In general, I have found that people with heat rash have gotten it because of the clothes they wear; tight clothing, such as underwear made of synthetic fabrics which do not breathe properly, is often a cause. See our *Preventive Medicine* chapter for more information on clothes.

205

SUNBURN

Symptoms:

Painful, hot, red areas on sun-exposed skin

Blistering	Nausea
Peeling	Chills
Fever	Fatigue

Physical Exam: On examination you will see red, swollen areas in sun-exposed places, occassionally with small blisters. The person may or may not have a fever or other symptoms.

What's Going On?: The sun's rays cause a direct toxic reaction in the skin, greatly increasing the blood flow to the skin, and causing the release of natural chemicals. These chemicals are released to protect the body and they can cause a total body reaction. The total body reaction is fever, chills, nausea, and fatigue. People become frightened of this because they don't expect it of sunburn; but it's all part of the sunburn condition, and need not be feared.

Treatment: The best treatment for the red swollen areas on the skin is to place towels soaked in cold water gently over those areas. The treatment for the fever, chills, and fatigue is bed rest, in order to turn a maximum amount of your energy to the healing process. Your body will heal itself within a short period.

Your Doctor As A Resource: In cases of sunburn with extreme discomfort a doctor may prescribe lotions, pain drugs, or other medications for symptomatic relief.

Prevention: Fair-skinned people and people taking certain drugs, such as tetracyclines (generic name) and people with certain chemicals on their skin such as perfumes, cosmetics or soap residues, should be especially careful of sun exposure. Most people get sunburned when they're in places they've never been before, and where they don't understand the sun conditions. They get burned on vacation trips, especially on trips to beaches and southern regions.

A general rule for preventing sunburn is to pay attention to your skin's reactions to the sun, and to protect yourself from exposure. A sun "tan" is one way your body protects you from the whole sunburn syndrome. So on the first days of exposure limit your time in the sun, and increase your exposure only after you have a protective tan and can go out without burning.

Some protective lotions may be helpful. But we feel that it is important to keep yourself open to your body's messages and limit your exposure time until your skin has developed a protective tan on its own.

WARTS

Symptoms:

Solitary or clustered protrusions or nodes of flesh, most often seen on the hands, fingers, toes, or genitals

Physical Exam: Upon examination you would see hard, solid, cluster-like protrusions on fingers, hands, toes, or genital areas. They may look like growing things, like miniature fleshy broccoli.

What's Going On?: Warts are known to be caused by a virus. They are mildly infectious, but many people never catch them even though they are exposed. It is believed that the virus is on the person's skin and suddenly breaks out for unknown reasons. Warts often appear in body areas of lowered resistance, along with other infections. They disappear as spontaneously as they appear, but it is difficult to predict when they'll disappear. They can be there for a week or a month or several years.

The lowly wart hasn't been given much attention in medical circles. But some *Homeopathic* doctors believe that warts, like other illnesses, are part of a person's total body picture of themselves, and that the wart will tell as much about a person's health and general approach to life as a severe illness would tell.

Treatment: Try to get in touch with that part of you that causes the wart. Use your imaginary doctor for this. If you are not successful at first, keep at it, and you eventually will be. You will discover that you can have a great deal of control over getting or not getting warts. Doctors have found that both hypnosis and "positive suggestion" can cure warts. We have found the following exercise to be effective in curing warts:

> Sit in a comfortable position. Relax your whole body, especially the part of your body that has the warts, using the technique you use to get your imaginary doctor. Look at and feel a part of your skin that you feel is absolutely healthy and beautiful. Close your eyes and imagine that the skin in the area of the warts looks and feels like the healthy area of skin. Imagine healing energy going to that area. You may or may not feel this as numbness or tingling in the part of your body that has the warts.

Understand that your warts will not disappear immediately. It takes your body a while to change the environment of your skin so that the wart virus will not want to live there any more. Your success will occur with your continued, positive feed-in to the affected area. For some people this will take days, for others it will take longer.

Some over-the-counter preparations to remove warts seem to work well for many people.

Your Doctor As Resource: Doctors can remove your warts with chemicals or by burning them with an electrical device (relatively painless), or by simple surgery. Doctors advise removal of warts because they sometimes become irritated or knocked off and then become infected. Warts are removed from the feet and toes, of course, because they hurt when you walk.

Prevention: Same as *treatment* described above.

HERPES SIMPLEX
(Also called "Fever Blisters, or "Cold Sores")

Symptoms: Small blisters on the mouth, genital areas or skin
Affected areas may itch or be painful

Physical Exam: You will see, in the mouth genital areas or skin, small raised blisters which turn into "punched out" sores. They may look like round sores with little holes punched out, which then become scabbed over. You may find them singly or in clumps. They can crust over and "weep" (become runny) toward the end of the herpes infection. Swollen lymph nodes in the area may be more disturbing to the person with Herpes than the actual disease itself.

What's Going On?: Herpes is a viral infection. Some people believe that the virus is on the skin from early childhood; others believe that you catch it from other people who have it.
     Herpes infections are known to be aggravated by certain things: another infection somewhere in your body that lowers your resistance (like when you have a cold), windburn, or nervous tension. In my experience, Herpes occurs and reoccurs for a certain period of time in a person's life, and then the person simply stops getting it, and is not troubled with it again.

Treatment: I've found that drying agents such as cornstarch or baby powder work to relieve symptoms on external infections. Herpes is self-limited (stops itself) and usually lasts from one to three weeks. If you find Herpes-type sores in the genital area, I'd advise getting a blood test to make sure its not Syphilis. The symptoms of Herpes and Syphilis often appear the same, and can be difficult to differentiate. Look upon Herpes as your body's message to you asking you to pay attention. Then take care of it the best way you know how.

Your Doctor As a Resource: Your doctor can give you a blood test for Syphilis if Herpes appears in your genital area (or mouth).

Prevention: Herpes takes place most often in times of tension and stress. Relaxation is an essential part of prevention. Avoid touching Herpes sores on other people.

ACNE

Symptoms: Soreness
Itching
Pimples, over the face, back and shoulders
Self-consciousness, shame and embarrassment can be the most
      disturbing "symptoms"

Physical Exam: Upon examination of the skin you will find pimples, red, pus-filled spots over the face, back, shoulders, etc. You may also find hard areas, called *cysts*, and some scar tissue.

What's Going On?: Acne is a very common skin disorder. It is seen most often in adolescence. Hormonal balances affects acne. Small skin folicles become plugged with oil, then become secondarily infected with bacteria that normally lives on the skin. The pimples which result are miniature infections.

Certain emotional factors of acne are well known to people who have it; it often gets better when things are going well in their life, and gets worse when things are going poorly. There is very little known about it medically and there is no instant cure for it. Most acne disappears as the adolescent moves into adulthood.

Treatment: It was once thought that diet — specifically foods like chocolate and nuts — aggravated acne. Doctors are now beginning to wonder if these foods have any significant affect at all. People who have acne report that certain foods do make it worse and certain foods tend to make it better. For each person it is a bit different, and once you find which foods aggravate it for you you should obviously avoid them.

Recently, doctors have been giving *tetracyline*, a broad spectrum antibiotic, orally, as a long term therapy for acne. This helps prevent small secondary infections. We recommend that you read the section on antibiotics, in the chapter called *Drugs Are Helpers*, before you consider this form of therapy.

Cleaning your skin with soap helps to prevent the bacterial secondary infection, so this is very valuable as both prevention and treatment. Drying agents, such as rubbing alcohol, are sometimes prescribed. Some doctors use exposure to sunlight and ultraviolet radiation lamps to treat acne. Women who take oral contraceptives have reported that their acne improves, but this should certainly not be considered as a therapy for acne in itself, since the oral contraceptives are female hormones. (See "Hormones" in the chapter called *Drugs Are Helpers* if you want to know more about this.)

Your Doctor As Resource: There are as many treatments for acne as there are skin doctors. Some work better than others. As with most treatments, your faith in the treatment and your attitude toward yourself and your skin will greatly determine how well the treatment works. Some people report relief from their acne with over-the-counter acne treatments.

Prevention: Loving your skin may be the first principle in preventing acne. Acne is a normal reaction in your skin to hormonal changes in your body, especially during the years of adolescence. Almost everyone has some sort of acne at some time in their life. When you become extremely afraid of acne, and ashamed and embarrassed about having it, you're probably affecting the blood flow to your skin and rather than cleansing out the infections you inhibit healing. (For more information on prevention, see *Preventive Medicine*, on diet, bathing, and relaxation.)

BOILS

Symptoms: A hot, red, swollen, and painful area on the skin similar to an overgrown pimple

Physical Exam: Upon examining the area of the complaint, you will see a swollen, pimple-like area on the skin, with some redness surrounding it and sometimes a white "head" on top of it. You will most commonly find boils in hair areas which are exposed to irritation, such as neck, armpits, breasts, face, buttocks, and genital areas. If you find red lines going away from the boil, also read *Lymphangitis* in this chapter.

What's Going On?: A boil is a bacterial infection involving a plugged hair follicle and the tissue around it. When the hair folicle gets plugged and doesn't drain, the body fluids *stand* in that place, and they become a perfect media for bacterial growth, just as a stagnant pool of water in a forest becomes a perfect media for bacteria and insects to breed.

The pus that you see inside a boil is made up of white blood cells coming to clear the infection away. The redness is caused by blood bringing nutrients and antibodies to the area. The pain which occurs is due to pressure on nerve endings because of the swelling. This is the thing that bothers most people even more than the boil itself. Scratching the boil can carry the bacteria of the boil to healthy areas of skin and cause new boils.

Treatment: Soak a wash cloth in hot water and place it directly on the boil. Keep it there for fifteen minutes. When the cloth cools, put it back in hot water and repeat the process. This brings increased blood flow to the area, which carries away the pus cells; swelling is reduced, thus taking pressure off the nerve endings. This treatment is most effective in the very first stages of the boil, when it first appears, or when you first notice it.

Your Doctor As a Resource: After a boil develops a "white head" a person can get instant relief by having the boil drained. This is done by the doctor with a sharp, sterile scalpel. A doctor can do it with relative ease and painlessness.

If a boil becomes very large and deep, a doctor should probably be sought to clean out the boil by draining it. Occasionally doctors recommend antibiotic therapy when boils are very severe. Boils are usually not wholly responsive to this form of treatment.

Prevention: You can prevent boils from growing larger with the treatment that we outline above. Prevent boils in general by loving your skin. Take care of it by cleaning and by not applying chemicals. (See *Preventive Medicine* for more on this.) Doctors often see boils on skin areas where a person has applied deodorants or antiperspirants which have plugged the hair follicles.

IMPETIGO

Symptoms: Itching and pain on areas of the skin anywhere on the body
Small pustules or "pimples" are sometimes seen

Physical Exam: You will find small pustules with white heads, crusting, or draining, with small amounts of clustered, yellow material surrounding the area.

What's Going On?: Impetigo is a bacterial infection: usually *staphylococcal,* or *streptococcal.* The bacteria is often carried under dirty fingernails, and thus is transmitted in that way. It spreads easily from one person to another, especially among people living in the same house. You can pick it up under your fingernails, scratch a small area of your own skin, and thus start or spread an impetigo infection on your own body.

Treatment: A commonly prescribed treatment is to rub soap, three times a day, vigorously into the affected area until the scab comes off. This soap treatment is the main part of the cure, but some doctors then apply an antibiotic cream.

Your Doctor As Resource: Your doctor can help you diagnose what you have. They can also prescribe drugs in severe cases where secondary infection is present.

Prevention: If a person in your house has Impetigo, you can prevent its spread to others by cleaning your house with an antibacterial disinfectant. Pay particular attention to cleaning bathroom and kitchen areas. But understand that person to person contact is the main way it is spread. All members of the family should get into the habit of frequent bathing, and children's fingernails should especially be given extra cleaning attention. Children should be told not to scratch sores or pick their noses since these are the most common ways that Impetigo is spread. Each person in the household should have their own washclothes and towels. Impetigo occurs most frequently where there is no running water and where personal cleanliness is neglected.

BLOOD POISONING (LYMPHANGITIS)

Symptoms: Throbbing pain in the area of an infection
Red streaks moving away from the site of an infection
Tender and enlarged lymph nodes in the area of an infection
Sometimes tiredness and fever

Physical Exam: You will see a red streak — which may be definite or faint — going from the infected site to the nearest lymph nodes. (See page 341 for a chart showing the locations of the lymph nodes.) You will find the nodes serving that location to be enlarged and tender.

What's Going On? Lymphangitis takes place in the lymph channels, which are like veins going from one lymph node to another throughout your body. These channels carry lymph, a substance which helps you defend yourself against disease and fight infection. Ordinarily, if you get an infection, such as a small boil, the lymph carries away white blood cells that contain decayed bacteria. But if live bacteria enters the lymph channels, the channels themselves and later the lymph nodes become inflamed and swollen. These inflamed channels are the red lines that you see in the skin.

It is important to recognize lymphangitis because it means that your body has been unable to handle the infection and that the infection is now spreading to the rest of your body.

Treatment: Your body needs outside energy to help it cure lymphangitis. Antibiotics will stop the spread of infection. Bed rest, elevating the obviously infected area, and heat applied to the infected area will all help. *But antibiotics are essential because the infection is spreading to the rest of your body.*

Your Doctor As A Resource: Your doctor is really helpful if you get lymphangitis. They can prescribe an antibiotic to help your body kill the bacteria. Commonly, lymphangitis responds quickly to antibiotics, but it should be stressed that early treatment is essential.

Prevention: Early treatment of boils, wounds and other skin infections is the best preventive medicine.

RINGWORM

Symptoms: Itching
Small, scaley, ringed patches
Patches may also appear gray and ringed

Physical Exam: Upon examination of the skin you see round, gray, scaley patches. These may be ringed, with a clear fleshy center. They are usually very symmetrical. The person's chief complaint may be "intense itching."

Upon examination of the person's scalp you will see scaley patches with broken hairs.

What's Going On?: Ringworm is a fungus. It is frequently transmitted by people who have been exposed to cats which carry the *dermaphyd* fungus causing the disease. It is relatively easy to cure.

Treatment: You'll need a prescription, so you'll have to use your doctor as a resource for this.

Your Doctor As Resource: Ringworm is one disease that your doctor can really help you with. They will usually prescribe an antifungal drug which you take orally. There also is a cream which can be applied to the skin. The ringworm responds promptly to this treatment and there are usually no further problems.

Prevention: The way to prevent ringworm from spreading is to cure it rapidly in everyone in your household, especially the children, and to avoid further exposure to people who have it. Avoid cats that may be infected with ringworm, and have a veternarian treat any cats in your own household that you suspect of having it.

JOCK ROT

Symptoms: Severe itching and moistness in the genital area.

Physical Exam: You'll find spreading, sharply demarcated red, raised areas and "weeping" (dripping) areas on the skin in the genital area, in and around the testicles and the insides of the thighs. Person may complain of itching and discomfort.

What's Going On?: Jock Rot is often caused by a fungus. Sometimes it's caused by friction with clothing, especially clothing that doesn't breathe well. It occurs in people who perspire heavily and who have not bathed enough to wash away the perspiration. The fungus grows best in moist areas of the body.

Treatment: In the *Last Whole Earth Supplement* there's a picture of Ken Kesey holding a box of cornstarch which is, in my opinion, a specific treatment for jockrot. In the very early stages, when you first see weeping red areas in the skin around your crotch, dip your hand right into a box of ordinary cornstarch and rub the fine powder over your genitals, being sure to cover your entire scrotum, and the inside surfaces of your thighs. The cornstarch acts as a lubricant, will dry the moist areas, thus preventing fungal growth, and will reduce or stop the chafing. Change your clothes frequently and wear cotton underpants. Then your body can go about the business of curing itself.

Fungicidal preparations also work, but I don't think they are necessary except in very severe cases.

Your Doctor As Resource: A doctor is rarely necessary in the treatment of Jock Rot except if you need an antifungal preparation by prescription. Consult a doctor if you are in question about diagnosing what you have.

Prevention: The most important thing in preventing Jock Rot is cleanliness. When it does occur, prompt treatment will prevent its spread, and will cure it before it causes discomfort. Wash your clothes frequently, bathe frequently, and wear clothes that don't rub and chaff. Keep yourself dry in the genital areas.

ATHLETE'S FOOT

Symptoms: Itching, burning, and/or stinging between the fingers or toes
Red areas on skin
Scaling areas
Tiny blisters on skin areas
Cracks in skin

Physical Exam: Upon examination of the person's feet or hands you see red areas, scaling areas, and any of the above symptoms, especially between fingers and toes. If you have difficulty diagnosing it, see physical exam section for *Contact Dermatitis.*

What's Going On?: Athlete's foot is a microscopic fungal infection of the feet and hands. It is spread in community showers and other wet areas where bare feet come in contact with floors and other surfaces shared by many other people.

Although you can "catch" athlete's foot, some people seem to have a resistance to it and never get it. When I was in medical school, a group of people stuck their feet directly in athlete's foot fungus for two hours. Only one person out of this group ever suffered the symptoms of athlete's foot as a result of this exposure.

Treatment: Antifungal drugs or powders are the usual cures for athletes foot. Over-the-counter foot powders, are often just as effective as prescription treatment.

Your Doctor As A Resource: Seldom necessary unless you want confirmation of your own diagnosis, or the Athlete's Foot is so severe you feel you need a prescription for an anti-fungal preparation to cure it.

Prevention: Cleanliness and the use of antibacterial disinfectants when cleaning showers and other wet areas plays a significant part in preventing the athlete's foot fungus from growing. Keep your feet clean and dry.

MONILIA INFECTIONS — "YEAST"

Symptoms: Severe itching around the vagina, anus, body folds, or
crotch areas
Itching around the mouth

Physical Exam: Upon examination you will find red, raw areas of flesh with smaller but similar red areas surrounding it. You may also see whitish, curd-like flecks on the red areas.

What's Going On?: Monila is a yeast-like fungus which is normally present in women's vaginas, and in both women's and men's mouths. When people are treated with antibiotics, normal bacterial flora is disrupted. This allows the yeast to multiply more quickly, and in greater abundance than is normal. Monilia may also multiply as a result of hormonal changes during pregnancy or during your body's introduction to birth control pills. Nylon underwear, worn in hot, moist climates or during heat spells, can also disrupt the normal bacterial balance of a woman's vagina and cause Monilia to multiply more quickly than is normal.

Treatment: The best treatment is prevention. Keep genital areas clean, dry, and cool, especially in hot weather. Especially do these things if you are taking antibiotics, birth control pills, hormones, or during pregnancy.

Your Doctor As Resource: Use your doctor to confirm your diagnosis, and/or to give you a prescription to heal it. The usual treatment is a anti-fungal cream. (If the infection takes place inside the vagina, anus, or mouth, see *Diagnosis and Treatment* sections on genitals and mouth.)

Prevention: Keep anal and genital areas cool, dry, and well bathed.

SCABIES
(Also called "The Itch")

Symptoms: Itching, most often at night, affecting genital areas, insides of buttocks, and nearly any other area of the body

Physical Exam: You will see tiny vesicles, red bumps, burrows and tunnels that look like lines or exclamation points (a dot and a line). These will be found between fingers, on the palms of the person's hands, on the scrotum, breasts, genitals, along the belt line, or in the armpits.

What's Going On?: Scabies is a *mite* (microscopic insect) infection. The mite's full name is *Sarcoptes scabiei*. They are seldom seen, however, because they live in the burrows they make under the skin. Scabies spread rapidly from one person to another, and are usually acquired by sleeping with a person who has them or through actual physical contact with clothes, blankets, etc., of a person who is infected with scabies.

Treatment: Launder your bedding and other cloth articles, including all clothes, to kill the eggs of the mites. On your body, scabies are quickly brought under control with *Kwell lotion.* Your whole family group has to be treated if anybody in your house has scabies, otherwise you'll be leaving eggs and mites to start the whole infection all over again.

Your Doctor As A Resource: Show your doctor the affected area of your body, describe your *present illness* and ask for a prescription of *Kwell lotion.*

Prevention: General cleanliness will prevent scabies infections. Avoid people with scabies, and promptly treat any symptoms of scabies that appear in members of your household.

LICE
(Also called "Crabs," "Pediculosis," and "Nits")

Symptoms: Itching
                  Tiny bugs seen at the bases of hair shafts
                  Itching may be intense in affected areas
                  Scratching may result in deep scratch marks or secondary
                  infections causing small pus-filled areas around hair
                  shafts and surrounding areas

Physical Exam: You will see small red dots, deep scratch marks, or pus-filled areas in the parts of the body affected.

What's Going On?: There are three different types of lice: the type found on the scalp, the type found on the body, and the type found in pubic hair areas. Occasionally you see the egg cases around the hair follicles. They look like little wax balls. Lice are spread rapidly by people who live in overcrowded dwellings or where cleanliness is lacking. Crabs and body lice are quite common. Mobility and frequent changes in life styles increases the spread of lice from one geographic region to another. Lice are *not* carried by dogs. Pubic and scalp lice live on hair and skin, while body lice actually live in the seams of clothing.

actual size

Body Louse
(magnified)

Treatment: Use *Kwell Shampoo* for the scalp, and *Kwell* lotion for the body and pubic areas. Kwell is a prescription drug so you'll have to get it through a doctor or clinic. It's also important to launder your clothes at high temperature in a laundromat. Also have bedding cleaned or washed. The eggs can stay alive in articles of clothing, and then bring about reinfection after you think you've gotten rid of the lice. If several people are living in the same house at the time of infection, everyone in the house should go through the entire treatment so that you're sure you get rid of the lice.

Your Doctor As Resource: A doctor is seldom necessary in treating lice, except to get a prescription for Kwell, if secondary infection is present, or if you want help diagnosing what you have.

Prevention: Pay attention to your body — especially where cleanliness is concerned — and you'll reduce the chances of ever getting lice.

MOLES

Symptoms: Small pigmented areas on the skin which are sometimes raised and hairy.

Physical Exam: Same as symptoms.

What's Going On?: Moles are made up of special skin cells which contain a pigment called melanin. They often are present at birth but can develop later in life. The reason we discuss them here is that many people seem to be under the impression that they are often "pre-cancerous." The truth is that common moles are rarely pre-cancerous. The time to consult a doctor about a mole is if it increases in size or changes its pigmentation. *During pregnancy, however, increase in the size of moles is normal and fairly common.*

Treatment: None necessary for common moles unless they increase in size or change color. See your doctor if this happens.

Your Doctor As A Resource: Your doctor can run tests (biopsy) on questionable moles to rule out cancer. Understand that even if malignant, such a mole can be healed with early treatment. But we'd like to emphasize that moles becoming cancerous are *not* common.

Prevention: Some doctors believe that moles exposed to constant irritation, such as on a belt line, have a higher chance of becoming either infected or malignant. So if you have such a mole, see a doctor if it changes size or color. But remember that man has had moles for millions of years, and common moles are made up of healthy living tissue, a part of your body as worthy of love as any other.

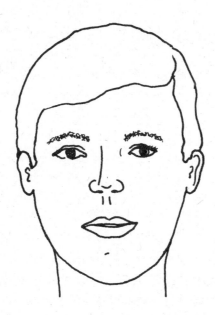

HEAD

Look upon your head as containing other organs besides your brain and skull. In the Head section, we deal with Eyes, Ears, Mouth, and Sinuses. Since a person's nose and throat are actually parts of the Respiratory System, we have chosen to deal with diseases such as Common Colds, Sore Throats, and Tonsilitis in the Respiratory System section.

HEADACHE
(Also called "Tension Headache")

Symptoms: Headache
There may also be a feeling of pressure, tightness, or constriction, often described as like a band around the head.
May also be described as a dull, pressing, and burning above the eyes

Physical Exam: Sometimes the person may look tense, upset, frightened, or anxious.

What's Going On?: Usually a headache is caused by muscle tension. Muscles contract, causing spasms of the blood vessels that run through them. This cuts down blood flow to other muscles which then send out signals that they're not getting enough blood. These signals are recorded in your brain as pain and discomfort.

Treatment: Pain medications such as aspirin sometimes help. Sometimes they don't do much good at all. Sometimes even potent pain medications fail. We feel that the best treatment for headache is rest, relaxation and relief from stress. Heat applied with a hot water bottle or a heating pad is one way to relax the tense muscles causing the headache, and thus affords some relief. Massage is another excellent way to bring relief.

Here's an exercise which we've found helpful in relieving a headache:

Relax your body using the same exercise you used to get your imaginary doctor. Concentrate especially on relaxing your head and neck muscles. A good exercise for relieving neck muscle tension is to imagine that your head is balanced on a point at the end of your spine, and if you tip your head even slightly it will fall in the direction you tip it. To relax your jaw, just let your mouth drop open. Close and relax your eye muscles. Then relax the muscles in your forehead. As you feel muscles relaxing imagine this feeling of deep relaxation spreading directly into all the areas that hurt.

Now imagine a hole in your head near the area of your headache. As you exhale your breath imagine that the pain is going out through that hole. Pain is going out through that hole and is colored a murky, muddy color. Continue breathing and relaxing until you begin to feel relief. Say to yourself "I am feeling better and better, more and more relaxed."

Understand that this method does not work instantly. It takes time for the blood flow to your muscles to get back to a normal, healthy state. The exercise works better if you practice visualization (see page 4) and relaxation exercises regularly. (See relaxation exercise in the *Preventive Medicine* chapter.)

Doctor As A Resource: If ordinary treatments don't relieve the headache, or if the headache has come following an accident, a blow on your head, or other trauma, use your doctor to help you diagnose and treat it.

Prevention: Understand that a tension headache is a message from your body telling you to change something in your life to relieve tension. For methods on doing this see the *Preventive Medicine* chapter, especially the parts on rest-work cycles, sleep, environment, and relaxation exercises.

MIGRAINE HEADACHE

Symptoms: A pulsing, throbbing headache
May be preceded by changes in vision, such as spots before
    your eyes, etc.
Sometimes nausea and vomiting

Physical Exam: You may or may not observe pulsing of arteries on the person's temples.

What's Going On?: One theory of migraine is that the main blood vessels to the head partially constrict. This is followed by an opening of the blood vessels inside the head. The wide-open vessels produce a throbbing pain, and muscle contraction and tension contribute to the pain. Migraine often begins in childhood, before fifteen years of age.

Treatment: There are potent sedatives and drugs which help to relieve migraine pain. Recently doctors have found that muscle relaxation techniques and positive body image techniques such as those we describe elsewhere in this book, have worked well in treating long-time sufferers of migraine pain. (See the treatments for *Tension Headache,* the "disease" directly above this one, for some specific techniques that relieve headache pain.)

Your Doctor As A Resource: A doctor can prescribe drugs for treating migraine, and psychotherapy for prevention of further attacks.

Prevention: Same as for tension headaches. Understand that migraine headaches can be prevented by you.

FOREIGN BODIES IN THE EYE

Symptoms: Pain and feeling of intense discomfort in the eye

Physical Exam: You can sometimes readily observe an object in the eye as you face the person with this complaint. Sometimes the eye has to be illuminated from the side with a flashlight. If it's not readily obvious where the foreign body is, draw the eye open as in the picture. Then have them look down, look to the left and look to the right. If you still do not see the foreign body, flip down the lower eyelid (see Physical Exam section on how to flip the lower conjunctive down). Often a foreign body can hide in the upper, outer part of the eye. Have the person pull out the outer part of the upper eyelid and look there.

What's Going On?: The eye is acutely sensitive, and tears will immediately flow to wash out a foreign body. Tears are a signal that it's essential to remove the foreign body to stop the irritation.

Treatment: Sometimes just grabbing the upper eyelid and pulling it down over the lower one, then moving the eye up, down and around will get the foreign body to come down onto one of the eyelids where it will come out by itself. If the foreign body is on the white part of the eye, it can be removed easily with a cotton Q-tip. Put the Q-tip very, very lightly over the white part of the eye where the foreign body is. This will pick up the foreign body. Sometimes irrigation with water can wash out a foreign body. Have the person lean their head over a sink and splash water gently into the open eye.

Your Doctor As A Resource: If you are unable to remove the foreign body or if it sticks in the *cornea* it's especially important to have it removed by a doctor. (The *cornea* is the transparent part over the colored area and the pupil.) The cornea can be ulcerated and that can lead to severe eye damage.

Prevention: Protect your eyes when you are in dusty or windy places. Wear goggles when you work around machines that can throw out particles like sawdust or plastic or metal shavings.

EYESTRAIN

Symptoms: Burning
Itching
Tearing of the eyes

Physical Exam: On physical exam you will see tiny blood vessels in the white part of the eye giving it a red appearance. Possibly the eyes will be tearing.

221

What's Going On?: Eyestrain is a common complaint caused by overwork in activities such as reading, driving, or watching television. It is also caused by exposure to smog. Blood vessels in the white part of the eye open and tears flow to wash out toxic particles and provide nutrients to the area.

Television commercials which show red eyes due to dilation of blood vessels and advise using a miracle drug to stop this redness are dangerous, in my opinion. Some of these drugs cause constriction of the small blood vessels. This produces a cosmetic effect; it does not cure the cause or treat the disease. But it prevents the eye from healing itself.

Treatment: Bathe the eye with water. Rest the eyes by closing them and relaxing the eye muscles. (For more on this see the eye exercises in *Preventive Medicine*.)

Your Doctor As A Resource: It is usually not necessary to consult a doctor. If discomfort persists, you may want to get a complete eye exam by an eye doctor.

Prevention: Avoid overusing your eyes. Pay attention to early signals such as tearing. If you can avoid smog, do so.

CONJUNCTIVITIS

Symptoms:
    Itching
    Tearing
    Discharge from the eye
    Sometimes the discharge can cause the eyelids to stick together, especially in the morning
    There may be some pain

Physical Exam: When the lower lid is pulled down (see Physical Exam chapter on the eye), instead of the mucosa being pink and healthy looking, you will see that it is bright red and swollen. Many blood vessels can be seen and there may be a yellow-green discharge on the mucosa.

What's Going On?: Conjunctivitis is one of the most common eye diseases seen by doctors. It is a bacterial or viral infection of the conjunctival mucosal membrane. *Bacterial* conjunctivitis is often called pink eye. It is highly infectious. The disease is self-limiting — lasting ten to fourteen days if untreated. But healing of bacterial conjunctivitis may be sped up by using antibiotic drops or ointment. *Viral* conjunctivitis does not respond to antibiotic therapy. It usually does not have a yellow-green pussy discharge. Often times conjunctivitis can be caused by a simple irritation, especially in people who live in dusty areas, areas where automobiles run on dirt roads, desert areas, or smoggy cities.

Treatment: *Bacterial* conjunctivitis is usually treated with antibiotic ointment or drops. *Viral* and irritative conjunctivitis are treated by irrigation of the eyes with saline or plain water three or four times a day.

Your Doctor As A Resource: Your doctor can prescribe antibiotic drops or ointment for bacterial conjunctivitis.

Prevention: A person who has bacterial conjunctivitis can prevent spreading it by using their own wash cloth and towel. They should also wash their hands after touching their eyes. To prevent irritative conjunctivitis, avoid exposure to blowing dirt and sand.

STY

Symptoms: Tearing
               Pain
               A foreign-body-in-the-eye sensation, though nothing can be found

Physical Exam: Initially you will see a small round pink swollen area on the eyelid. This progresses to a yellow spot discharging pus.

What's Going On?: A sty is a local bacterial (staphylococcal) infection of the small glands in the eyelid. The gland ducts become plugged and the trapped fluid is a perfect site for bacteria to live.

Treatment: Keep the area clean. Apply hot soaks (see section on treatment of Boils) to the area three times a day for fifteen minutes each.

Doctor As A Resource: A doctor should be seen if the sty does not respond to treatment or if the eye socket becomes swollen and red. They can prescribe medication to help your body heal itself.

Prevention: Stys are probably mildly communicative. The person who has the sty should use their own wash cloth and towel.

IMPACTED EARWAX

Symptoms: Feeling of fullness in the ear
               Sometimes ringing in the ear

Physical Exam: You will see yellow-brown to black wax, which is sticky and soft, blocking the person's ear canal. (See the chapter on *Physical Examination* for details on examining ears.)

What's Going On? Earwax, or *cerumen,* is a normal, protective secretion of the external ear canal. It normally dries and falls out by itself and doesn't need any care other than regular bathing. Sometimes, due to the fact that your ear canal has many normal twists and turns, or to over-production of the earwax, it may accumulate and cause minor hearing loss or a feeling of fullness in the ear.

223

Treatment: Some doctors have a small currette-like spoon which can be used to gently scoop out the wax. It takes some care, otherwise the ear drum can be injured. An easier way for a non-medical person to remove the wax is to wash the ear out with an irrigating syringe and water. Or you can use a very mild (1½%) solution of peroxide. The peroxide sold in the drugstore is usually 3%. So dilute it by half or ask your druggist to dilute it for you.

Fill a glass about ¾ full of the 1½% peroxide solution. Now lean your head over a sink or a bathtub. Fill your ear syringe with the peroxide solution. Squeeze the bulb of the syringe and direct the flow into your ear, allowing it to run out freely from your ear into the sink or tub, as you do so. (This is known as "irrigation.")

Gently irrigate your ear three to four times a day for three days. This treatment will cause the wax to dissolve, and in turn run out of your ear as you irrigate it. Irrigating with peroxide solution can irritate your ear canal, so it should not be done routinely.

Your Doctor As A Resource: The doctor can help if you are unable to remove the impacted wax yourself.

Prevention: Keep your ears clean and do not allow large amounts of wax to build up. Do not use sharp objects to clean the wax out because they can cause damage to the ear drum or the canal.

INFECTION OF THE EAR CANAL
(Also called "External Otitis")

Symptoms: Itching in the ear canal
Scaling
Possibly a watery discharge from the ear
Possibly some hearing loss
Pain — which can be extreme if the canal becomes blocked with
    skin or debris.

Physical Exam: You will see scaling, red, swollen and possibly pus-covered areas in the tube leading to the drum. You may also find enlarged lymph nodes in the neck. If you pull the person's ear up and out (See *Physical Exam* chapter on examining the ear) it will hurt.

What's Going On?: *External otitis* is an infection of the ear canal. The canal is the tube leading into the ear: not the drum itself or the area behind the drum. It's actually a skin infection rather than an ear infection because skin lines the canal, and this is the part that's infected. It is usually caused by a bacteria, less often by a fungus. It's important to differentiate External Otitis from a middle ear (See *Infections of the Middle Ear,* below infection. Make sure that a middle ear infection isn't accompanying it.

Predisposing factors are a warm, moist climate in the ear, or trauma to the ear. It frequently follows fresh water swimming. It can also be caused by scratching the canal while you are cleaning your ear. This scratch can become secondarily infected.

Treatment: Local treatment is all that's necessary. The objective of it is to keep your ear dry and clean and to protect it. Antibiotic drops are used to treat bacterial infections; alcohol-acetone drops are used to treat fungal infections. A warm to hot washcloth or towel, wrung dry and placed over your ear will increase blood flow to the area and may relieve pain. Aspirin can also be used to relieve pain.

Your Doctor As A Resource: Your doctor can clean the canal if you are unable to. They can tell whether the infection is caused by a bacteria or a fungus and prescribe the proper drops.

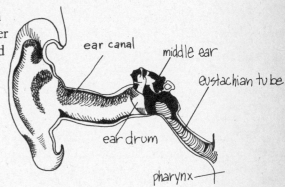

Prevention: Keep your ears clean and dry. Do not use sharp objects to clean your ears. Make sure children do not scratch their ears with their finger-nails — especially if they have impetigo or boils.

INFECTIONS OF THE MIDDLE EAR — OTITIS MEDIA

Symptoms:
Pain in the ear
Fullness in the ear
Hearing loss
Fever
Chills
Discharge from the ear containing blood or pus or both

Physical Exam: The normal light reflection and metallic grey quality of the ear drum are not seen. The drum can be red or dull grey and bulging. (See the *Physical Exam* chapter for complete instructions for ear exam.) You may also see a bloody discharge, or pus.

What's Going On?: Otitis Media is what people commonly call an earache or an ear infection. It is a bacterial or viral infection of the middle ear, which is the area *behind the ear drum.* Streptococci, pneumococci, and staphlococci are the most common bacterial causes. An ear infection usually follows an upper respiratory infection or cold when the cold hasn't been fully cured.

The middle ear is a closed area drained only by the Eustachian tube, which leads from the middle ear to the back of the throat. (See drawing in *External Otitis.*) The Eustachian tube normally equalizes pressure between your middle ear and the outside world, and this causes your ears to "pop." The tube can become blocked due to swelling of the tissues in the throat caused by a cold. When the tube is blocked, the pressure cannot equalize and a vacuum is produced in the middle ear. Fluid then comes into the middle ear from surrounding tissues and is trapped. The trapped fluid becomes a perfect media for the growth of bacteria from the throat. White blood cells and body fluids coming to fight the infection cause pressure to build. The pressure against the sensitive ear drum is what causes the pain of the earache. If the Eustachian tube remains blocked, the pressure in the middle ear often increases until the ear drum ruptures. This rupture is helpful because it relieves the pressure and allows some of the pus and blood to drain out through the ear canal. The drum heals itself in four to eight hours.

The pain goes away as your body heals the infection, does not produce more fluid, and absorbs the fluid, present in the middle ear, back into the tissues. Antibiotics do not remove the pain of an earache because they act on the bacteria; the pain is caused by the fullness and pressure in the middle ear. The antibiotic lowers the number of bacteria until your body can heal itself. This prevents the spread of infection to the skull bones or brain (mastoiditis, which is an infection of the bone behind the ear, used to be seen a lot before antibiotics). Now ear infections rarely have dangerous complications.

Some hearing loss often accompanies a middle ear infection because the fluid trapped in the middle ear dampens the conduction of sound waves. A hearing loss can persist for up to four or six weeks as the fluid in the middle ear is slowly absorbed by the body. A continued slight loss of hearing does not mean that your body is not healing the infection.

Treatment: Otitis media is treated by a doctor with antibiotics which work on your whole body. Penicillin is often the drug of choice for adults. Antibiotic ear drops don't do any good because the infection is *behind* the ear drum. It often helps to apply dry heat, such as a hot water bottle or a warm dry towel, to the area. Even cupping your hand over your ear can help. This increases blood flow to the area which helps fight the infection. Heat may also help relieve the pain. Relaxation and concentration on something else help to take your mind off the pain (see *Preventive Medicine* section on relaxation). Also, aspirin can be taken to relieve pain. A decongestant or antihistamine is useful because it causes the mucosa of the Eustachian tube to shrink. This opens the tube and allows the middle ear to drain.

Your Doctor As A Resource: Your doctor can prescribe the proper antibiotic to treat the Otitis Media. They can follow the course of the infection to see that it responds to the antibiotic chosen. They can also prescribe antihistamines to help promote drainage. If a hearing loss remains after four to six weeks it indicates a possibility of fluid still in the middle ear which may have to be drained by a doctor.

Prevention: Rapid treatment of a cold, especially if you know you are susceptible to ear infections, will decrease the chances of your getting an Otitis Media (see section on the *Common Cold*). Blow your nose gently to prevent spreading bacteria from your throat to your middle ear. If you feel like an ear infection is developing, turn all your healing energy to its treatment. Rest in bed and keep your ear warm.

SINUS INFECTION

Symptoms:
Pain in the face
Swelling and tenderness of the sinus area
Fever
Runny nose
Postnasal drip
Possibly a sore throat and cough
Headache — typically worse during the day
Toothache or a feeling of "long teeth"

Physical Exam: You may find tenderness over the sinus areas when you press on them (see *Physical Exam* chapter for diagram of the sinuses). A red pharynx with a discharge dripping down the back of the throat is sometimes seen. To help differentiate sinus infection from toothache, have the person jump up and down, landing on their heels. The person will feel pain in the sinus areas above the teeth if it is a sinus infection. With a toothache, you usually have pain in a particular tooth. In sinus infection, pain will probably be felt in all the teeth on one or both sides of the upper jaw. Dental pain usually produces swelling locally around the tooth.

What's Going On?: The sinuses are pockets in the bones of the face. In an infection the membranes inside the sinuses swell up and produce fluid. The tubes that lead out of the sinuses may become blocked and the fluid does not drain into the back of the nose. This produces a static site, perfect for infection. Pressure builds up inside the sinuses and the swollen membranes press on local nerves, causing pain.

A sinus infection occasionally occurs after an upper respiratory infection or an allergic situation. It sometimes can occur by itself. It's important to differentiate a sinus infection from tooth problems since they require different treatment.

Treatment: Hot soaks, bed rest, and antibiotics are usually helpful. Steam inhalation helps open the tubes and promotes drainage by liquifying the mucous. Antihistamine pills, nose drops or sprays are often given by doctors to shrink the membranes of the nose and sinuses. Antihistamines must not be used excessively. Overuse can result in a rebound effect in which the membranes expand after they have shrunk. This expansion causes nasal blockage and sometimes increased pain. (See the chapter *Drugs Are Helpers*.)

An exercise that may help you is called "Open-Drain." Get comfortable, relax your body by the exercise that you used to get your imaginary doctor. Picture clearly (visualize) the tubes leading from your sinuses to your nose. Relax the area around the sinuses. Imagine the tubes opening and fluid draining out from the sinus. This will cause relaxation of the muscles around the sinuses. Blood flow will increase and will help to heal the infection.

Your Doctor As A Resource: Your doctor can prescribe antibiotics especially if you have a fever. They can also prescribe antihistamines. If you have a chronic sinus infection, your doctor may x-ray the area and possibly do more to promote drainage.

Prevention: Early treatment of a cold or allergic situation is important, especially if you know you are prone to sinus infections.

ORAL MONILIA

Symptoms: Pain anywhere in the mouth
                  Possibly a fever

Physical Exam: You will see creamy, white, curd-like patches in the mouth. (The mucosa of the mouth is usually bright red.) If the curd-like patches are scraped off, bleeding occurs. You will also feel enlarged lymph nodes in the person's neck.

What's Going On?: Monilia is a micro-organism, a yeast-like fungus. It lives normally in some people's mouths. Many organisms normally live together in ecological balance in the mouth. When the balance is upset, monilia can become much more numerous. When antibiotics are taken, all the bacteria in the mouth that are sensitive to that antibiotic are killed. This gives more food to the monilia which can then overgrow, causing the symptoms. Obviously, monilia overgrowth does not always occur when someone takes antibiotics.

Treatment: Monilia is treated with an anti-fungal mouth rinse. A very mild salt water solution used as a mouth wash can give local relief from pain.

Your Doctor As A Resource: Your doctor can diagnose monilia and prescribe an anti-fungal mouth rinse.

Prevention: Some doctors believe that eating yogurt or acidophylus foods or food supplements (available at health food stores) while you are taking antibiotics will help prevent you from getting monilia.

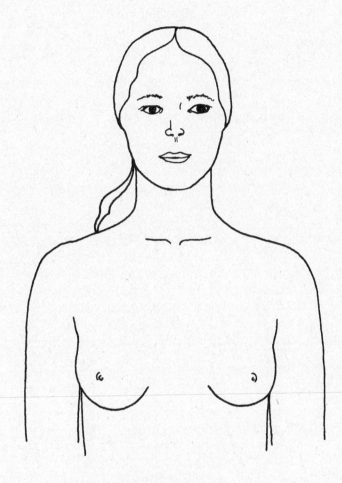

BREASTS

We're including in this section two breast problems for which women consult doctors. These are Breast infections and Breast lumps. We would like to stress here the fact that actual diseases requiring treatment in these categories are far less common than the *fears,* created in our society, which bring thousands of healthy women to doctors' offices. Read this section with the purpose of dispelling fears and developing a positive and realistic attitude toward your breasts.

BREAST INFECTIONS

Symptoms: Pain in the breast   Soreness
                  Heat   Swelling

Physical Exam: You will find a swollen, red, hot, and tender area on the breast. If the area is solid and has a whitehead, then it's possible that an abcess is present.

What's Going On?: During nursing, a duct in the breast can become plugged, producing a closed area where milk is trapped. This provides a site where bacteria can grow and produce an infection. Bacteria on the skin can get into a plugged duct through a crack in the nipple. Cracks are most often caused by a baby biting at the nipple. Breast infections can occur in women who are not nursing, but are much more common in nursing mothers.

   The heat is caused by increased blood flow to the area which carries away the bacteria from the site. The swelling is caused by body fluids and white blood cells coming into the area to fight the infection. A whitehead, if it's present, consists of pus, which is actually white blood cells which have stayed in the area and not drained.

Treatment: It used to be thought that the mother should stop nursing at the infected breast or stop nursing altogether. Many doctors treating nursing mothers now advise that the mother continue nursing. The *La Leche League* also says that emptying the breast is very helpful. They suggest either allowing the baby to nurse if it's a mild infection, or, if it's a severe infection, manually expressing milk from the breast.

   Hot soaks, which increase blood flow and bring swelling down, are the best treatment for superficial breast infections. Wash cloths should be put in hot water, then applied to the breast. When they're cool, they should be put back in hot water and reapplied to the area. You should do this for fifteen minutes to a half hour at a time, three or four times a day. Rest is also important because it takes a tremendous amount of energy to produce all the proteins, antibodies, and white blood cells necessary to fight the infection, and fully heal your body.

Your Doctor As A Resource: If the area of heat and redness begins to expand and becomes worrisome to the mother, she should consult her doctor. They may put her on antibiotics. The antibiotic will come through the breast milk, but many doctors advise that the mother continue nursing even though the baby will be getting small amounts of the antibiotic. If an abcess develops, it may have to be lanced so that the infection can drain. This does not necessarily mean that the mother and child will have to give up nursing.

Prevention: It's important to establish a good nursing pattern to keep the breast from becoming engorged. Also, the baby should not be allowed to chew on the nipple and abrade it. Relaxation is crucial in nursing. (See the section on relaxation in the *Preventive Medicine* chapter). If you're tired or tense, the milk doesn't come down and your breasts can become engorged. When the milk doesn't come down soon after nursing begins, the baby is more likely to become frustrated and chew on your nipple.

BREAST LUMPS

Symptoms: Lump in the breast
Pain occasionally associated with the lump

Physical Exam: You will feel a lump in the person's breast. (See *Physical Examination* chapter for how to examine the breasts.)

What's Going On?: There are several different causes of breast lumps in women. The most common type of breast lump is the cyst. These are not cancerous and are often fluid-filled. Another common type of breast lump is the fibroadenoma. It is a firm growth and is also not cancerous. Breast cancer is an uncommon cause of breast lumps in women under forty years of age.

Most young women who find a lump in their breast immediately assume that they have cancer. In actuality, it's much, much more likely that they have a cyst or a fibroadenoma. (See the chapter on *Rare Diseases, Heart Disease, and Cancer.*)

Treatment: Presently the treatment of breast lumps varies from doctor to doctor. It also depends on the characteristics of the lump. In young women, some doctors check the lump occasionally to make sure that it is not changing. Other doctors surgically remove (biopsy) the lump to examine it under a microscope to determine what type of lump it is. If the lump is fluid-filled, the doctor can drain it with a needle.

Your Doctor As A Resource: If you have a breast lump you should have it examined by a doctor. They can diagnose what type of lump it is and treat it appropriately. The value of diagnosis is that it can often remove any lingering worries that you might have.

Prevention: Some doctors believe that breast lumps, like many other diseases, can be related to a person's emotional life. If this is true, it may be possible to prevent and cure breast lumps by getting in touch with your areas of anxiety and tension.

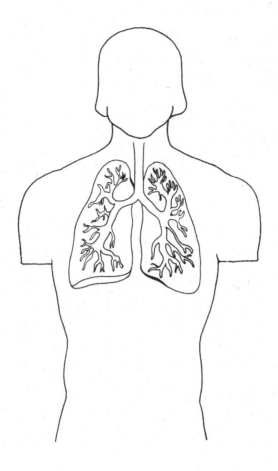

RESPIRATORY SYSTEM

Your respiratory system includes all the parts of your body directly involved with bringing fresh air and oxygen into your body and getting rid of the body's waste products (carbon dioxide) through the air. This means everything from your nose and throat all the way down to your lungs. We feel it is important to look upon your nose, mouth, and lungs as belonging to a whole system. This is an excellent preventive medicine orientation ... to think in terms of healing your cold or sore throat before the infection spreads to your bronchial tubes and lungs. You can prevent serious diseases by learning to recognize small infections and take responsibility for healing them quickly. Thus we start, here with discussions of minor infections, such as the Common Cold and Hay Fever, then work toward the more serious diseases such as Bronchitis and Pneumonia. Hopefully, by taking care of the minor ones you'll never have to deal with the more serious infections.

COMMON COLD

Symptoms:

Tiredness	Fever
Headache	Nasal discomfort
Runny nose	Watery discharge from nose
Sneezing	Blockage of nose
Dry or sore throat	Hoarseness
Muscle aches	Some pain under the sternum
Cough which brings up a small amount of sputum	

Physical Exam: You will find the nasal mucosa swollen and red, the pharynx swollen and red, and the tonsils often slightly swollen and red. The lymph nodes in the person's neck may be slightly enlarged and tender. You may find all or some of the symptoms listed here.

What's Going On?: Colds are caused by viruses. Viruses are tiny living things that can only reproduce inside cells of other organisms. They are "pure information;" they contain the same substance (DNA) that is found in chromosomes (DNA passes on the information, from one generation to the next, that determines such things as sex, eye color, hair color — and the myriad of other factors that make us who we are.)

One way to look upon a cold is to see that viruses are using the cells of your body for the energy and materials they need to reproduce. The viruses come to live in your nose and throat when the environment there is perfect for them: meaning a particular temperature, a particular acid base, a particular moisture, and a particular *aura* or energy level. You control these levels by sending messages from your mind which tell blood vessels in mucosal tissue to open or close. You also control chemicals in your body, such as histamines, hormones, and saliva which affect the acid base of mucosa. In essence, your body and mind have the knowledge to welcome or reject cold viruses.

When you are out of harmony with yourself and Nature, the mucosa becomes perfect for the viruses to move in. The *out-of-harmony* can be: lack of sufficient rest, tension and anxiety, unhappiness, nutritional lacks, mucosa irritated by tobacco or other chemicals, conflict about your place in life, or problems of cleanliness. There are as many reasons for dis-harmony with yourself and Nature as there are people or colds.

When a virus moves into your nose, your body protects itself by trying to wash the virus away. Blood flow increases to your nose and throat, causing them to become red. This flow brings in white blood cells and antibodies to kill the viruses. The nasal mucosa produces mucous to flush away the virus. All these are what you recognize as "local symptoms" of a cold.

Other chemicals are produced in your body which cause fever and tiredness, and other discomforts, which you recognize as "general symptoms." These symptoms are evidence of your body's healing processes, and are signals to your mind to correct the disharmonious factors in your life.

If you don't allow your body to heal itself, the swollen wet, mucous-covered mucosa becomes a perfect place for bacteria to grow. These bacteria can produce

Tonsil Infections, Strep Throat Infections, Ear Infections, Bronchitis, or Pneumonia. (For more information on these, see the specific disease in *Diagnosis and Treatment.*)

☆   ☆   ☆

There must be two conditions present to get a cold: the presence of viruses, and the proper environment (your nose and throat) to provide a good living situation for them. This means that if someone in your household has a virus you know that one of these conditions is present, and to prevent the virus from spreading you will have to put out some extra effort and energy. If you feel disharmonious, the second factor is present and you should take care to avoid viruses.

Treatment: Begin treatment by taking on an attitude of healing: know that you have the power to heal yourself. Look upon your life as including the whole universe, meaning that your life includes your body, the virus that is causing a cold in you now, and all other beings and elements that make up the universe. Understand that your body is now interacting with a particular virus, producing a reaction which prods you to change activities to improve your life and strive for greater harmony. The first thing a cold virus asks you to change is your activity level. The symptoms almost force you to slow down and rest. Look upon these symptoms as a natural sedative. Rest, where a cold is concerned, means sleep and relaxation. It means pausing in your life to get in touch with yourself. Thus, the first part of the treatment is to let go of your usual routine and allow yourself to *go with* the cold: you're tired, you ache, things are difficult for you to do. So sleep, relax your muscles, and slow down. Slow way down. If you have a difficult time slowing down, ask yourself and your imaginary doctor if that may be the very reason for your present illness — that you have been going too fast or too hard and you need to slow down to improve the harmony of your everyday life.

Rest will give you the energy necessary to synthesize proteins for antibodies to kill the virus, and relaxation will increase blood flow to bring antibodies and white blood cells to the infection. (For specific instructions about rest and relaxation methods, see the *Preventive Medicine* chapter. The information on bio-rhythms and rest-work cycles will help you find out why you got sick.) Relaxation exercises will also give you relief from muscular aches associated with the cold, and by increasing blood flow to muscles that have been tense due to discomfort these exercises will help bring nutrients to cells that are sick, and will carry away waste products.

To relieve the symptoms of fever, drink large quantities of fluids. But understand that you do not have to treat the fever of a cold. The fact is that the fever often helps cure the cold by speeding up the activities of some body chemicals.

Aspirin can be used for relieving fever and muscular aches, but read the chapter *Drugs Are Helpers* first.

☆   ☆   ☆

Understand that drugs prescribed by doctors for colds are given to relieve symptoms only. They do not affect the course of the cold. Antibiotics are *not*

234

effective against the viruses that cause colds, so they will not help at all in the treatment of a simple cold.

Doctors usually prescribe antihistamines to stop runny nose and nasal discomfort. Again, understand that these drugs only relieve symptoms. You will find that rest and relaxation will ease these same symptoms tremendously, and will allow the mucosa to heal itself at its own rate. Sometimes introducing foreign chemicals to the body takes away energy that might otherwise go to the natural healing process. For example, antihistamines cause shrinking of nasal membranes, but after the drug wears off the membranes can become more swollen than they were before the drug was used. Doctors call this penomenon "rebound." What it means to you is that antihistamines *can* both prolong the cold symptoms and make the cold worse.

The best way to relieve the cough or tightness in your chest caused by a cold is to drink plenty of fluids. This means *doubling* or *tripling* your normal fluid intake. For most people this will take effort. Make a point of drinking a full glass of something you enjoy about every two hours or more: water, fruit juices, vegetable juices, or herb teas. All the cells of your body will take up water and water will go to areas where there is mucous. This will thin the mucous and help you free it from your throat through coughing. The water will literally *wash away* the cold. If you wish to do so, do any of the exercises at the end of *Drugs Are Helpers* called "Increasing The Positive Energy of Drugs," to increase the benefits of the liquids that you drink.

Another way to relieve congestion caused by mucous is to use a vaporizer for steam inhalation. Very tiny particles of moisture are absorbed by mucous which causes it to liquify. A small amount of pine or eucalyptus oil added to the vaporizer water will speed up this process. Hot water running into a sink, or steam from a hot shower or bath will help, but are not as effective as a vaporizer. Breathing vapors from a pan of boiling water, however, can result in burning the delicate mucosal tissue in your nose.

Your Doctor As A Resource: A large part of a general practitioner's time is taken up treating the common cold. The doctor is not necessary in treating the cold itself but can be helpful in treating and diagnosing any complications resulting from the cold.

Complications from the common cold include: Sinus Infections, Tonsilitis, Strep Throat, Laryngitis, Bronchitis, and Pneumonia. These diseases come about when mucous membranes injured by a virus become infected with bacteria. A doctor can diagnose these infections and then prescribe an antibiotic, if necessary, to help your body heal itself.

Prevention: The best way to prevent getting the common cold is to learn to pay attention to activities and situations in your life which cause tension or disharmony in your life or which put extra stress on your body and mind. This means keeping in touch with how the foods you are eating affect you, how your environment affects you — and all the other factors we discuss in *Preventive Medicine*.

Much has been written in the past couple of years on vitamin C and the common cold. Most of the books written on the subject present good cases for its use. From our experience, we feel that vitamin C, taken regularly as a food supplement, is a helpful preventive technique. Higher than normal dosages of vitamin C, taken when the first symptoms of a cold appear, may help you to heal the cold in the first stages.

INFLUENZA (FLU)

Symptoms:

Chills	Fever
Tiredness	Muscular aches
Headache	Cough
Runny nose	Anxiety

Physical Exam: Same as for *Common Cold.* You may find all or some of the symptoms listed here for flu, or also for the *Common Cold.*

What's Going On?: Flu is a very contagious virus infection. It usually occurs in epidemics, meaning that many people from the same region and at the same time get similar symptoms. The disease is often identified when a doctor sends a sample culture to a laboratory. Then when the same symptoms occur in many other people, the doctors assume it is an epidemic. When flu occurs in isolation it is difficult to differentiate from a common cold and might be diagnosed as such. However, influenza characteristically has a much more rapid onset than the common cold, often appearing and manifesting symptoms within minutes. A person also experiences muscle aches, exhaustion, and anxiety seemingly out of proportion to the other symptoms.

Flu is spread by coughing which transmits the virus in the droplets of saliva from the nose and throat. The period between exposure and the first appearance of symptoms is very short: usually 1 — 4 days. Usually the illness lasts 1 — 7 days.

Flu can lead to sinus infections, ear infections, bronchitis, and pneumonia. This occurs because the flu damages the delicate mucosa of the nose, throat, and lungs, and becomes a perfect environment for the growth of bacteria which cause these more serious illnesses.

Treatment: Turn to the *Common Cold* section for what to do.

Your Doctor As A Resource: See the *Common Cold* section. In addition, if the fever lasts for more than five days or the cough begins to bring up mucous, be sure to consult your doctor so they can rule out bacterial infections such as bronchitis, strep, or pneumonia.

Prevention: Same as for *Common Cold.* In addition we suggest that you turn to the *Preventive Medicine* chapter, page 42 for how to prevent the spread of airborne infections. Since influenza is highly contagious the more the person is isolated the less will be the chance of spreading it to other people.

Polyvalent influenza vaccine can give you fair, temporary protection against influenza. However, keep in mind that it does not work if you have already been exposed to the disease.

SORE THROAT – PHARYNGITIS

Symptoms: Sore throat   Dryness
                 Hoarseness   Fever
                 Person may feel depressed and ill

Physical Exam: The mucosa of the person's throat is red and slightly swollen. You may see sticky mucous in the throat. You may find that lymph nodes in the person's neck are swollen.

What's Going On?: Pharyngitis is an inflammation of the mucosa of the pharynx in the back of the throat. It's usually part of an upper respiratory infection. The inflammation is commonly caused by a bacterial or viral infection. However, it can be caused by the inhalation of irritants such as tear gas, by excessive smoking, or by excessive use of the voice.

Treatment: Rest in bed, drink plenty of liquids to help dilute the mucous, and keep warm to prevent energy loss. Gargling with warm salt water will soothe your throat and will wash away mucous. Swallowing small amounts of honey will also help to soothe your throat. Your body can usually cure a sore throat with just rest and relaxation. However, if the sore throat is caused by streptococcal bacteria which you can discover only by doing a culture, (see section on *Strep Throat*), it should be treated with antibiotics. If your throat is not responding to your treatment have a culture done.

Your Doctor As A Resource: By doing a throat culture your doctor can differentiate a streptococcal pharyngitis from the other causes of a sore throat (see section on *Strep Throat*). They can prescribe antibiotics for you if necessary.

Prevention: Avoid irritating the throat by too much talking or smoking, or by inhalation of irritants such as tear gas or ammonia. Begin treatment at the first sign of a sore throat, especially if you know you are prone to pharyngitis.

STREP THROAT – ACUTE STREPTOCOCCAL TONSILLITIS

Symptoms: Rapid onset of a sore throat   High fever
                 Lack of appetite   Chills
                 Difficulty swallowing   Muscle aches
                 Pain in the neck (sometimes)   Headache

Physical Exam: When you look at the person's throat you will see very swollen and red tonsils. There will be pus or white plaques (patchy spots) on the tonsils and in the little areas between the tonsils (the crypts). The back of the throat will also be red, swollen and pus-covered. You will find enlarged lymph nodes in the neck.

What's Going On?: The infection is caused by streptococcus bacteria growing on the tonsils and the throat. The body is reacting to the infection by bringing more blood into the area; this causes the redness and swelling. Strep throat can follow an upper respiratory infection or it can occur by itself.

The only sure way to diagnose strep throat is to have a culture done. A swab is put in the back of the throat and touched to the tonsils to pick up bacteria. The swab is rubbed on a media plate which will grow streptococci if they are present. Cultures usually cost more than five dollars and some doctors don't have the equipment to do them. When doctors don't have equipment available, they often treat throats that they suspect are strep infections to prevent complications. They may treat for a strep throat when any four of the following symptoms are present: fever, a painful sore throat, enlarged tonsils, plaques on the tonsils, lymph node swelling in the neck.

Doctors treat strep throat with penicillin, an antibiotic, not primarily to cure the sore throat, but to prevent heart and kidney disease. In a streptococcal infection, substances are produced which cause rheumatic heart disease and glomerulonephritis, a kidney disease. It has been found that ten full days of antibiotics are necessary to prevent subsequent heart and kidney complications. Since the advent of penicillin, the incidence of rheumatic fever, rheumatic heart disease, and glomerulonephritis has decreased significantly. Therefore, it's essential to seek medical treatment if you suspect a strep throat or tonsillitis.

Doctors who do cultures feel it's not beneficial to prescribe antibiotics unless a culture shows the presence of streptococci, because antibiotics are not effective against viral sore throats and because antibiotics have their own side effects (see section on antibiotics in *Drugs Are Helpers*).

Treatment: The primary treatment for strep throat is antibiotics. If you are taking antibiotics, take the full ten-day course; do not stop when your throat feels better (see explanation in *What's Going On?*). Rest in bed and keep warm because it takes a large amount of healing energy to fight the infection. Fluids help dissolve the secretions and bring more blood into the area. Drink plenty of them; drink a full glass of fluids every hour or so. Gargling may be soothing. Relaxing your throat will help relieve the pain and speed healing.

Your Doctor As A Resource: Your doctor is very valuable in treating strep throat. They can take a culture to diagnose the infection and prescribe antibiotics for treatment.

Prevention: Strep throat is a highly communicable disease. It is spread by droplets from the nose and mouth containing the bacteria when a person sneezes or coughs. A person who has a strep throat should cover their mouth and nose when they cough or sneeze. They should wash their hands after coughing and before handling food If possible, avoid exposure to the person who has the strep throat. Early treatment of cold symptoms may also help prevent a strep throat.

LARYNGITIS

Symptoms: Hoarseness   Pain and cough
                Constant urge to clear your throat
                Fever and tiredness

Physical Exam: The larynx can't be seen without special tools. Hoarseness is usually enough to diagnose laryngitis.

What's Going On?: Laryngitis is a viral or bacterial infection of the larynx — your voice box. It often results from an untreated common cold, tonsillitis, or other upper respiratory infection. Using your voice a lot, smoking, or breathing irritating materials can be contributing factors. The characteristic hoarseness is the result of the mucosa swelling around your vocal chords.

Treatment: Rest in bed. Also rest your voice, and avoid smoking and breathing irritating materials. Steam inhalation with a vaporizer and heat applied to your neck will loosen mucous and relax the infected area. If tonsillitis, a common cold, or other respiratory infection preceded the laryngitis, those illnesses must be treated at the same time (see *Diagnosis and Treatment* sections on common cold and tonsillitis for how to treat them).

Your Doctor As A Resource: A doctor can give you a prescription for antibiotics if the laryngitis is caused by a bacterial infection such as strep (see the *Diagnosis and Treatment* section on *Strep Throat* for more information). If symptoms of hoarseness persist for more than two weeks, you should have your doctor examine you for other treatment.

Prevention: If you have a cold or other respiratory infection, take the time to treat it so that the infection doesn't spread to your larynx. Don't use your voice excessively, and avoid breathing or inhaling irritating substances.

BRONCHITIS

Symptoms: Tiredness   Fever
                Muscle pains   Sore throat
                Runny nose   Cough

Physical Exam: The person may have a fever. You may see swollen, red mucosa in their throat and you may find swollen or tender lymph nodes in their neck. You may hear *rhonchi* or the sound of tiny bubbles popping in the affected areas when you listen to the person's back, chest and sides with a stethoscope. See the *Physical Examination* chapter, page 167, for complete instructions of how to do this part of the exam.

What's Going On?: Bronchitis is an inflammation in the lower wind pipe in your throat and in the larger tubes (the bronchial tubes) carrying air to and from your lungs. It often results from an upper respiratory infection or a common cold that doesn't get completely cured.

The first thing that happens is that the blood flow increases to the mucous membranes of the bronchial tubes to protect them from the upper respiratory infection. White blood cell activity increases and the mucosal tissue swells. Cells in the bronchial mucosa which have been injured by the cold virus or bacteria begin to secrete a sticky mucous. This mucous prevents the *cilia* — like hair-like projections that normally act as part of a sophisticated filtering system — from doing their job. As a result, the normally sterile bronchial tubes become an ideal environment for bacterial growth. Irritating substances, including tobacco smoke, prevent the cilia from doing their normal job in the necessary filtering process.

The cough, which is such an unpleasant symptom in Bronchitis, is actually your body's reflex to get the thick mucous out of your lungs. This coughing is essential if you are to heal yourself, so trust your body's reflex and let yourself cough freely and openly. You will want to cough deeply, loosening the mucous from your bronchial tubes and forcing it up. Shallow, raspy little coughs are of no value and will even irritate your throat, possibly causing further infection.

Treatment: Rest in bed. It takes a lot of energy to cure yourself of Bronchitis so you will want to turn as much energy as possible to the healing process. Stop smoking so that you won't further damage the already injured bronchial tubes and cilia. Drink a large amount of fluids — as much as a gallon a day. The fluids will be absorbed into all the cells of your body. These fluids will be released by the cells in the bronchial tubes to thin out the mucous and make it easier to cough up. You will have to make a conscious effort to drink as much fluid as necessary — say, one half glass of water per hour. That's a lot of water but it is one of the most essential parts of treating bronchitis.

Steam inhalation from a vaporizer is extremely beneficial. The microscopic water vapor mixes with the mucous, dilutes it, and makes it easier for you to cough it up.

An old but still good treatment for draining the bronchial tubes is to lie flat on your stomach and hang your head over the edge of the bed so that it's lower than your chest. Do this for one minute, twice a day at first. Increase the time if you like it, but be warned that it does make some people dizzy. This position promotes drainage of the mucous. It may also be helpful to have someone pat you sharply on the back, over the lungs, to loosen mucous.

Vicks Vapor Rub, Mentholatum, Ben Gay or other, similar, over-the-counter drugs will help relieve the soreness in your chest. "Expectorant" cough medicines will help you to cough up the mucous. Some very effective ones are available without prescription. Ask your druggist specifically for a simple expectorant cough medicine.

Have someone massage your chest and back. This will help you to relax your muscles, bringing increased, beneficial blood flow to your chest area. It will also help you to breathe more deeply in order to clear your bronchial tubes.

Your Doctor As A Resource: If you have a high fever that persists or if you feel very sick, your doctor may prescribe antibiotics to treat the infection. You may also wish them to help you diagnose what you have in order to rule out pneumonia.

Prevention: Take care of yourself —especially when you have a cold or other upper respiratory infection. Help your body heal itself completely whenever you have a cold. If you smoke, understand that the tobacco irritates your bronchial tubes and actually damages your cilia, making you more prone to bronchial problems than non-smokers. If you don't wish to stop smoking entirely, at least do so when you have even minor respiratory infections so that you lessen the chances of bronchitis.

Vitamin C taken when you have a cold (see *Common Cold*) can help your body protect itself from bronchitis.

PNEUMONIA

Symptoms: Sudden onset of chills and fever
Cough, bringing up rusty-colored mucous
Pain in chest

Physical Exam: The person appears very ill. Their respiratory rate is very high: 30-40 breaths per minute. Each breath that the person takes will be labored, and often times they will moan or grunt as they breathe. On your visual examination of the chest, chest expansion will be less on the side of the pneumonia infection. When you percuss the person's back it will sound *dull* in the areas affected. On the stethoscopic exam, the person's breath sounds will be very low in volume, and you will hear *rales.* If you need help doing any part of this exam turn to page 167, *Physical Exam*, for complete, detailed instructions.

What's Going On?: Pneumonia is an infection of the smallest air passages (the alveoli) in your lungs. It is usually caused by *pneumococcus* bacteria. It can also be caused by other bacteria and various viruses. It often follows untreated common colds, upper respiratory infections, or bronchitis, especially in elderly people or in people who neglect their bodies through inadequate diet, overexposure to the cold, or fatigue.

The bacteria spreads to the lungs through the bronchial tubes, and then to the smallest air passages. Injured tissue cells in the small air passages release body fluids which provides an ideal environment for bacterial growth. A few hours after bacteria begin to grow, white blood cells come to the area and start consuming the bacteria, and the body begins to heal itself. The problem is that the white blood cells moving to the area can become so numerous that they actually block the tiny air passages.

The *alveoli*, the tiny air passages, are the places where the oxygen brought into your lungs is absorbed into your blood to feed all the cells in your body. In this same place your blood gives off carbon dioxide waste products which you then normally exhale. If your *alveoli* are blocked, you breathe faster in an attempt to get enough oxygen and to get rid of enough carbon dioxide to carry on the life process in your body.

Coughing is important in pneumonia, just as it is in *bronchitis*. It is necessary to clear your lungs of mucous (see *Diagnosis and Treatment* section on Bronchitis).

Treatment: Your body will need help in curing itself of penumonia. Antibiotics are the best way to do this. They lower the number of bacteria down to a point where your white blood cells can handle the rest without blocking your *alveoli*. We believe that if a person has pneumonia they will have to seek outside their own body for the energy necessary to heal themself. This is because the disease itself draws off so much energy. When you have pneumonia, antibiotics and your doctor represent the most effective sources of this healing energy for most people.

Your Doctor As A Resource: Doctors can really help you when you have pneumonia. They can do chest x-rays to see the solid areas of the pneumonia. They can also do white blood cell counts to tell if there's an increase in the white blood cells, which is an indication of infection. They can do a culture of the mucous to determine the specific strain of bacteria causing the pneumonia; they can prescribe an antibiotic to which that particular bacteria is sensitive.

If what you have proves to be pneumonia, and you are taking antibiotics, the rest of the treatment is the same as we describe for bronchitis.

Prevention: Taking care of yourself is clearly the way to prevent pneumonia. This means giving your body good food, adequate rest, exercise, relaxation and pleasure. It's especially important not to neglect a cold, other respiratory infections, or bronchitis.

TUBERCULOSIS

Symptoms:

Tiredness	Loss of appetite
Weight loss	Easily fatigued
Slight fever in afternoon	
Cough, and person may spit up blood	
Slight pain in chest	Night sweats

Physical Exam: You may hear rales upon stethoscopic examination of the upper part of the chest but this finding is not common. The person with TB often looks gray, weak, and thin.

What's Going On?: TB is an infection caused by a bacteria called *mycobacterium tuberculosis*. The bacteria form little hard lumps which get bigger, if untreated, and

242

the bacteria then spreads to other parts of the body. Due to skin tests and lung X-rays, TB is now uncommon in the United States. But some cases are still found where there are poor sanitation, poor medical facilities and malnutrition.

Treatment: Your body will need the extra energy of antibiotics to heal itself of TB.

Your Doctor As Resource: Your doctor can find out if you have been exposed to TB. They do this by injecting a small amount of protein from TB bacteria under your skin; if you have been exposed to TB, that area will become red and raised. A doctor can also do a chest x-ray to confirm a diagnosis of TB. If you do have TB, the therapy includes the use of special antibiotics to heal you, and isolation to prevent its spread to others. Bed rest is also part of the therapy. TB responds to treatment best when treated early.

Prevention: Avoid exposure to people with TB, maintain a good diet, and get a skin test or chest x-ray every year or so.

HAY FEVER
(Also called "Allergic Rhinitis")

Symptoms:
- Nasal congestion
- Itching of the nose
- Itching of the eyes and tearing
- Runny nose
- Occassionally violent sneezing

Physical Exam: The mucosa inside the nose will be pale, bluish, and swollen. The conjunctivae of the eye will be swollen and sometimes tears are seen.

What's Going On?: Your body is recognizing substances in the external environment that it feels are a threat. These are most commonly pollens, animal *danders* (a substance in animal fur), household dust, and fungus. These substances are called "antigens." Very often, with Allergic Rhinitis, the person's body is responding to these antigens in an exaggerated way; the body is misreading the threat.

I feel that the body leans an allergic reaction in the same way that it learns a phobia such as the fear of heights, or cats, or flying in an airplane. But with an allergy your body learns a biochemical reaction instead of reacting with fear; it produces a protein antibody which reacts with the antigens of the specific substance to which you are allergic and thus produces the allergic symptoms. Injured body cells release histamines to protect themselves, and all the organs that react to histamines go through chemical changes causing swelling and increased or decreased blood flow.

You may not know or remember why your body learned to react in the way it does to the substances which cause your allergy. Understand, though, that at some time in your life your body did have a reason to fear that substance, or something associated with that substance. The reason for your body's fear may no longer be applicable, however; realizing this you can go ahead and un-learn the mechanism which causes you the discomfort of the allergic reaction, if you wish.

☆   ☆   ☆

A history of the allergy in a person will help you to distinguish Allergic Rhinitis from a cold. Hay fever is often the cause of repeated "colds" in people who get colds only during a particular period or season of the year. For example, ragweed pollinates between August 15 and September 1 in parts of the United States. So if a person gets a "cold" each year at about that time of the year, it is logical to suspect Allergic Rhinitis as a cause.

A family history of allergies can also give clues to diagnosing a person's allergy.

Treatment: There is no specific treatment in Western medicine for Allergic Rhinitis. The most common "treatment" is antihistamines, but their action in your body only serves to relieve symptoms. They do *not* act to change the cause of the allergic reaction nor to prevent further episodes of the allergy.

An exercise which we've found effective for people with allergic rhinitis is as follows:

Do the complete exercise for getting in touch with your imaginary doctor. Let yourself be comfortable with your imaginary doctor in your imaginary room. Ask your doctor if they feel that you are ready to heal yourself of your allergy. (If you are not ready, discontinue this exercise but try it again in a few days or weeks. You may also wish to ask your imaginary doctor why they feel you are not ready.) If you are ready, ask your imaginary doctor what method they would suggest to free you of the allergy. Again, there are as many methods as there are people. Understand, too, that this exercise takes practice and that some peoples' imaginary doctors ask them to go through many different steps on the way to curing their allergies.

One person's imaginary doctor told her to take an imaginary pill instead of an antihistamine, and to wash it down with actual water whenever she felt the symptoms of her allergy coming on. After several days of this treatment, the imaginary doctor told her that she was now in control of the reactions which had been taking place in her nasal mucosa, and it was time for her to heal herself without the imaginary medicine. She was then told to pay attention to the feelings of her nose and throat throughout the day, and to learn how to read her body's messages from these areas. When she did this she learned to detect early tensions in these areas and by relaxing them she learned to prevent the symptoms of Allergic Rhinitis from occuring. She relaxed her nose and throat by sitting down, closing her eyes, and telling those parts to relax.

In the beginning she did these things consciously and deliberately. But as she repeated the process day by day her body slowly learned new mechanisms for dealing with the antigens that had previously caused uncomfortable reactions. One way to look at this is that the woman consciously set about to teach her body a mechanism for effectively dealing with the allergy, and once learned, she turned the new behavior patterns over to her body's *Three Million Year Old Healer* to maintain on its own.

Another person learned that his allergy was always worse when he was doing things that he really didn't want to do — such as entertaining his relatives when they came to visit. The imaginary doctor told this person to do the thing that he most enjoyed doing, instead — which, for this person, was painting. As the person learned to make his choices on this basis, the allergic reaction became less and less severe until it eventually disappeared altogether.

Your Doctor As A Resource: Your doctor can take skin tests to determine the exact cause of your allergy. They can also "desensitize" you with specific antigens. This can be useful in treating ragweed allergies. They may also prescribe antihistamines or steroids to suppress your symptoms. We suggest that you read our chapter *Drugs Are Helpers* so that you can make a choice of treatments if these drugs have been suggested for your use or if you are now using them for your allergy.

Prevention: Find the things in your life that cause your allergy, and then avoid contact with them. For example, leave your house while it is being cleaned — vacuumed, swept, or dusted — if you know that you are allergic to house dust. Use foam rubber pillows, since they do not collect dust as other padding materials do, and they contain no allergic-causing materials. (Feather pillows contain dander.) Remove from your house all carpets and drapes that collect dust. Use synthetic blankets instead of blankets made of materials that might contain antigens. If you are allergic to household pets such as cats, dogs, or birds consider getting rid of them.

As you can see Allergic Rhinitis can greatly limit your life. There is no reason to believe that you will always have allergies. Allergies are curable. It has been our experience that as a person's life changes their allergies tend to disappear.

ASTHMA

Symptoms: Recurring attacks of tightness in the chest, difficulty breathing, wheezing, and coughing up mucous
Attacks usually start abruptly

Physical Exam: You'll notice as the person breathes out that that part of the breathing cycle will be longer than usual. The person will look as though they're fighting for air, and you will often be able to hear their breathing from across the room. They will have *greater difficulty exhaling* than inhaling.

With your stethoscope you'll hear musical-sounding wheezes over lung areas.

What's Going On?: Asthma is most often found with people who have a history of allergies to such things as pollen, dander, and house dust. A history of allergies in their family is found in half the people who have asthma.

Between attacks the person usually is in harmony with the world around them. However, emotional stress, minor infections or changes in the person's hormonal balance can upset that harmony. When this takes place, the person may have allergic reactions to substances which do not ordinarily bother them. Their body recognizes these substances (antigens) as a threat and produces its own substances (antibodies) to protect itself. The antibody-antigen reaction damages cells in the medium-sized lung

245

passages (small bronchi), and these cells then release thick mucous and body fluids. Then the smooth muscles in the walls of the small bronchi go into spasms and the air passage becomes narrowed. This narrowing of the air passages is what makes it difficult for the asthmatic person to exhale.

The changes which cause the narrowing of the air passages are reversible. Your body can widen these tubes just as it can narrow them, by relaxing the smooth muscles in the small bronchi, reabsorbing the body fluids and coughing up the mucous. This is the way your body actually stops an asthma attack by itself, a process which you can witness in yourself every time you get over an asthma attack.

Many people who have asthma know that they get asthma attacks when they are anxious or tense. They also know that the fear that they may stop breathing during an attack *increases* the severity of the attack. Understand, though, that it is extremely rare for a person who has asthma to stop breathing during an attack.

We have found that as people's lives change their need for the asthma often diminishes and they are freed of the discomfort of attacks. (See our discussion of *Hay Fever — Allergic Rhinitis* for more on allergic reactions.)

Treatment: An acute asthma attack is usually treated with a drug called *epinephrine*. This drug is now commonly used in "inhalers." It is a body hormone which your adrenal glands normally secrete. Epinephrine usually is secreted during times of fear and is known as the hormone of "fright and flight." In ancient times when man was defending himself from Mastadons and Saber Tooth Tigers, this hormone was probably responsible for his survival. In your body this hormone normally helps to reroute the flow of your blood to the muscles in your arms, legs, back and heart, bringing tremendous energy to these parts. At the same time it relaxes the smooth muscles in the small bronchi of your lungs so that air can pass more freely in and out. Epinephrine also causes a greater amount of *glucose*, the body's energy substance, to be released into the blood.

Relaxation of your mind and your body is extremely important in stopping an asthma attack. If you have asthma, learn to do one or more of the relaxation exercises which we describe in this book. Learn how to do them, and practice them at times when you are healthy and free of the discomforts of asthma. Once you have acquired these body skills, and can do them with ease, you will be able to relax your body and mind during an asthma attack. This relaxation will allow your body to stop the attack. (See *Hay Fever* section for further treatment relevant to asthma.)

Your Doctor As A Resource: Most people with asthma need help from a doctor to get relief during an acute attack. The doctor can give you an injection of *epinephrine* to stop a severe attack. They can also give an injection of *aminophylline* to relax the bronchial muscles. Sedatives can be given to reduce general anxiety.

Prevention: Avoid the causes of allergic reactions; this means pollens, animal dander, and house dust. Understand that emotional tension and stress help create the situations within your body which cause you to react to these substances. Thus, you can look upon asthmatic attacks as your body's messages to you to resolve tension and stress and do things to bring greater harmony into your life. In this book we suggest several paths to accomplish this: meditation, body relaxation, and the environment exercises in the *Preventive Medicine* chapter are all good places to start. Daily breathing exercises, also in the *Preventive Medicine* chapter, have been found to prevent asthma attacks.

People with asthma often have attacks during or after colds or other respiratory infections. Prevention of cold by adequate sleep, good diet, and avoiding fatigue, will also prevent asthma. (For more information on preventing colds, see the *Common Cold* section of the *Diagnosis and Treatment* chapter.)

Early and assertive treatment to heal colds is essential for people with asthma.

Smoking irritates bronchi and can bring on asthma attacks. So if you smoke and have asthma . . .

We have found that many people who do the things we describe in this section have cured themselves of asthma.

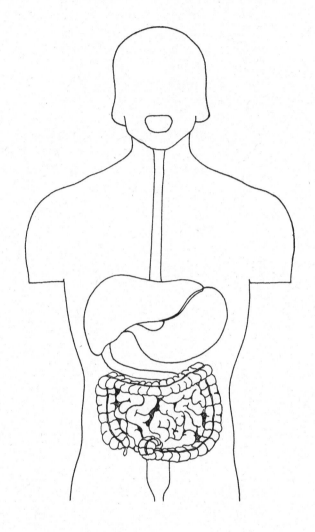

GASTROINTESTINAL

This section includes organs of your body which have to do with digesting food. In reality, the first digestive organ of your body is your mouth. We don't, however, deal with the mouth here. (See our chapter *Going Further* for the description of a book that does.) In this section we tell you about diseases and disorders that most people associate with their stomach and intestines: Diarrhea, Vomiting, Constipation and Worms, etc.

HICCUPS

Symptoms: Hiccups

Physical Exam: Not applicable.

What's Going On?: Hiccups is a reflex involving rhythmic spasms and other reactions in your throat, lungs, and diaphram. The messages to cause these reflexes go through your mind, and are at a fairly conscious level, so it is possible to control hiccups consciously.

Treatment: Most remedies for hiccups involve distracting the person who has them. When the person's attention is distracted to other things, their mind forgets about the hiccups and they stop. Common distracting methods are: interesting conversation, sex, fright, or having the person perform a ritual which someone has convinced them will really stop the hiccups. Rituals are: drinking ice water, standing on your head, holding your breath, etc.

Relaxation exercises, directed especially to your lungs and diagram, are probably the most consistantly successful methods that we know of to stop the hiccups. Use the relaxation exercise which we describe for getting your imaginary doctor.

Your Doctor As A Resource: Doctors can prescribe tranquilizing drugs and sedatives for hiccups that won't stop. But this is rarely necessary.

Prevention: If you are prone to getting hiccups, you may find that doing the breathing exercises in the *Preventive Medicine* chapter will help you. Practice these exercises before you have a hiccup attack so that you will have these skills when you need them.

DIARRHEA

Symptoms: Passing liquified stool or watery stool

Physical Exam: You may find some tenderness in the abdomen. Listen for sounds in the abdomen with your stethoscope. The sounds will be overactive if compared to normal bowel sounds.

The person with diarrhea will also have symptoms of whatever illness is causing the diarrhea. For example, with an intestinal virus infection the person may have fever, chills, vomiting, and cold symptoms.

What's Going On?: The intestines are tremendously active with diarrhea. They are passing food from the top to the bottom without absorbing much food value, and without absorbing water from the stools. The intestines are irritated, they're upset. If you listen to them with your stethescope they will sound like water bubbling in a teakettle.

Diarrhea is often caused by viral infections which are spread by the fecal/oral route. This means that if a person has diarrhea and doesn't wash their hands, then touches a food preparation surface, the virus can be spread to whoever eats foods prepared on that surface.

Other causes of diarrhea are: food poisoning, bacterial dysentary, and anxiety. People often get diarrhea when traveling, which some doctors attribute to the person's body being subjected to changes in diet, nervousness, etc.

Treatment: Avoid solid foods but drink bland liquids. Water and weak teas are best for this condition. Avoid milk. After your body becomes accustomed to the liquid diet, and the diarrhea slows down, bland solid foods can be eaten. Avoid raw vegetables, fruits, fried foods, bran, syrups, spices, and coffee. Avoid all dairy products. The best things to eat are toast and tea. (For more on a bland diet, see the chapter on *Preventive Medicine*.) Relaxing your body is important in treating diarrhea because it helps slow down bowel activity.

The most important thing in diarrhea is to maintain the balance of fluids in your body. A person can pass a large amount of liquid in the stool with diarrhea, so it is important that they replace the fluids they lose or else they will become dehydrated. In adults this is less serious than with children because an adult has a higher fluid volume than a child. The treatment is to drink a lot of fluids to replace the fluids lost in the diarrhea.

In babies, diarrhea can be a very serious problem. Diarrhea can quickly drain the baby's store of fluids. A doctor should be notified if the baby has diarrhea. Generally it will be recommended that you take the baby off milk — unless the baby is breast-feeding. The baby is then given mild tea, apple juice, and water. Usually the diarrhea will stop, the baby will get adequate fluids by mouth, and everything will be okay.

Your Doctor As A Resource: A doctor can help you if you are unable to stop the diarrhea yourself of if severe pain, dehydration, or bleeding occurs.

☆　☆　☆

If your baby has diarrhea the doctor will probably want to make sure the baby is not becoming dehydrated. If in several days, fluid taken by mouth cannot maintain the baby's fluids, the doctor might prescribe intravenous feedings for a short time. This, fortunately, is rare.

A doctor can prescribe drugs to slow down or stop diarrhea if they think it is necessary.

See the Treatment section of Vomiting for a simple test that you can do to test for dehydration.

250

Prevention: The prevention of diarrhea includes cleaning toilet and food preparation areas, and avoiding exposure to people who have diarrhea. Find out which foods, if any, cause you to have thin and watery stools, and then avoid those foods in your diet.

VOMITING

Symptoms: Nausea and vomiting

Physical Exam: The person may show symptoms of the problem which has caused them to vomit. For example, if they have a stomach virus infection, the person may have some fever. They may also have cold symptoms and/or they may have diarrhea.

What's Going On?: Something happens in your stomach that your body recognizes as unusual. The brain receives a signal that something is wrong in the stomach or G.I. tract. It sends a signal back which causes muscles in the stomach to contract in order to empty out the contents.

This reflex can be consciously controlled to some extent, but most of the time your body is telling you to vomit for a valid reason. So you will usually be more comfortable in the long run if you relax and let your body do what it wants to do.

Vomiting is caused by irritation of the stomach and G.I. tract, which can have different causes. It can be due to a viral infection (one of the most common causes) or it can be due to dietary indiscretions. It can be due to morning sickness during pregnancy. Vomiting can have emotional causes such as anxiety.

Vomiting is your body's way of purging it of things that it doesn't want, or need, or which it feels are a threat to it. Indian witch doctors use it as a way of purging their body of evil spirits. So you can think of vomiting as something positive, rather than something to be afraid of. It is your body's way of cleaning itself out, of allowing it to heal itself more quickly.

Treatment: If the vomiting has been caused by overeating or drinking, pregnancy, or a viral infection, no specific treatment is necessary except that relaxation exercises will help you to be more comfortable during this time. Any of the relaxation exercises in *Preventive Medicine* or elsewhere in the book will help. The most important thing is to maintain your intake of fluids. In the beginning avoid eating solid foods until the vomiting and nausea have stopped. Then eat only very bland foods: dry crackers, bread, toast, and clear broth.

If you are vomiting, and you lose a glass full of water (or fluid) every ten or fifteen minutes, it is essential that sooner or later you replace that fluid in approximately the same amount. Otherwise you may become dehydrated, which is a serious condition.

To test for dehydration: Pinch a small amount of skin on the soft part of your forearm. Hold it up for a second, like a little tent of flesh, and then release it. Normally the skin pops down instantly to its previous position. If a person is dehydrated their skin will remain raised and will *slowly* return to its previous position.

Water, weak herb tea, diluted juice or a very small amount of carbonated beverage can be drunk to help your body maintain its fluid level. Carbonated beverages may have a settling effect for people who have been vomiting. In severe nausea or vomiting a teaspoon or a tablespoon of a carbonated beverage every couple of minutes, gradually increased to twice that, can prove very soothing.

There are anti-nausea and anti-vomiting drugs that are often quite helpful. Relaxation is extremely important in that it interupts the nausea-vomiting cycle. What happens is that a person may become tense and afraid with nausea. This added stress lowers their threshold so that less stimuli is necessary to cause them to vomit. When this stress is added to the discomfort of nausea and vomiting, the person may continue vomiting even long after there is nothing to empty from their stomach. Complete body relaxation, using whatever technique the person can manage at the time, will usually raise their threshold and allow them to stop vomiting. If you practice relaxation exercises when you are fully well, these skills will make it easier for you to gain control of your reflexes whenever you are sick, in order to aid your body in healing itself.

Your Doctor As A Resource: It's usually not necessary to see your doctor unless you are frightened about vomiting, or you have other symptoms such as pain or bleeding or dehydration. However, in the case of babies, this is a different matter. Babies have a very low amount of total body fluids, and vomiting can deplete their fluids quickly. A doctor will be of great help if you have a baby who is vomiting, or if the baby looks very sick. They will usually recommend that you discontinue milk unless the baby is breast feeding, and that you feed the baby very small amounts of mild fluids: very weak tea, apple juice, or water.

A doctor can prescribe anti-vomiting drugs if you are unable to control your vomiting through relaxation.

Prevention: Get in touch with your diet — especially if you are drinking alcoholic beverages or overeating. (See the diet section of the *Preventive Medicine* chapter for more information on how to do this.) If the vomiting is due to morning sickness in pregnancy, the woman should be especially careful about eating foods which are definitely appetizing to her and to avoid foods which she dislikes.

Vomiting in a viral infection is not harmful and there is no need to prevent it. Your body is purging itself. If you relax yourself after the first time you vomit and you avoid solid foods for several hours, or until your nausea completely passes, the nausea-vomiting cycle will pass and you will be much more comfortable.

CONSTIPATION

Symptoms: A feeling of fullness in the bowels
                      Not having bowel movements with the regularity that is customary
                      Inability to move your bowels

Physical Exam: Usually nothing is seen on the physical exam. If the person is extremely constipated, a hard mass of feces may be felt in the anus. The person's chief complaint will be constipation.

What's Going On?: The lower intestines have what is called "peristalsis" — a natural massage-like action which moves the contents of the bowels through the intestines and eventually out of the body. If peristalsis is inhibited, the stool won't move.

Normally your body absorbs water from the stool in your lower intestines. If the stool remains in the lower intestine too long, more water than usual is absorbed and the stool becomes pasty and hard. The harder the stool, of course, the more difficulty you will have moving it out of your body, since the normal peristalsis will be inhibited.

Understand that a bowel movement every day is not essential. For one person a normal bowel movement cycle can be twice a day; for another person it can be once a week. When a person's normal bowel pattern changes radically, and suddenly, this is constipation; the fact that you don't move your bowels every day is not, in itself, a sign of constipation.

In most cases constipation is due to diet, anxiety, or pregnancy. Other causes are lack of food intake, and lack of fluids.

Doctors know of no relationships between constipation and lack of "pep" or energy, being "out of sorts," or "being unresponsive to your family."

Treatment: Fluids are extremely important in overcoming constipation. The more water you drink the more will be present to be absorbed by the stools in your intestines; thus the more likely the stool will be of the right consistency to be easy moved. If you are troubled by constipation, double or triple your usual intake of fluids.

Adequate bulk in your diet: raw vegetables, salads, wheat roughage, or bran, can help bowel movements by providing stimulus for the peristaltic action. Raw fruit, stewed prunes, dates, apple juice, and cantaloupe all aid in loosening the stool.

If you find that you are slowly constipated, increase your intake of fruits and liquids.

Nancy's method for curing constipation is to eat six cantaloupes in two days. She calls this "the-six-cantaloupes-in-two-days-method."

Other foods that aid in relieving constipation are honey, and molasses. Increasing your intake of olive oil, or vegetable oils, in salads, and then drinking the fluid left over in the salad bowl, is also helpful.

Here's a recipe for cookies which will probably end your constipation and which are delicious too. (Don't eat more than four unless you are really constipated — less for kids.)

Grandmother Pelton's Chocolate-Molasses Cookies

1 cup light brown or raw sugar
1 cup equal parts butter and
    vegetable shortening
1 pint Molasses
1 tsp. cinnamon
1 tsp. cloves

3 egg yolks, beaten
3 squares of bitter chocolate, melted
½ cup hot water with 1 tsp
    baking soda
3½ cups of pastry flour, or enough
    to make a soft dough

Drop the pastry dough onto a greased cookey pan. Bake for 12—15 minutes in a 350° oven. Yield is about 4 dozen large cookies.

Relaxation is important in relieving constipation, because you can work yourself up into a fear of not being able to move your bowels, which brings tension to the abdominal muscles. Tension changes the blood flow and slows down the normal peristaltic action.

Here's an exercise recommended by women who have had trouble with constipation during pregnancy: When you sit down on the toilet, put your legs out straight, supported by a box or a chair which is the same height as the toilet seat. Then lean back against the toilet. This allows the bowels to move more freely and eliminates the need to strain. Straining during constipation is said to help create hemorrhoids.

We do not recommend the use of laxatives or enemas in the treatment of normal constipation unless specifically prescribed to you by your doctor. The laxatives interfere with your bowels' normal reflexes. (See *Drugs Are Helpers* for more information about the use of laxatives.)

Your Doctor As A Resource: Your doctor is essential only if you are an elderly person with a sudden change in bowel habits. The doctor can make sure that there isn't any other problem causing the constipation. They can also help you if your constipation doesn't respond to the treatments which we describe, or if you feel like you are impacted. (Impacted means the stool has hardened in the rectal area and must then be removed by hand.)

Prevention: Diet is the most important factor in prevention of constipation. When you first notice your stool becoming hard add more raw vegetables, oils, and fluids to your diet until the consistency of your stool is satisfactory. Get sufficient exercise to keep your abdominal muscles elastic and strong.

Most people have a particular time of the day when they are accustomed to moving their bowels. It may be in the morning, afternoon, or evening. Whatever time it is, you will find that your bowels move more easily at that time than at other times of the day. If you can't have your own time to have a bowel movement, and the structure of life around you keeps you from doing it, this often leads to constipation. If you are about to have a bowel movement and then your boss calls you, probably your intestines will continue absorbing water from the stool and you may end up being slightly constipated by the end of the day. So take the time to move your bowels at the time of day to which your body is accustomed.

FARTING
(Also called "Timpanitis" and "Flatulence")

Symptoms: Passing gas from the rectum

Physical Exam: Nothing is usually seen.

What's Going On?: Gas from the eating and digestive processes builds up in the bowels and has to come out some way; so it comes out either from the bottom or from the top.

In the gas gets in the bowels because people swallow air when they eat, swallow it when they are anxious, or because they eat gas-producing foods such as carbonated beverages, cucumbers, beans, etc.

It is important to know that farting has no medical stigma attached to it; the stigma is strictly social. Some people attempt to hold the gas in their bowels because they are embarrased — which probably does them more harm than good. It is really quite good for you to pass the normal gas that is in your bowels from normal food digestion.

Treatment: Not applicable.

Your Doctor As A Resource: Not applicable.

Prevention: Avoid foods which you have found to cause you to fart alot. Eat slowly, not "gulpingly," and relax after eating.

GASTRITIS — ACUTE INDIGESTION

Symptoms: Poor appetite
Fullness and pressure in the stomach
Occasionally nausea and vomiting
Uncommonly, vomiting up blood
Mild stomach pain

Physical Exam: There may be some tenderness over the stomach area. The person may look tired and sick.

What's Going On?: Gastritis is an irritation of the stomach. It is most commonly caused by excessive consumption of alcohol. It can also be caused by hot or spicey foods. To help you understand what gastritis is, put some alcohol on your finger,

255

especially on a cut. It burns. The mucosa of the stomach is even more affected by alcohol than the skin. Alcohol directly injures the cells of the mucosa by drawing the water out of the cell. When there are large amounts of alcohol in the stomach, whole patches of mucosal cells can be killed. Neighboring damaged cells produce mucous to protect themselves. The body increases its blood flow to the area to bring nutrients to damaged cells. Patches in the wall of the stomach can become so irritated that they bleed. These raw, bleeding, mucous-covered patches can take days for your body to heal.

Treatment: Eat and drink nothing until the acute pain is gone. Then drink liquids such as water, mild teas, bouillon, or thin soups. When you feel comfortable drinking these liquids, you can eat bland foods such as buttered toast, cooked cereals, soft-boiled eggs, milk, mashed potatoes and jello. When you can tolerate these foods well, you can eat broiled meats, not fried. They should be well chewed. It may be necessary to adhere to this diet for two weeks.

Relaxation exercises are valuable in curing gastritis. Tense, anxious states cause increased stomach acid secretions which prolong the gastritis.

Here is an exercise to help you heal your stomach:

Lie down in a comfortable position, and do the exercise you use for getting your imaginary doctor. Especially concentrate on relaxing your abdomen and the muscles around your stomach. Visualize your stomach, and its mucosal lining. Imagine that the mucosa is pink, vibrant, and healthy.

This exercise will relax your stomach, increase circulation to the mucosa of your stomach, and will bring healing energy into the area to heal you.

Your Doctor As A Resource: A doctor can help you if the pain is severe by giving you pain medications. They should be consulted if you vomit blood, to make sure it is caused by the gastritis. Often people with gastritis symptoms think that they have an ulcer. (see *Diagnosis and Treatment* section on Ulcers). Your doctor can help you differentiate between the diagnosis of gastritis or an ulcer.

Prevention: Avoid excessive consumption of alcohol or eating spicey foods, especially if you are prone to gastritis symptoms. Be aware of messages from your stomach; eat only foods that agree with you. At the first signs of gastritis, start treating yourself by eating a bland diet. This will prevent further irritation of the lining of your stomach and help the mucosa heal more rapidly.

ULCERS

Symptoms: Pain, described as steady, aching or gnawing located over the
                      stomach area.
                   There may be heart burn or vomiting

Physical Exam: You may find slight or moderate tenderness over the stomach area.

What's Going On?: An ulcer is a small, crater-shaped hole in the mucosal tissue of the stomach or on the top part of the small intestine (duodenum). Doctors believe that ulcers may be caused by over-secretion of hydrochloric acid in the stomach. There is no doubt that emotional tension and stress is extremely important in creating ulcers. The tension or stress is literally "eating you up." So look upon ulcers as your body's message to you to resolve sources of tension or stress in your life. Ulcers can lead you to seek and discover greater harmony and thus greater pleasure in life.

The pain of ulcers is noticed one to four hours after eating a meal. This pain is relieved by eating food, drinking milk, or taking antacids. It is made worse by alcohol and spicey foods. The pain can be described as like a steady hunger pang over the stomach and it may seem to move to your back or even shoulder.

Treatment: A treatment prescribing changes in diet will cure the ulcer itself but will not remove the situation that caused the ulcer. (For a bland ulcer diet see the *Preventive Medicine* chapter on diet.)

Doctors usually prescribe two to three weeks of rest. The person is advised to stop working at their job, and during this period of rest they should be in a relaxed atmosphere. The use of tobacco, aspirin and alcohol is stopped. A typical ulcer diet should be nutritive and given in frequent, small feedings. Bland foods such as milk, cottage cheese, eggs and boiled potatoes are often suggested.

A person with an ulcer should not eat foods such as coffee, tea, carbonated beverages, and foods that the person knows will disagree with them; these cause increased production of stomach acids which prevent the ulcer from healing.

Antacids can help relieve ulcer pain but do not help your body heal the ulcer. Neither do they prevent further ulcers from starting.

☆   ☆   ☆

Body and mind relaxation is important in treating an ulcer. For more information on this read the *Antacids* section of *Drugs Are Helpers,* and the *Preventive Medicine* chapter.

Your Doctor As A Resource: Your doctor can help you diagnose ulcers. Complications of ulcers such as bleeding ulcers, or *perforation* (an actual hole in the bowel) are medical emergencies for which you'll need your doctor's help.

Prevention: Prevention consists of resolving emotional situations in your life which give rise to the condition in your body that cause the ulcer. Understand that you have the ability to control the secretions of stomach acids and you can, therefore, create or heal an ulcer yourself. The complications of ulcers can be serious so we feel that the symptoms of ulcers represent messages which you must heed. You may find it helpful to consult your imaginary doctor and ask them to assist you in locating the situations in your life causing your tension, and to suggest ways to resolve them. (See the chapter, *Disease As a Positive Life Force* for more information on this.)

GASTROENTERITIS
(sometimes called "Stomach Flu")

Symptoms:

Tiredness	Poor Appetite
Nausea	Vomiting
Diarrhea	Stomach ache or abdominal cramps
Fever	Chills

Physical Exam: The abdomen may appear slightly bloated. Tenderness is usually indefinite and the areas of tenderness shift from one place to another in the abdomen. Bowel sounds, heard with a stethoscope or putting your ear against the person's abdomen, will be loud, constant, and overactive. They will be unusually active.

What's Going On?: *Gastroenteritis* is usually caused by a virus. It is less commonly caused by a food allergy, food poisoning, or bacterial dysentery infection. The virus affects the mucosal lining of the bowels and causes irritation. The disease usually runs its course in 2 or 3 days. The discomfort comes about because the normal intestinal activities are completely disrupted, resulting in gas, vomiting, and diarrhea.

Treatment: See the section on *Common Cold* for bed rest and general relaxation. See sections on *Vomiting* and *Diarrhea* for treatment of these symptoms.

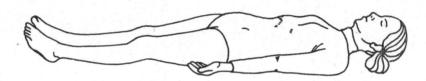

Your Doctor As A Resource: A doctor should be consulted if the symptoms do not improve within three days, or if dehydration occurs.

Prevention: Viral gastroenteritis is spread by the fecal-oral route. See page 91 for how to prevent infections that are spread in this way.

APPENDICITIS

Symptoms: *First Stage:*   Pain around the navel with loss of appetite, nausea and vomiting
             Second Stage: Pain in right lower quadrant of abdomen, made worse by coughing

Physical Exam: You will find tenderness in the right lower quadrant if person is in the second stage. The person may have a low fever and also be tense over their right lower quadrant. (See *Physical Exam* chapter for complete instructions on examining the abdomen.)

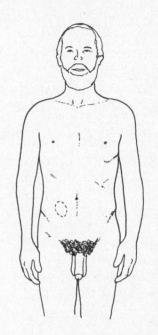

What's Going On?: The appendix is a small, hollow, finger-like projection of tissue that is a part of the large intestine. It usually is found in the right lower quadrant of the abdomen but is occasionally found elsewhere in the abdomen. The opening of the appendix can become blocked by a small piece of feces. When this happens the appendix cannot drain its contents into the intestine; it becomes a stagnant area where bacteria, which normally live in the intestines, can grow and multiply abnormally. These multiplying bacteria, and fluids produced by the body to protect itself, increase the pressure inside this condensed finger of tissue and causes the appendix to swell in size. The swollen appendix presses on blood vessels and impedes the normal flow of blood to the membranes around the intestines. These membranes are full of nerve endings which send pain messages to the brain.

Treatment: The diseased and swollen appendix must be removed surgically. If this is not done, the swelling can increase, rupture the appendix and the bacteria will be released into the abdomen causing serious infection throughout your body. *Never take laxatives, seltzers or pain medications if appendicitis is suspected.* Laxatives and seltzers can further damage the appendix, and pain medications will only mask the problem.

Your Doctor As A Resource: A doctor is necessary to help you cure appendicitis. They can do a white blood cell count to confirm the diagnosis. They can remove the appendix to prevent further problems in your body. In emergencies where a doctor is not available to remove the appendix, such as in remote wilderness areas or on an ocean voyage, large dosages of antibiotics can reduce swelling and prevent further problems until proper medical help can be gotten. The surgery for appendicitis is common and is very safe.

Prevention: Not applicable.

HEPATITIS

Symptoms:
Early phase (prodomal phase):
Tiredness
Muscle pains
Running nose and sore throat
Poor appetite
Nausea
Low fever
Possibly some mild abdominal pain in the right upper quadrant
Possibly a distaste for smoking
Middle phase (acute phase — clinical jaundice):
The person's eyes and skin turns yellow — five to ten days after the early symptoms
Urine turns dark brown
The stool turns light yellow to white
Healing phase:
Return of appetite

Physical Exam: You may feel a swollen liver (see *Physical Examination* chapter on liver). It may not be very large, and this is absent in over half the cases. It may be slightly tender. The person's temperature may be up from normal.

You can detect *jaundice* (yellowing of skin and eyes) by looking at the whites of the person's eyes in normal, outdoor light. Most incandescent lamps are slightly yellow and prevent you from really being able to recognize jaundice. So either use fluorescent lights or take the person next to an outside window to look at their eyes. Sometimes jaundice is difficult to detect.

What's Going On?: Hepatitis is a viral infection of the liver. There are two basic types: *Infectious Hepatitis* with a short incubation period (the time from exposure to appearance of symptoms) and *Serum Hepatitis* with a long incubation period. Infectious Hepatitis is a common disease in young people today.

Infectious Hepatitis occurs occasionally in isolated cases, sometimes in epidemics. The transmission of the virus is fecal/oral. This means that if a person has a bowel movement, wipes themself, and then doesn't wash their hands afterwards, the virus can be spread to other surfaces in the house that they touch. Kissing, smoking the same cigarette, drinking out of the same glass or eating from the same plate can also spread Hepatitis. Infectious Hepatitis tends to occur in crowded places ... colleges, military bases, communes. The virus is present in the faces during the early and middle phases of the disease.

Serum Hepatitis —long-incubation Hepatitis — is a different virus found in the blood and not usually excreted in the feces. The incubation period is six months and the disease is usually spread from one drug addict to another when they share the same syringe. Serum Hepatitis is actually a different disease than Infectious Hepatitis and is much less common.

Treatment: The treatment for both forms of Hepatitis is bed rest in the acute phase and low activity in the healing phase. It takes a tremendous amount of energy to recover from Hepatitis. The liver is a biochemical factory necessary in producing *glucose*, the energy substance of the body. So if a person's liver is sick, they need to conserve their energy much more than usual.

Nutrition is especially important: a difficult situation since people with Hepatitis usually have poor appetites. A high-protein, high-carbohydrate diet helps the liver heal itself (see *Preventive Medicine* chapter on diet). Brewers Yeast or B-complex vitamins can be taken to help stimulate the appetitie. Alcohol should definitely be avoided because it makes the liver work harder.

Relaxation and mellowing yourself out are very important in treating Hepatitis (see *Preventive Medicine* chapter on relaxation). Sometimes Hepatitis can be a disease with a long recovery time; it can even last four months. Lots of people with Hepatitis become very upset at the idea of being sick for so long. The fact that they're upset can impair their healing because they're constantly tense, uptight, and angry. We feel that if people can relax and enjoy the "vacation," an illness provides they're much more likely to get something out of their illness and be cured faster. We have known people with Hepatitis who use the vacation to think about their lives in creative ways and who come out of it having changed their lives for the better. Hepatitis is rarely a serious disease in young, healthy people.

Your Doctor As A Resource: Your doctor is valuable in treating Hepatitis. They can order tests to determine the severity of the illness. The two most common blood tests are the *SGOT enzyme test* which measures tissue damage and the *Bilirubin test* which measures the substance which causes the person to look yellow with jaundice. These tests tell a lot about how severe the Hepatitis is and about how well the healing is progressing. They're not essential — they don't make the person better — but they aid in telling the person how much energy they have to conserve. And they aid in diagnosing very mild cases. In rare cases of Hepatitis the doctor can help by feeding the person intravenously until he or she is well enough to eat by themselves. If severe nausea occurs, a doctor can prescribe anti-nausea drugs.

Prevention: Preventing Hepatitis can be more troublesome than treating it. The most important thing is cleanliness. Everyone should wash their hands after going to the bathroom. If there's a separate bathroom in the house, the person who has Hepatitis should use it; if not, everyone should wash their hands carefully. The person with Hepatitis should eat off their own plates and these plates should be cleaned separately. Also bed sheets should be laundered separately. This is usually enough isolation to prevent its spread. The risk of getting Hepatitis from a person in your home when these things are done (and it's understood that the transmission is fecal/oral) can be quite low.

There's a tremendous amount of paranoia and fear associated with having a person with Hepatitis in the same house. This fear can be worse than the Hepatitis. It can also lower your resistance. By creating muscle tension and abnormal blood flow it can increase a person's chances of getting the disease.

An injection of gamma globulin (GG), the antibody fraction of the blood, can lower the chance of a person getting Hepatitis or can make the case milder. GG is taken from the donated blood of many people. It is assumed that some of the donors have been exposed to Hepatitis and have formed antibodies to it. It's amazing to think of GG as antibodies from many unknown people helping you to stay healthy! GG shots are usually given to close household contacts or intimate contacts of known cases as soon as possible after the case is diagnosed. GG does not cure Hepatitis; it just gives the body some extra anti-bodies in addition to the ones it may already have.

HEMORRHOIDS
(Piles)

Symptoms: Itching, pain, and/or a small amount of bleeding around the anus

Physical Exam: Hemorrhoids appear as small, round, purple-colored growths or "tabs" of skin around the anal area. (See *Physical Examination* chapter for more details on examining the anus.)

What's Going On?: Hemorrhoids are widened veins around the anus. They may be inside the anus where they can't be seen, or they may be external where you will be easily able to see them. Essentially, they are varicose veins. See the *Varicose Veins* section of this chapter for details about what they are and how they are formed.

Constipation (straining to defecate), pregnancy, and possibly prolonged sitting make hemorrhoids more likely to occur.

Treatment: Avoid constipation by using the methods we describe in the section on *Constipation*. Warm baths — sitting a half hour in a warm tub once a day — relaxes the affected areas and allows your body to naturally shrink the hemorrhoids.

Your Doctor As A Resource: Hemorrhoids that don't respond to the above treatments can be surgically removed by a doctor. But this usually is not necessary.

Prevention: Avoid straining the anal area by using the methods described in the section on *Constipation*. The exercise in that section is especially helpful. Pregnant women and people who are suceptible to hemorrhoids, should especially do this exercise.

PINWORM INFECTION — ENTEROBIUS

Symptoms: Itching in the anal area, particularly at night
Possibly mild abdominal pain
Nausea
Poor appetite

Physical Exam: Pinworms can occasionally be seen in the anal area, but the diagnosis is not usually made visually.

What's Going On?: Enterobius vermicularis (pinworm) is a spindle-shaped round-worm. It's the most common worm infection in the United States. It is seen in all economic groups. Eggs are deposited in large numbers near the anus. They are infectious and can be transferred to other people by the anal/oral route. If a person goes to the bathroom, wipes themself, and then doesn't wash their hands, they can spread the eggs. Also, if a person handles clothing containing the eggs, and does not wash, they can become infected. The eggs are resistant to household disinfectants and can remain active in dust for a considerable time. Usually if one person in the house has pinworms, the other people in the house will get pinworms. There are generally no complications from it; it's not a dangerous disease. But the infection is annoying and for that reason it's valuable to treat it.

Treatment: Pinworms are usually treated with a prescription drug which rapidly kills the worms. The house — especially the bathroom — must be cleaned thoroughly to make sure that the eggs don't re-infect people. Underwear and sheets should be laundered in very hot water. People should wash their hands after going to the bathroom and they should carefully wash the anal area when they bathe.

Your Doctor As A Resource: The doctor is helpful in that he or she can definitely diagnose pinworms by putting a piece of scotch tape next to the infected person's anus to pick up the eggs which can be identified under the microscope. Some doctors will treat pinworms without an actual microscopic examination.

Prevention: Pinworms can be prevented by cleanliness and by avoiding exposure to people who have pinworms.

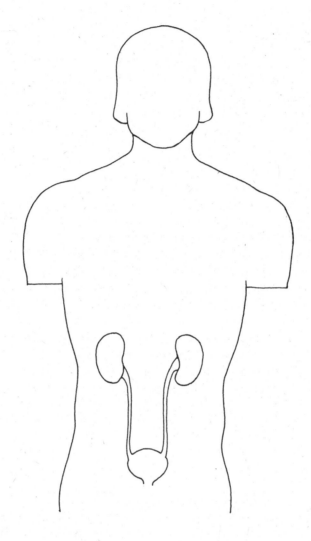

GENITOURINARY

In this section we include discussions of diseases which involve both men and women. Some of these are very minor, some are more difficult to heal. In considering this section understand that we are talking about both external and internal organs, all of which help to make up the Reproductive System, and/or the Urinary System.

VAGINAL DISCHARGES — VAGINAL INFECTIONS

Symptoms: Fluid coming out of the vagina in a greater than normal amount
Itching
Pain during intercourse
Rash on the outside of the vagina
Burning on urination

Physical Exam: When doing the external vaginal exam you will see a discharge present on the vulva. You may possibly see some inflammation and redness in the area. There may be a rash or sores in the area of the vagina. On internal vaginal exam (speculum exam) you will see a discharge and redness and swelling of the mucosa in the vagina. (See the *Physical Exam* chapter for full instructions on examining the vagina.)

What's Going On?: Many organisms normally live in the vagina. When healthy, the vagina is like a village living in ecological harmony. Bacteria, monilia (a yeast-like fungus), and trichomonas (a one-celled organism) co-exist in amounts that normally produce no symptoms. Temperature, moisture, surface tension, and acid-base balance usually keep the numbers of the organisms in balance. Several glands in the body secrete hormones which affect these factors. The secretions of the glands are directly influenced by the mind. When hormonal balance, or other environmental factors change, one organism in the vagina can over-reproduce at the expense of the others. This disturbance of the normal balance produces the symptoms of a vaginal infection.

The most common organisms that grow excessively in young women are monilia, trichomonas, and a bacteria called hemophilus. It is difficult to differentiate between the different types of vaginal infection on physical exam. For this reason, a smear is usually taken by the doctor. When a sample of the discharge is examined under the microscope, the different organisms can easily be identified.

Vaginal infections often occur when the normal bacterial balance is upset. This can be due to antibiotic therapy, which kills sensitive bacteria in the body. It can also be due to frequent douching with antiseptic preparations. Vaginal infections may be more likely to occur in women taking birth control pills because oral contraceptives alter the body's normal hormonal balance. Pregnant women are also susceptible to vaginal infections for this reason.

Monilia grows best in warm, moist areas of the body. It is often seen in women who wear nylon underwear, which does not breathe. It is also seen in women who wear leather pants.

Anxiety and tension make it much more likely for some women to get vaginal infections. Emotional factors influence hormonal balance and muscle tension in the vaginal area. Muscle tension decreases blood flow, which changes the vaginal environment, encouraging one organism or another to overgrow.

Treatment: Monilia is treated with an anti-fungal agent in the form of suppositories. Vinegar douche (two tablespoons of white vinegar to a quart of water) can be used in mild infections. Vinegar changes the acid-base balance of the vagina to acid which makes it more difficult for the monilia to grow. Trichomonas is usually treated with a pill containing anti-trichomonal chemicals. Some doctors also treat the woman's mate because trichomonas can be carried by the man and given back to the woman. Douching with water helps your body heal itself of mild trichomonas infections. Hemophilus is usually treated with antibiotic vaginal creams. Non-prescription douches, which druggists can suggest, are helpful in mild cases.

Relaxation of the muscles around the vagina is very helpful in curing vaginal infections of all kinds. An exercise we find effective is:

Lie down and make yourself comfortable. Do the relaxation exercise that you used to get your imaginary doctor. Concentrate on relaxing the muscles around your vagina; let your muscles feel loose. Imagine blood flowing into the area, bringing healing energy. Imagine that your vagina feels vibrant and tingles. Picture the mucosa in your vagina as pink, slightly moist, and healthy. Do this each day, with or without other treatment, until healed.

Another useful exercise is:

Lie on the floor on your back, with your head and shoulders on two pillows. Bend your knees up, keeping your feet on the floor. Let your knees spread as far as you can, with the soles of your feet touching each other. Relax the muscles in your vaginal area. Place your hand over your vagina so you can feel the muscles relax. Rest in this position as long as you wish. This exercise stretches the muscles and tendons in the vaginal area and helps you loosen up.

Resolution of emotional conflict is extremely important in curing vaginal infections. One doctor we know treats chronic vaginal discharges with psychotherapy and hypnosis. He gets excellent results.

Your Doctor As A Resource: Your doctor can do a smear and identify the organism causing the vaginal infection. They can prescribe a suppository, pill, or cream to treat the particular organism causing your infection. They can also do a test for gonorrhea, which is another common, more serious cause of a vaginal discharge (see section on *Gonorrhea*). If you are sexually active, you should have a test done to be sure that your discharge is not caused by gonorrhea. Your doctor may also want to do a urine analysis to make sure that burning on urination is not caused by a urinary tract infection (see section on *Urinary Tract Infections*). They can do a speculum exam to make sure that the infection does not involve the cervix (see section on *Cervicitis*). If you have an intra-uterine device, the doctor can check it during the speculum exam. An infected intra-uterine device can also be a cause of vaginal discharge (see section on *Tubal Infections*).

Prevention: You should avoid nylon underwear and leather pants if you are prone to vaginitis. Avoid excessive douching and douching with strong chemical preparations. Most doctors now recomend douching only for treating vaginal infections, not for routine cleanliness. Early treatment of a mild vaginal infection by the methods discussed in the treatment section can prevent a more serious infection.

Learning how to relax the muscles in the vaginal area is helpful in preventing vaginal infections. Relaxed pelvic muscles help maintain the vaginal flora (normal bacteria) at a healthy balance. To prevent getting a vaginal infection following antibiotic treatment it may be helpful to eat acidophilus yoghurt, a bacteria (available at health food stores). One doctor we know even recomends douching with diluted yoghurt while you are taking antibiotics.

CERVIX INFECTION — CERVICITIS

Symptoms: Vaginal discharge
Some back pain (occasionally)
Sometimes pain during intercourse
Sometimes burning upon urination

Physical Exam: You will see a discharge on the external vulva. On internal exam the cervix will appear red and swollen with a great deal of discharge. Sometimes white plaques may be seen on the cervix and the discharge may contain pus and blood. (See the *Physical Exam* chapter for instructions for vaginal examination.)

What's Going On? Cervicitis is an inflammation of the cervix, which is the lower part of the uterus. It is the most common gynecological problem women can have; it is said that over 50% of all women eventually get a cervix inflammation. Cervicitis can be due to infections following the delivery of a baby. Gonorrhea and other bacteria can cause cervicitis in non-pregnant women. Birth control pills produce a mild, chronic cervicitis.

Treatment: Cervicitis is treated with antibiotics. If the inflammation doesn't respond to antibiotic treatment, the doctor may cauterize the cervix with a silver nitrate solution or freeze it, which brings about healing.

Your Doctor As A Resource: Cervicitis should be treated by a doctor. They can do a culture to determine what bacteria is causing the infection and treat it with the appropriate antibiotic. In a chronic infection they can cauterize the cervix.

Prevention: Early treatment of minor vaginal infections may help to prevent cervicitis. Good hygiene may also help, but routine douching is not recommended. You should see your obstetrician after the birth of a baby. They may find and treat you for a mild cervical inflammation.

GONORRHEA

Symptoms: **Female:**   At least half of the women who have had gonorrhea
report having no symptoms
May have green, pus-like vaginal discharge.
Burning sensation on urination.

267

Urinating more than usual
Pain in lower abdomen
Pain during intercourse
Swollen lymph nodes near vagina

Male: Occassionally, males have no symptoms
Green, pus-like discharge from penis
Burning on urination
Itching feeling in the penis (urethral itching)
Swollen lymph nodes in genital area

Physical Exam: Female: On the external examination of the vagina usually nothing is seen. Sometimes you may see swollen, red mucosa, especially around the urethral opening. On internal examination, using a speculum, you will see a green, pus-like discharge around the vaginal walls and the cervix. In some cases nothing will be seen. There may be tenderness in the lower abdomen. (See the *Physical Examination* chapter for complete instructions for doing pelvic exams.)

Physical Exam: Male: The tip of the urethra — opening of the penis — may be red and swollen. The testicles, or tubes, may be tender.

What's Going On?: Gonorrhea is an infectious disease caused by the bacteria *neisseria gonorrhorea*. It is a bacterial infection similar to a strep throat or pneumonia infection. Neither your body nor the bacteria make a moral judgment about it. The infection involves the mucous membranes of the genital and urinary tract. This is the environment in which the gonorrhea bacteria grows best. It can also grow in other mucous membranes of the body, such as mouth and rectum. It is spread only through sexual contact. It is not caught from contact with toilet seats.

The period between exposure and the appearance of first symptoms (incubation period) is 2 to 10 days. At the present time (1973) gonorrhea infections are so widespread that we must consider it an epidemic. Anyone who is sexually active, who is having sex with more than one person, and with people who are having sexual relations with more than one person, should consider themselves highly susceptible to getting gonorrhea.

In an untreated gonorrhea infection the bacteria will spread to other areas of the person's body. In a woman, bacteria will spread from the vagina to the cervix, uterus, and the tubes leading from the ovaries to the vagina. (See *Tubal Infection* in this chapter for more on this.)

In a man, the infection can spread from his penis to his prostate gland, tubes and testes.

In both male and female the bacteria can be carried in the blood to the person's joints, lungs, and heart. These complications can be dangerous, so gonorrhea should always be promptly treated.

People who have had sex with a person who has a case of *diagnosed* gonorrhea should get treatment to prevent the bacteria from growing in their own system.

Treatment: Gonorrhea must be treated with antibiotics. Your body can easily heal itself with the help of these drugs.

Your Doctor As A Resource: Your doctor can really help you with gonorrhea. In a man, the doctor can diagnose gonorrhea by examining a sample of the discharge (a smear) with a microscope. In a woman, the doctor can diagnose the gonorrhea by taking a sample of the discharge from her cervix. He puts this sample on a "nutrient plate" and grows it in a special incubator for two days. This is what's known as a "culture." If gonorrhea is present, the doctor will prescribe antibiotics to help your body heal itself.

After treatment for gonorrhea, a man should not have sexual intercourse for one week. A woman should abstrain until she has had a second culture to show that the bacteria is no longer present in her body.

Prevention: Few cases of gonorrhea are seen with people who have only one sexual partner who, in turn, has only one sexual partner. This is the surest way to prevent gonorrhea.

If you are having sexual relations with more than one person, or your sexual partner is having sex with people other than you, then *condoms* (rubbers) will be of some use in helping to prevent gonorrhea infection.

Keep in touch with your body's messages, especially messages from your genitals. Early diagnosis and early treatment of gonorrhea, and other infections in the genital area, can prevent its spread and complications.

Most county health departments throughout the United States have VD Clinics which will give free tests and treatment for gonorrhea and other venereal infections. They are also happy to give free counseling and information on any and all aspects about venereal disease.

TUBAL INFECTION — PELVIC INFLAMMATORY DISEASE (P.I.D.) — SALPINGITIS

Symptoms: Severe, cramp-like pains in the lower abdomen (see drawing below)
Often chills and fever
Vaginal discharge
Lymph node swelling

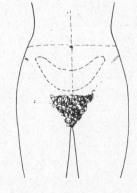

Physical Exam: You will find that the person is very tender to the touch in the tubal area of the belly. The back wall of the vagina will also be tender to touch.

What's Going On?: Salpingitis is an inflammation and infection of the Fallopian tubes which lead from the ovaries to the uterus. It's also called Tubal Infection and Pelvic Inflammatory Disease (P.I.D.). It is most often due to a bacterial infection such as gonorrhea. Streptococcus and mixed bacterial infections can also cause salpingitis. It can also result from an infected intra-uterine device; this is most frequently seen in women who have not had children.

Many women are afraid that a tubal infection will make them sterile. The infection can "wall" itself off in a tube, thus blocking the tube. After the infection drains down into the vagina, the "walls" can remain. These walls are what doctors call *membranous adhesions,* which can block the tube and prevent eggs from reaching the uterus. This happens in some severe cases of tubal infection, certainly not all. I think it is important for a woman who has a tubal infection to have a positive attitude toward curing it and not be afraid of becoming sterile. Worry produces tension and cramping in the area where the infection is and reduces blood flow to the area. This prevents both the body's own antibodies and antibiotics from reaching the site of the infection.

Treatment: Systemic (administered for the whole body) antibiotics are used to treat the bacterial infection. They kill off the bacteria, thereby assisting the body's normal healing mechanisms. Pain is controlled with aspirin or stronger medicines if necessary. Heat applied to the lower abdomen may make the person feel more comfortable and speed the healing. Bed rest is important because it takes a great deal of energy to cure a tubal infection.

We find that it is very helpful to do relaxation exercises. They can relieve worry and eliminate muscular tension. This will bring greater blood flow and antibiotics to the area and relieve pain. The following is an exercise that we suggest for relaxing:

> Make yourself comfortable. Do the relaxation exercise that you used to get your imaginary doctor. Concentrate on relaxing the area around your Fallopian tubes. Imagine that the area is warm and pulsing with energy. Think about an area of your body that feels perfectly healthy to you; now imagine that feeling is spreading down to the area of the infection. Picture the Fallopian tubes themselves; imagine that they are open and draining and lined with pink, healthy mucosa.

Your Doctor As A Resource: A doctor is helpful in diagnosing salpingitis. They can take a culture and determine which bacteria is causing the infection. Then they can treat you with the proper antibiotic. They may do a white blood cell count which, if it is high, indicates an infection.

Prevention: Early treatment of gonorrhea and other pelvic infections is most important in preventing tubal infections. If you have an intra-uterine device, it's important to have it checked if you notice any symptoms of infection. You are in control of preventing tubal infections and keeping your body entirely well.

BARTHOLIN CYST

Symptoms: Painful swelling on either side of the lower part (labia) of the vagina

Pain on intercourse

Fatness in the bottom of the labia

Physical Exam: The bottom of the vagina will look distorted. You will see a swelling that is red and hot and feels fluid-filled. The swelling is often tender to the touch.

What's Going On?: There are two small glands, called Bartholin's glands, in the lower sides of the vagina. The ducts of the glands can become blocked. Then stasis can occur and bacteria can grow, causing an infection.

Treatment: An infection of Bartholin's glands is treated with a "broad spectrum" antibiotic. (See the chapter *Drugs Are Helpers*.) Local heat on the infected area is very important — hot soaks increase the blood flow and bring the body's antibody healing mechanism to the site. This helps to relieve the blockage and allows the gland to drain normally. Usually antibiotics and heat are enough to cure the cyst.

Your Doctor As A Resource: Your doctor can prescribe an antibiotic to treat the infection. Sometimes the cyst has to be surgically removed by a doctor after the infection cures. This completes healing.

Prevention: Prompt treatment of all vaginal infections is the best prevention.

SYPHILLIS

Symptoms: **First Stage:**   A sore in genital, anal or mouth area

Second Stage: Rash anywhere on the body

May be sore throat, loss of hair, runny eyes

Physical Exam: *The first stage:* You will find a red, raised area which turns into an open, red sore. It often is not tender to the touch. This sore is often found on a hardened area of skin. The lymph nodes nearest to the sore will be enlarged and may be tender.

In the second stage: Raised, flat, red sores can be found anywhere on the person's body. They often look like a total body rash. The person's throat may look inflamed and red. Patchy hair loss may be seen on their head and/or body. Mucous membranes around their eyes may be red and swollen.

What's Going On: Syphillis used to be known as "the great imitator" because its symptoms were so much like so many other diseases. It is caused by a spiral shaped organism called *treponema pallidum* spread by sexual contact. After exposure to a

271

syphillis sore, the spiral organisms multiply slowly on the skin. Then 2 to 10 weeks later the first stage sore appears, and spiral organisms enter the person's body to remain there until treated. If untreated, the sore disappears by itself and 6 or more weeks later the second stage symptoms appear. If untreated, these symptoms also disappear, but the spiral organisms are still in the body. Years later, these organisms cause severe damage to the person's heart, brain and eyes. A pregnant mother who has syphillis will pass it on to her child.

Because the symptoms of syphillis are much like the symptoms of other diseases, they are accurately diagnosed only by laboratory tests. There are two tests: in one, fluid from the first stage sore is examined under a microscope to detect any spiral organisms; the second is a blood test (VDRL), to test for the presence of antibodies which your body produces if the organism is present.

Treatment: Syphillis is easily cured with antibiotics.

Your Doctor As A Resource: A doctor can accurately diagnose syphillis and can prescribe antibiotics to cure it. After this antibiotic therapy they should do a repeat blood test (VDRL) to make certain that the spiral organism is no longer present in your body.

Prevention: Most county health departments throughout the United States have VD Clinics which will give free tests for Syphillis and Gonorrhea. They are also happy to give free counseling and information on any and all aspects about venereal disease. Condoms may be of some value in preventing the spread of Syphillis.

ACUTE URINARY TRACT INFECTION

Symptoms:
Chills and fever
Burning on urination
A desire to urinate more often than usual
Urinating more often than usual
A feeling that you want to urinate sometimes when you can't
Pain or tenderness in the flanks
Backache
Occasionally bloody urine
Sometimes nausea and vomiting

Physical Exam: The person's lower back may be tender. To test for this, "punch" lightly in the area indicated by the drawing. This is the area over the kidneys. Also, the person's temperature may be elevated.

What's Going On?: Urinary tract infections are caused by bacteria, most commonly by *E. coli*, the bacteria normally present in the intestines. The infection usually involves the bladder, the tubes leading to the bladder and kidneys, and sometimes the kidneys themselves. This infection is most common in young women. It can be caused by a partial blockage in the urinary tract. The blockage causes an irritation, and the area around the irritation becomes swollen. This makes the blockage worse and causes the urine behind it to become partly stagnant. The stagnant urine is a place where bacteria can breed easily. The urine, which is completely sterile in a healthy person, becomes full of bacteria and pus (white blood cells fighting the infection). The bacteria and blood cells in the urine cause the burning sensation when you urinate.

Treatment: Urinary tract infections are always treated with antibiotics. Drinking a lot of liquids helps remove the stagnant condition and wash out the urinary tract. Bed rest helps you conserve your energy for healing the infection.

Your Doctor As A Resource: A doctor can help you heal yourself of a urinary tract infection. They can examine the urine under a microscope and identify bacteria and blood cells, which are not present in normal urine. They can culture the bacteria to determine the type it is and which antibiotic it is sensitive to. They can then prescribe the proper antibiotic. They can do a culture two weeks after treatment to see that you are healed.

When a person gets several urinary tract infections in a short time, doctors often take an x-ray of the urinary tract to see if there is a definite obstruction causing the infections.

Prevention: Some doctors believe that not urinating for a long time after you feel the urge makes it more likely that you will get a urinary infection. Drinking a lot of fluids may also help prevent urinary infections. Early treatment of a urinary tract infection and cultures after treatment can help prevent permanent kidney damage. If you have ever had a urinary infection, be especially alert to messages from your urinary tract.

NONSPECIFIC URETHRITIS (N.S.U.)

Symptoms: Burning on urination
Itching or pain in the urethra, the tube leading from the bladder
     to the penis or vagina

Physical Exam: You may see red, swollen mucosa around the tip of the urethra. (See *Physical Examination* chapter on examining the male and female genitalia). You may also see a discharge at the tip of the urethra. Often you may see nothing.

What's Going On?: N.S.U. is an inflammation of the urethra. It is called "nonspecific" because it is usually impossible to identify the organism causing it. It may be caused by bacteria which normally live in the genital tract, in a nonspecific urethritis, these organisms would become much more numerous. It may be caused by mycoplasma, an organism which is neither a virus nor a bacteria.

A male may show symptoms of N.S.U. after contact with a person who has trichomonas (see *Diagnosis and Treatment* section on Vaginal Discharges). Nonspecific urethritis may be caused by irritation from frequent sexual activity. Heavy alcohol consumption may be related; the alcohol is passed in the urine and can irritate the urethra. N.S.U. often follows a treated gonorrhea infection, possibly due to damage in the urethra caused by the infection. Urethritis can be caused by a narrowing of the urethral tube (a stricture); sometimes these can be anatomical, or they may be caused by a gonorrhea infection, both of which are correctable.

Treatment: N.S.U. will often respond to treatment with the antibiotic tetracycline. Your body can usually heal itself from a nonspecific urethritis if you prevent irritation to the urethra. To do this, avoid drinking alcohol or coffee, and eating spicy foods. Also avoid frequent sexual activity until the N.S.U. is healed. Drinking a lot of fluids probably washes the urethra and helps to cure the infection. The infection can take as long as a month to heal completely.

Your Doctor As A Resource: Your doctor can help you in diagnosing N.S.U. by doing a smear and a culture (see *Diagnosis and Treatment* section on Gonorrhea). If no organisms are found (especially gonorrhea) with these tests, the diagnosis of nonspecific urethritis is confirmed. If this is the case, the doctor can prescribe tetracycline for you. Due to the present epidemic of gonorrhea, you should have your doctor do laboratory tests for any symptoms of N.S.U. In cases of repeated N.S.U. infections you should consult a urologist who can check to see if you have a narrowing in the urethra (stricture).

Prevention: Early diagnosis and treatment of gonorrhea can prevent strictures that will cause N.S.U. If you are prone to urethritis, try to avoid excessive alcohol consumption and very frequent sexual contact.

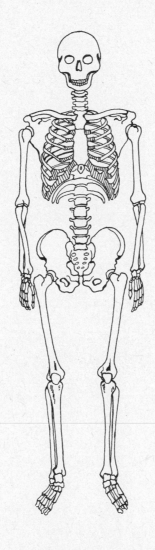

EXTREMITIES

In this section we deal with complaints associated with bones and muscle, with things that go wrong when the energy exchanges between blood, muscle, and bone are not completely harmonious. Actual breaks in bones and bleeding are not dealt with here. But we tell you how to deal with them in the *Emergency Medicine* chapter.

LOWER BACK PAIN

Symptoms: Pain in the lower back, made worse by movement
Pain sometimes shooting down the legs
Sometimes tingling feeling in legs

Physical Exam: You will find tense muscles in the person's back and legs. You may find these areas tender to the touch as you examine the person. The person's back may appear to be bent to one side or another.

What's Going On?: The back is a very complicated structure. There are cartilaginous (tough, fibrous tissue) discs between the vertebrae (small bones in the back) which allow the vertebrae to move. Spinal nerves come out between the vertebrae and go down to the legs and to other areas of the body.

Sometimes, while picking up an object while your back muscles are tense, or during unexpected twisting, the muscles that surround the nerves will become stretched and will cramp. The cramping causes poor blood supply to nerves and muscles, and this produces the pain of back ache. Some people can even get a low back pain by getting out of bed the wrong way.

In my experience, the pain can take place when a person is in a tense situation, rushing, or not paying attention to what they're doing. It can take place when doing things improperly: lifting improperly, or bending improperly. People who exert themselves when they are not accustomed to using their muscles are prone to lower back pain.

Treatment: Rest in bed in the position which gives you the greatest relief and comfort. The most comfortable position is often lying on your side. The bed should be firm, and if you have a soft bed you should use a board under the mattress for extra support.

Total body massage, concentrating on the lower back areas, will also help relax muscles and make the person more comfortable. For more information about doing a total body massage, see *The Massage Book*, by George Downing and Anne Kent Rush, published by Random House/The Bookworks.

Understand that the middle and upper part of the back can be affected in ways similar to what we describe in lower back pain. The treatments, too, are similar.

☆   ☆   ☆

The following are techniques used by chiropractors and doctors to relieve mild back pain. Note that there are three different techniques: for upper, for middle, and for lower back pain.

If the pain is in the person's upper back or neck have them drop their chin to their chest. Tell them to relax and let it drop, but to not force it in any way. Now stand behind them and cup their chin in your right hand; at the same time spread your left hand over the back of their head.

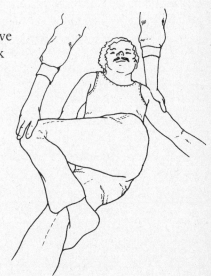

Support their head fully so that they can relax their muscles. Then gently turn their head 90 degrees to the left, then 90 degrees to the right. Go back and forth slowly. This usually brings relief in a short time. One or more treatments may be necessary.

If the pain is in the person's middle back, stand behind them and wrap both your arms around their chest. In order for this to work you will have to be at least as tall as the person with whom you are working. If you are not, try standing on a step above them or on a telephone book as you lift.

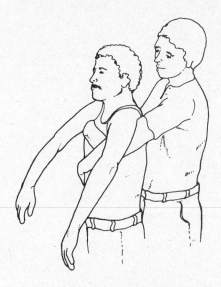

Tell the person to relax. Now squeeze and lift. Sometimes you will hear some popping as you do this.

If the person's pain is in their lower back: Have the person lie on their back on the floor, and ask them to lift one leg, flexing it at the knee. Then have them hook their toes under the straight leg.

Let's say that the person has lifted their left leg. Now kneel down at the person's right side and place your left hand on their left shoulder to hold their shoulder down firmly against the floor. At the same time draw their flexed knee over their right leg until that knee touches the floor. Do one side of their body and then do the other side. By rotating the lower part of the back from right to left in this way you can bring relief almost immediately.

In most cases of lower back pain it is difficult to tell if the pain is actually emanating from the middle or lower back regions. So we recommend doing both the lift technique and the roll technique whenever lower back pain is experienced.

Aspirin may be used to relieve some of the symptoms of lower back pain.

Your Doctor As A Resource: Your doctor can prescribe muscle-relaxing drugs to relieve the symptoms of lower back pain. In cases of severe, unrelenting back pain the doctor can take x-rays to rule out other, rarer causes.

Prevention: Pay attention to your body, especially the way you use your back to lift. Use your leg muscles to do the lifting, rather than lifting from a touch-your-toes position. Your spine is not structurally designed to lift heavy objects from this latter position. Pay particular attention to the way you are using your back whenever you are tense, rushed, or are doing a task which you do not enjoy doing. People with histories of back pain would do well to pay particular attention to how their backs feel as they lift and move.

The next most important factor in preventing back pain is to strengthen the back muscles. You can do this by regularly doing the exercises which we have described in the exercise section of *Preventive Medicine*. Understand that you should do these exercises only when your back is feeling good — *not* during an episode of back pain. Doctors now believe that regular exercise of the back, such as we describe, can prevent back pain even in people who have had many episodes of pain throughout their lives.

VARICOSE VEINS

Symptoms:
Swollen legs
Leg cramps
Visibly widened veins in the legs
Fatigue or pain in the lower legs after long periods of
standing up

Physical Exam: You will be able to easily see thickened veins and perhaps swelling in the person's leg or legs when they stand.

What's Going On?: *Veins* are blood vessels that carry the blood from your feet and legs (and elsewhere) back to your heart. (*Arteries* are blood vessels that carry your blood from your heart to your extremities and all other parts of your body). The veins in your legs have tiny valves that prevent blood from returning to the lower parts of your legs, drawn toward the earth by gravity. Deeper veins in your legs are surrounded by muscles which support them and aid in returning blood to your heart. Veins close to your skin are surrounded only by a thin layer of fat which does not support them.

Pregnancy, being overweight, or many hours standing on your feet tend to increase the pressure in the veins of a person's legs. The veins close to the skin can then become stretched to the point that the valves cease to work. Then the weight of the blood in the veins actually stretches the veins themselves, causing the symptoms characteristic of varicose veins.

Treatment: Whenever possible, elevate your legs so that they are level with your heart. Avoid prolonged periods of standing. These measures are effective in people prone to varicose veins: people who are overweight, pregnant women, and people who spend hours on their feet. Elastic supportive stockings provide external support for the otherwise poorly supported veins.

Your Doctor As A Resource: A doctor can remove severe varicose veins if they cause you discomfort in your legs or if you are disturbed about the way they look.

Prevention: If you are prone to varicose veins be particularly careful about standing for long periods of time. Elevate your legs whenever possible. Elastic stockings will also help prevent varicose veins. See the exercises in the *Preventive Medicine* chapter for strengthening leg muscles. Such exercises will help increase circulation and support veins.

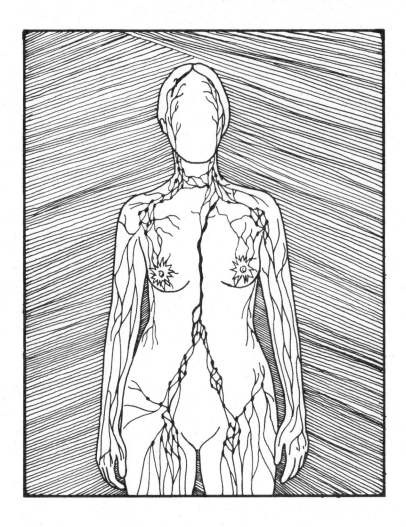

LYMPH SYSTEM

Your lymph system involves your entire body and is the system through which harmful bacteria are destroyed and rendered harmless. If you want to know more about lymph, see the explanatory drawing on page 341. The drawing above is a "map" of the lymph system, showing its main routes in the human body. We deal with only one disease in this section, *Mononucleosis. Lymphangtis* is another disease of the lymph system, but since its symptoms are usually associated with the skin we tell you about it in the *Skin* section.

INFECTIOUS MONONUCLEOSIS

Symptoms: Tiredness
                   Fever
                   Sore throat
                   Painful swollen glands in the neck, armpits, and groin
                   Pain in the left upper quadrant of the abdomen
                   Occasionally, yellow jaundice

Physical Exam: You will find enlarged lymph nodes in the neck, armpits, and groin, a red swollen throat, and sometimes a fine red rash over the body. The person may also have enlarged tonsils and a fever.

What's Going On?: Mononucleosis is an infection of the lymph system caused by the Ebstein Barr virus. It occurs most often in people between the ages of 10 and 35. The virus is probably spread in airborne droplets such as in coughing and sneezing. It may occur in single cases or in epidemics. In addition to affecting the lymph system, it can affect the nervous system (causing a headache), and the lungs, (causing a cough). Mononucleosis can also affect the liver, causing yellow jaundice. The illness can last from two weeks to two months.

Treatment: The person should remain in bed and rest while they have a fever. It takes a tremendous amount of energy to heal yourself from mononucleosis. A high-carbohydrate, high-protein diet is important. (see *Treatment* section of *Hepatitis*). Treat the fever and sore throat as discussed in those sections.

Your Doctor As A Resource: Your doctor can do an antibody test to diagnose mononucleosis.

Prevention: Mononucleosis is a communicable disease; avoid exposure to people who have it. The person is communicable from just before the symptoms appear until the fever and sore throat are gone. While they are contagious, the person should carefully dispose of tissues and they should wash their hands after coughing or blowing their nose. They should cover their mouth and nose when they do cough or sneeze to prevent airborne spread of the virus. People should avoid fatigue and keep themselves in a good state of nutrition, especially if someone in their home has mononucleosis. For more information, see the *Preventive Medicine* chapter on sleep, diet, and rest-work cycles.

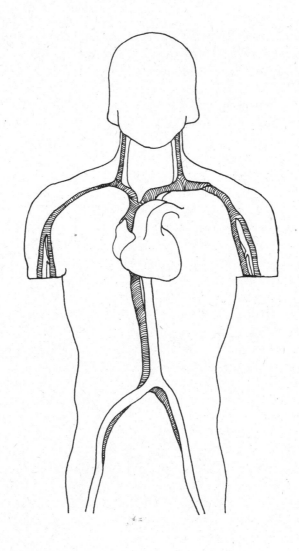

BLOOD SYSTEM

Your blood system involves your entire body and is the system through which nutriments are carried to every cell. If you want to know more about blood and what it does, see pages 339 to 340. We deal with only one disease in this Section, *Anemia*. For "Blood Poisoning" see page 211.

ANEMIA

Symptoms: Pale skin and pale mucous membranes
Weakness

Physical Exam: The person will look pale. Draw down their lower eyelid and examine the conjunctiva. (See the chapter on doing a *Physical Examination* for details.) In an anemic person, this conjunctiva will look whitish pink rather than a healthy vibrant pink.

What's Going On?: Anemia occurs when the number of red blood cells in your body is low, or when the chemical carrying oxygen in your blood (hemoglobin) is low. Hemoglobin contains iron, and the most common cause of anemia is iron deficiency. The most common cause of iron deficiency is loss of blood during menstral periods, or in childbirth, when people do not supplement their usual diet with iron. It can take as long as 3 months for a person's natural iron reserve in their body to return to normal after blood loss. In general, if a woman's diet contains iron-rich foods (such as liver) she will not need iron pills to supplement the iron lost in menstruation. With very heavy menstral bleeding she may need an iron supplement. With childbirth, women should take iron supplement pills for at least four months before and after delivery.

Television commercials have deluded many of us into believing that all people who are *tired* are anemic and need iron to restore their energy. The fact is that iron will not give you energy if you are not anemic. If you have symptoms of anemia, your doctor can give you a blood test to tell if you are anemic, and tell you how much of an iron supplement you need.

Treatment: Once you have determined that you are anemic, iron pills to supplement your diet slowly build your body's iron stores back to a healthy level. Supplementation must be extended over a period of several months in order to be effective. See *Your Doctor As A Resource,* below, for how to determine if you are anemic.

Your Doctor As A Resource: Your doctor can give you a blood test to determine if you actually are anemic. If you are, they then will determine the cause of your anemia. Anemia should not be treated without determining the cause since the anemia may be the result of uncommon conditions, such as slowly bleeding ulcers or hemorrhoids, which need treatment themselves.

Prevention: Supplemental iron in your diet for the whole term of pregnancy and for four months after childbirth will prevent iron deficiency anemias. Include enough iron in your diet (See the diet section of *The Preventive Medicine* chapter) to meet your normal body needs.

COMING OUT HEALTHY

Many people manifest the symptoms of diseases which they are studying as they first learn about them. It is a common experience in medical school for students to develop mild symptoms, of the very diseases they are learning to heal. This proves the power of your imagination to affect your health. We believe that since imagination can create disease you can also use it to create health. Here is an exercise to prevent your getting any of the symptoms that you read about, and to make you healthier than you were when you started:

> Make yourself comfortable. Do the relaxation exercise that you did for getting your imaginary doctor. Then let your ideas of all disease symptoms that you have read about, become bubbles in your consciousness. Now imagine that these bubbles are being blown out of your mind, out of your body, out of your consciousness by a breeze which draws them away from you, far into the distance, until you no longer see them or feel them. Watch them disappear over the horizon.
>
> Now imagine that you are in a place that you love. It may be the beach, in the mountains, on the desert, or wherever else you feel fully alive, comfortable, and healthy. Imagine the area around you is filled with bright, clear light. Allow the light to flow into your body, making you brighter, and filling you with the energy of health. Enjoy basking in this light for a moment. Then open your eyes, look around you, and either say to yourself, or feel, "I am coming out healthy. I am healthier and feel stronger than I have ever felt before."

This exercise will actually help you focus your healing energy in order to rid yourself of mild symptoms. Use it whenever you feel that you need it.

EMERGENCY MEDICINE

In this chapter we tell you how to approach emergencies calmly and effectively. We focus on how to deal with fear and panic, and what possibilities there actually are that you might ever have to face a medical emergency situation. We tell you what you can do and/or what medical people do in a number of emergencies in which relatively fast actions are helpful to the healing process.

However, the chapter is not intended to be used as a first aid manual, but rather as a supplement to one. If you want to study complete details on handling all types of emergencies, take a look at our list of books on the subject in *Going Further*.

☆   ☆   ☆

Here are the emergency situations we discuss:

287 — Bee Stings
287 — Bleeding
289 — Breathing: Blockage, choking, etc.
290 — Broken Bones
290 — Burns
291 — Dog Bites
291 — Drowning
291 — Electric Shock
291 — Head Injuries
292 — Neck Injuries
292 — Nose Bleeds
293 — Poisoning
294 — Resuscitation: Person has stopped breathing and/or person's
            heart has stopped beating
295 — Shock

Following the descriptions of these emergencies are directions for *Putting Together Your Own First Aid Kit*, (page 296), and an overview called *Preventing Medical Emergencies*. If you do not wish to read through all the medical emergencies, we suggest that you read only *Bleeding, Burns*, and *Resuscitation*, and then move on to read *Preventing Medical Emergencies*. This will give you at least a cursory overview of emergencies, and how to handle them.

EMERGENCY POSSIBILITIES:

Many people live in dread of a medical emergency. This dread has been instilled in them partly by television shows which depict emergency situations. In actuality, medical emergencies are uncommon. A study done by a magazine for doctors that deals with emergencies showed that a busy doctor didn't see more than four emergencies a month. If you think about how many medical emergencies you have been involved in during your life, you will probably find that there have been very few. And if you think of how many of those have been serious enough to dread, the number will be even smaller.

Many people think of a medical emergency as something that has to be dealt with in a split second. In actuality, in most medical emergencies you have plenty of time to administer first aid (if necessary) and get the person to a hospital.

HOW TO HANDLE EMERGENCIES:

The first thing to do in a medical emergency is to *relax*. Fear and anxiety in an emergency prevent you from dealing effectively with it. These are learned reactions, and they can be unlearned. *Being calm* is the most valuable skill you can have in treating an emergency. Your calmness will enable you to determine the extent of the injury quickly and thoroughly. Fear often causes people to overlook important findings or to run around, doing things in inefficient ways.

Your calmness is an important treatment for the injured person. When you are calm, it will help them to relax. Relaxation can slow down bleeding, make breathing easier and relieve pain.

Here is an exercise that can relax and calm you in an emergency:

Close your eyes for a moment. Take several long deep breaths.

Breathe slowly and rhythmically. As you breathe, imagine that your body is becoming more relaxed with each breath. Feel the relaxation spreading through your whole body. Let your mind be blank. Just count the breaths. Count *one* as you breath in and *two* as you breathe out, and so on. If you have a thought, let it come and go but do not hold onto it. When you feel relaxed, open your eyes. You are now calm and ready to help the injured person. You will do the very best you can. Realize that that is all you can do.

Any of the relaxation exercises in the *Preventive Medicine* chapter are valuable tools to help you deal with emergencies.

It is also helpful to relax the injured person. Do this when you feel it is most useful. There may be other things you want to do first. To relax the injured person, first imagine that your calmness is flowing to the person. It often helps to touch the person as you do this. Next gently and calmly tell them to relax. You can guide the injured person through any of the relaxation methods you have learned in the book. Remember that this relaxation is an important part of your medical treatment. It is especially valuable with children who are hurt.

After relaxing yourself and the injured person (if possible), *determine if the person is bleeding, having trouble breathing,* or *in shock.*

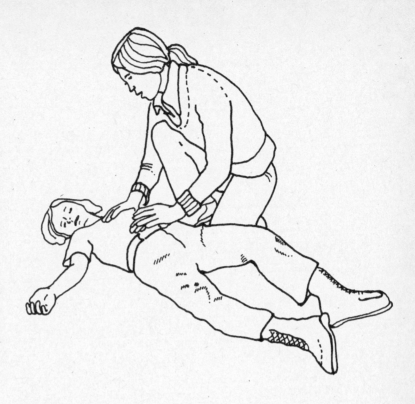

BEE STINGS — ANAPHYLACTIC SHOCK

Shock can occur within minutes after a person's body recognizes any substance as a threat. This occasionally occurs as a reaction to penicillin or insect bites.

The **symptoms of anaphylactic shock are**: fear, a feeling of pins and needles, a red rash over the body, swelling, difficulty breathing, a choking sensation, wheezing, nausea and abdominal pain, and occasionally loss of consciousness.

Anaphylactic shock is treated by laying the person down and making them comfortable. Then they are given *epinephrine* in an injection. Doctors have this medicine on hand for treatment of shock.

A person who has a known history of allergy to insect bites should discuss with his doctor whether it would be advisable for him to have a kit containing *epinephrine.* Anaphylactic shock is a medical emergency because the person in shock can stop breathing. (See section following on Resuscitation.)

BLEEDING

The most important thing for you to know about *bleeding* is that it can almost always easily be stopped by direct pressure on the site of bleeding. Doctors don't usually use tourniquets or pressure points any more because faulty use of a tourniquet can cause nerve and blood vessel damage. Direct pressure is almost always a better method and is easier.

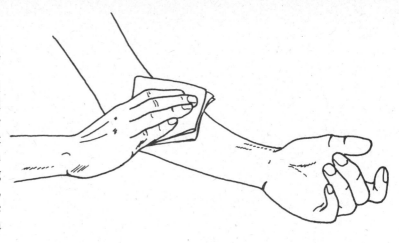

To stop bleeding, place sterile gauze pads or a clean cloth on the wound. Then put your whole hand firmly over the wound and press down hard. Keep your hand in this position for at least three minutes. Then check to see if the bleeding has stopped. If it hasn't, re-apply pressure until the person can be taken to a doctor.

Another way to apply direct pressure is to wrap roll gauze over sterile gauze pads. Wrap the gauze tightly, but not tightly enough to cut into the skin — you don't want to completely stop blood circulation to the area below the wound. Next wrap an elastic bandage around the gauze. The elasticity of the ace bandage will maintain pressure long enough for you to take the person to a doctor. A minor wound such as a small laceration will usually stop bleeding in a short time; a more severe wound will need the direct pressure maintained on it until the person can get to a doctor.

Understand that the heart is a pump. It pumps blood through the blood vessels at a low pressure. All you have to do is equalize that pressure and you will stop bleeding. It's just like putting your finger over a hole in a hose and stopping the water from coming out.

Many people are alarmed at the sight of blood. Blood is a natural substance; it's beautiful. When you stop bleeding by direct pressure, you rarely lose enough blood to cause concern. An adult has over five quarts of blood in his body; they need to lose a considerable amount for the loss to cause them any difficulty.

If you've ever been alarmed at the amount of blood that you thought someone was losing, try this: put a drop or two of red food coloring in a quarter cup of water (2 ounces). Splash the colored water over an old cloth or on the floor. It will probably look like a lot of blood, yet it is only 1/80th of the total amount of blood in your body.

If the wound is a minor one you can evaluate it to see if it needs stitches. If the cut does not *gape* open, only the top layer of skin has been cut and the wound can heal by itself. If this is the case you need only to wash the cut out thoroughly with clean water. A mild soap can also be used if you wish. Make sure that you get all foreign bodies such as dirt, sticks, glass, etc., out of the cut because your body cannot fully heal itself with these things in its way. Do not be afraid to use lots of water. Doctors in Emergency often use two quarts of water to clean out even a small cut. A small amount of bleeding from a cut is helpful, washing out foreign particles from the wound and bringing healing nutriments to the area. (See the drawing on page 340 for how your body heals a cut.)

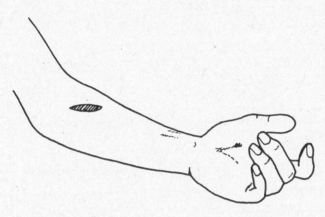

If the wound gapes (see drawing) it will be more difficult for the body to heal itself without some help. Your body will often heal a wound that gapes by filling in the open area with new tissue. This takes time and the wound is therefore more likely to become infected. The new tissue which your body forms in such a wound is "scar" tissue. For esthetic reasons and because a large scar near a joint can make movement difficult, wounds that gape are usually *sutured* (stitched). The sutures hold the two sides of the wound together. Your body can heal a sutured wound more quickly and easily because it doesn't have to form new tissue for such a large area. The length of the cut and therefore the number of stitches is usually not that important; the wound heals from side to side, not from end to end.

After a severe cut or puncture wound, especially if the cut has gotten dirt in it, you should get a Tetanus immunization from your doctor or clinic. Check with your doctor to see if your previous immunization is still good or if you need a "booster." This will depend on the type of injury and your doctor's own policy on providing protection from Tetanus. In general Tetanus immunizations last from five to ten years. Most doctors will give a booster after a severe injury.

BREATHING: BLOCKAGE, CHOKING

Sometimes in an emergency situation the injured person is having trouble *breathing*. If they are gasping for breath, you will be aware of this immediately. If they are unconscious, you will have to look at their chest to see if it's rising and falling. If there is any question in your mind, put your ear against their chest and listen for breath sounds.

Difficulty in breathing is often due to food blocking the windpipe. If the person is unconscious, their tongue may be blocking their air passage. Every effort must be made to remove the obstacle that is hindering breathing. Open the person's mouth and reach in with your fingers. Pull out the particles of food or straighten out their tongue. If you are unable to remove the obstacle, instruct the person to take small shallow breaths and to keep calm. They are often able to breathe around the obstacle in this manner, providing enough oxygen until you can get them some help. You can often dislodge an object from a child's throat by putting them over your knee, with their head hanging down; then pound on their back with the heel of your hand. (If the person is not breathing, see the section on resuscitation.)

289

BROKEN BONES

The most important thing to do if there is a broken bone is to immobilize it; to **prevent the injured area from bending or twisting.** This prevents the bones from damaging blood vessels and nerves in the site of the break. The best way to immobilize the bones is to use some sort of splint. (If you are interested in learning to splint or you want a book which shows you how to splint, for your medical library, see *Going Further*.) The important thing to realize is that any firm board and some adhesive tape or strips of cloth can make a splint. If necessary, you can even tie one leg to the other leg, or one toe to another toe, etc.

Once they are set by a doctor broken bones are mended by the three million year old healer. Before you get the person to the doctor they will probably be experiencing a great deal of pain. Concentrate on helping them with this by presenting as relaxed and confident a manner as possible, and by keeping in mind the things we tell you about pain in the *General Symptons* section of the *Diagnosis and Treatment* chapter.

Signs of broken bones are: swelling, discoloration, deformity, and pain when you press on the area. A fracture often prevents the person from moving the injured part in a normal manner without great pain. Doctors often find it difficult to differentiate between sprains and fractures without an x-ray. So if you are injured and have the symptoms above, it's a good idea to have an x-ray taken.

BURNS

There are three depths of burns:

First degree burns involve only the top layer of skin. They appear as red areas on the skin.

Second degree burns are a little deeper. They appear as areas of redness with blisters.

In **third degree burns** the full thickness of the skin is burned. Such burns appear raw and often white.

First and second degree burns should be washed gently with mild soap and water. Wash cloths soaked in ice water and applied to the burn will cut down the flow of blood to the area. This will make the person feel better and can reduce the damage done by the burn.

Because the skin is broken in a second-degree burn, you must take care to avoid infection. When the skin is broken, the body's normal protection is lost and bacteria that are normally on the skin can grow on the moist area of the burn. For this reason second-degree burns are usually covered with medicated sterile petroleum gauze. The gauze dressing needs to be changed once a week. When the dressing is changed, you will often see yellowish areas with dead skin around them. This is perfectly normal; the yellow areas are actually new skin growing. When the dressing is changed you can remove the dead blistered tissue and wash the area with mild soap again.

Due to the danger of infection, it's not a good idea to put butter or kitchen grease on a second degree burn.

Severe burns and all third degree burns should be seen by a doctor. Protect the burned area with clean towels or sheets. Relax: you have time to get the person safely to a doctor. Your relaxed mood and gentle reassurance are the best *First Aid* you can provide.

After second or third degree burns, especially if the burn has gotten dirt in it, you should get a Tetanus immunization. (See the last paragraph on *Bleeding* for more on this.)

DOG BITES

In general the emergency is not the dog bite itself, it is the possibility of *rabies*. Rabies is a viral disease transmitted in the saliva of an *infected* animal. If the dog is a household pet and has rabies immunization there is little likelihood that it could have rabies. The dog should be found and watched for 7 to 10 days by a veterinarian or by its owner. If the dog has rabies it will die within that time. So if you can locate the animal and it is not sick, it's only necessary to wash the wound thoroughly and have the person get a *tetanus* immunization from their doctor. The doctor will also know if rabies is a danger in your area.

DROWNING

Get the person out of the water as quickly as possible. First lay them on their back and remove mucous from their nose and throat with your hands. Turn them on their side and allow the water to drain out of their mouth. If the person is not breathing, immediately begin resuscitation. (See section following on resuscitation.)

ELECTRIC SHOCK

The first thing to do is to free the person from the electrical source. You must protect yourself when you do this. If possible, turn the electrical power off. Otherwise, remove the wire or electrical device with a dry wooden pole such as a broomstick or other non-conducting substance. If the injured person is not breathing, administer resuscitation. (See section following on resuscitation.)

HEAD INJURIES

An important thing in a head injury is whether or not the brain has been damaged. Brain damage may occur when the membrane that surrounds it is torn, causing tiny blood vessels to bleed slowly. Blood accumulates, causing pressure on the brain. If, after an injury, the person does not lose consciousness, you can almost always assume they are alright. If they become unconscious they may have a serious head injury and they should be taken to the hospital for diagnosis and treatment.

One way to tell if the membrane around the brain is torn in a person with a head injury is to observe them for several days. Have the person rest and relax. Check the pupils of their eyes every half hour. If the pupils react equally to light (see *Physical Examination* chapter), this is a good sign that the membrane has not been torn. Some doctors suggest that someone who knows the person well should be around them for a day or so. This friend can evaluate whether the injured person acts normally, thinks clearly, and knows who they are; if the person is acting normally then the membrane is probably all right; if the person loses consciousness again after the accident, the membrane may be torn. This is why doctors wake people up hourly after a head injury. They are making sure the person is simply sleeping and has not lost consciousness.

The person with head injuries should not take any alcohol, sedatives, pain medications or other drugs after the injury. These drugs can change a person's behavior and make it difficult to tell if they are acting normally, or are in need of special treatment to help them get well.

Many times after a head injury, **a person can feel somewhat "spaced out."** This is due to the brain being bruised when it bounces against the bones of the skull. It's a normal occurrence after a head injury and by itself does not mean that the membrane surrounding the brain has been torn.

Bleeding from the membrane is very slow bleeding; you have time to get the person to a doctor.

NECK INJURIES

If there is any chance that the person's neck has been injured, don't move them. Neck injuries can occur in falls, surfing or car accidents. They can also be associated with any head injury. **If you suspect a neck injury, ask the person to move their toes and fingers.** If they cannot, their spine may be injured.

Moving the person can result in further injury to the spine. **Immobilize their head and neck without moving them.** You can use rolled up towels or clothing placed close enough to prevent their head from moving. Then get help; an emergency ambulance is best.

NOSEBLEEDS

The same principle applies to stopping nosebleeds as applies to stopping any other external bleeding: direct pressure on the site. With a nosebleed you take your thumb and forefinger and firmly grasp the center of the person's nose, as shown in the drawing. Squeeze hard enough to cause pressure, but not hard enough to cause pain. Continue applying pressure for a full five minutes without letting go. This will stop almost all nose bleeds. If this does not work, try it two more times. If you are still unable to stop it, a doctor can help stop the bleeding.

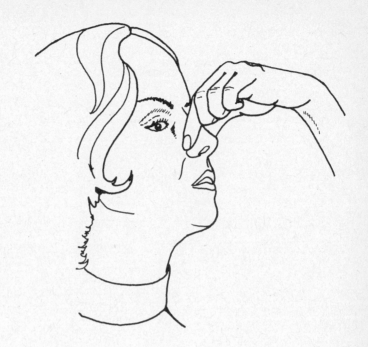

POISONING

If there's a question of a poisoning, see if you can **identify the particular poison** the person has eaten. Get the bottle or container and try to estimate how much the person has swallowed. **Call a nearby emergency hospital** and explain the situation. They will give you instructions on what to do. Since there are many different things in a house that may be poisonous and treatment varies depending on what the poison is, it is best to get advice before trying to make the person vomit or administering other first aid. For example, in cases of kerosene or gasoline ingestion, you *do not* want the person to vomit because the poison may further burn the person's throat as it comes up and it can also be inhaled by the person and damage their lungs.

Doctors who deal with emergencies have *ipicac syrup* or activated charcoal on hand. Ipicac syrup can make a person vomit when necessary; activated charcoal can absorb the poison in the person's stomach, without causing them to vomit.

In the case of **inhalation of poisonous vapors**, take the person to fresh air immediately and then call for medical help.

When a person gets **poisonous substances on their skin**, such as acid, flush the area immediately with huge amounts of water in a shower or under a hose. Do this even before the person's clothing is removed. Then remove their clothing. Then call for medical help.

RESUSCITATION

Resuscitation must be started within three or four minutes after the person has stopped breathing to prevent brain damage. If the person is not breathing, they should be placed on their back on a firm surface (do not use a bed). Tilt the person's head backwards; this keeps their airway open. Keep their head tilted backwards while you administer resuscitation.

Clear the person's mouth of mucous, vomit, or foreign bodies. Use your hands to do this. Separate the person's lips and teeth and press your mouth to theirs. Now forcibly blow air into their mouth from your mouth while you keep their nose closed with your fingers. The person's chest should rise when you blow in. If their chest doesn't move, their airway may still be obstructed. Check their mouth and throat again to see if they are blocked.

If their chest moves then the resuscitation is successful.

Feel the person's neck to see if a pulse is present (see drawing). If a pulse is present it means the heart is beating and it is only necessary to give breathing resuscitation.

Continue mouth-to-mouth resuscitation until the person's normal breathing returns.

Breathe 12 to 15 times a minute, blowing in for 2 seconds and allowing 3 seconds for the air to come out.

If you do not find a pulse and cannot hear the person's heart beating, place the heel of one hand in the center of the person's chest, in the area shown in

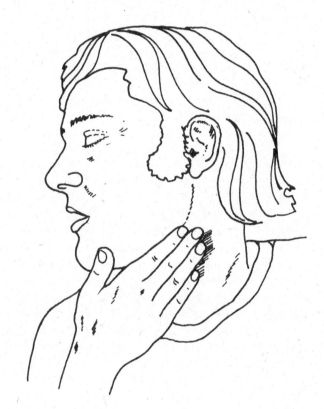

294

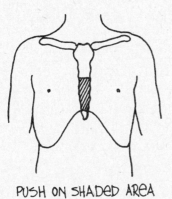

PUSH ON SHADED AREA

the drawing. Place the heel of the other hand on top of it and apply firm downward pressure. Apply enough pressure to depress the chest 2 inches (less in children). Then let up. Do this once every second.

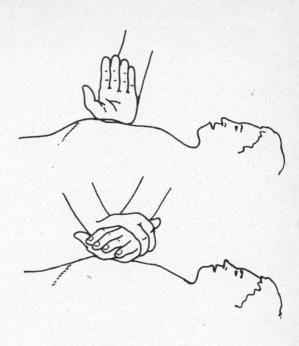

After 15 pushes, stop and blow into the person's mouth 5 times in the manner described above.

Continue this alternate breathing and chest pressure until medical help arrives or the person can be gotten to a hospital, or until the person begins breathing normally.

If a second person can help, have one person blow into the injured person's mouth 15 times a minute while the other person depresses the chest 60 times a minute continuously. If either person becomes tired, they can trade off.

The chances are extremely great that you will never have to do resuscitation in your life. If you ask the people you know chances are they have never had to do resuscitation either. But, this method can save a person's life, especially in drowning accidents or in electric or anaphylactic shock or drug overdoses.

SHOCK

When people are in shock they are pale and cool. Their skin is moist; they are often thirsty. They have a weak but rapid pulse.

Shock can be due to fainting or loss of large amounts of blood. In fainting, most of the body's blood leaves the head and goes to the bowels and muscles. A person who faints will recover by themselves in a few minutes without any help.

A person who is in shock due to the loss of blood should be taken to the hospital immediately. Keep them warm. Have them lie down and raise their legs slightly, so that their legs are higher than their head. This tends to send their blood back to their head. If the person is conscious, help them to relax. In any case, take them to the hospital without moving them unnecessarily.

Putting Together Your Own First Aid Kit

Most commercial first aid kits are useless in real emergencies. They usually contain only bandaids and an unnecessary antiseptic. The kit below is inexpensive and will handle all the medical emergencies we describe in this book.

Item	What It's For
Bandaids — assorted strips	To protect small wounds from dirt
Sterile gauze pads: Ten 4"x4" square pads	To control bleeding and to protect burns and large wounds.
Roller bandage: One 2" gauze roll	To hold gauze pads to control bleeding.
Elastic Bandage: One 4 inch roll	To hold gauze pads to control bleeding, and to immobilize sprains and fractures.
Adhesive tape: One 5 yard roll, 3" wide	To hold dressings, close small cuts, help make splints, etc.
Tweezers	For removing splinters.

PREVENTING MEDICAL EMERGENCIES

Many emergencies occur because people don't pay enough attention to themselves. Many accidents, as well as many diseases, are messages to you from your body telling you that there are things in your behavior or your environment that have to be changed. If a person is worried or preoccupied, they often lose track of what they're doing and create an emergency situation for themselves. A person worried about losing their job can run their car off the road. They may look upon this event as an accident, and feel sorry for themself. We think it's more helpful for such people to ask themselves why the accident happened and what they could learn about themselves from it. We think accidents are like disease. Just as one person gets recurring sore throats, another person is constantly having accidents. Our ideas about *target organs* apply to accidents as well. (See *Systems Review* page 30 and *Preventive Medicine* page 69.)

The main thing to realize is that you can have a great deal of control over whether or not you will be involved in a medical emergency.

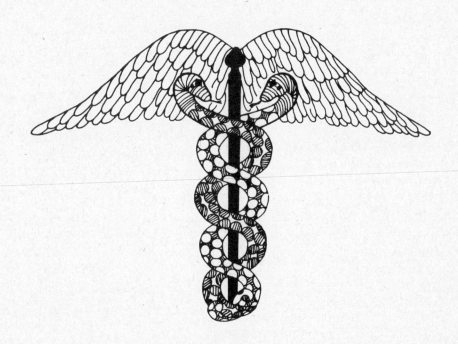

YOUR DOCTOR AS A RESOURCE

Sometimes your body needs extra energy from "outside" in order to heal itself. The medical doctor is usually the most available source of this energy.

A doctor can represent security where dealing with disease and injury are concerned. For many people the doctor becomes a dominant figure. The "sick" person feels helpless, passive, and that all the power for healing lies with the doctor. Many doctors, indeed, adopt the attitude that they (the doctor) must be in full control at all times. As a result people often feel ambivalent about going to the doctor's office. They may want help but be reluctant to allow themself to become dominated by the doctor. We suggest that in order to get the most from your doctor you get in touch with your feelings about them. Here's how to do that:

Sit in a relaxed position where you will not be disturbed for 20 minutes or more. (You may wish to do the relaxation part of the exercise for getting in touch with your imaginary doctor here.)

Visualize yourself going to your doctor. (Your real doctor, not your imaginary one.) Visualize yourself phoning for an appointment, driving to the office, approaching the door of the office, opening it, going inside. Imagine yourself in the waiting room. Then imagine the receptionist calling your name. Imagine yourself in the examination room. The door opens and your doctor enters.

Now visualize your doctor sitting down directly in front of you. (If you wish you can set up two chairs facing each other, for this exercise.) Tell your visualized doctor exactly what you feel toward them. These feelings may or may not involve: fear, hopefulness, anger, love, trust, resentment, etc. Talk to your doctor just as though they were there. Say to them, "When I am with you I feel _____ ." Then complete the sentence with whatever comes to your mind. Stay with your *feelings* about your doctor. Don't discuss anything else with them.

Imagine you are the doctor. Say whatever you, as the doctor, feel. You may wish to go back and forth several times, being your doctor and then being yourself.

As you do this exercise, understand that you are expressing feelings which you do not need to express toward your doctor in real life — unless you wish to do so. You are thus completely free to say or do whatever comes to your mind.

Understand that all the feelings you express are your own. The feelings you express when taking the role of your doctor are your own feelings, even though you see them as being expressed by your doctor.

People who do this exercise discover information which helps them to better relate to their doctors. Confronting your own feelings toward your doctor through this exercise will also help you understand basic feelings which you have toward disease and healing.

THE DOCTOR'S RESOURCES

Now that you have gotten in touch with your feelings toward your doctor, you can go on to assess what your doctor offers you as basic health resources.

Your doctor is a resource for:

Assistance in diagnosing and treating diseases: The doctor has extensive knowledge, specialized information, and has seen a lot of illness. For these reasons they are excellent sources for helping you diagnose and treat a disease you may have. Your doctor can help you diagnose an illness you may have and prescribe the most current treatments to help you to help your body heal itself.

Tests such as x-ray, cultures, blood analysis, urine analysis: to help diagnose certain diseases such as strep throat, venereal disease, etc., and to determine if bones are fractured following accidents.

Antibiotics or other prescription drugs: if your body needs additional healing help, such as for healing pneumonia and other bacterial infections, or for healing a disease which requires a prescription drug.

Emergency situations: to handle some emergency situations involving broken bones, deep flesh wounds, poisoning, and burns, a hospital Emergency Room is better equipped than your family doctor because it has oxygen, blood transfusion equipment, x-ray machines, etc. But some people contact their own doctors for advice when emergencies arise. Very often doctors are able to handle minor emergencies in their own offices.

Immunization: Your own doctor is a good resource when you want to get immunizations such as DPT, Polio Vaccine, and for Tetanus boosters when you need them.

Oftentimes when your doctor makes a specific diagnosis of a disease which you have, your worry and fear of the unknown are ended. This stops the drain on your energy caused by uncertainty and doubt, and it allows you to focus your energy more positively on healing.

☆   ☆   ☆

Because your body heals itself your doctor needs your help to help you. Healing is an equal participation situation — with healer and patient succeeding only if both actively participate in the process. To do this you need to take responsibility for yourself and participate in the healing in every way you know how or learn how to do through this book.

If you have doubts about your doctor's part in the healing process, you can slow down the healing processes which he or she prescribes. Your body can tense up muscles, causing blood vessels to narrow and preventing antibiotics or other drugs from reaching the area of your body that needs them. The doctor can give you the proper antibiotic to heal whatever infection you have, but you can determine how well it reaches the area of illness. Thus you are in control of your healing.

Trusting your doctor depends, in part, on how they communicate information to you. Most doctors do not volunteer information. You will have to take control of the situation if you wish to get the information you want. For you to participate in your healing in a positive way you will have to ask questions, and demand that you get all of your questions answered. The answers will enable you to understand the disease and the healing process and thus you can focus your energy on healing yourself.

People going to a doctor usually want to know:

What the doctor is doing as he or she examines them.

What's going on with their illness. (See the format for this that we present in the *Diagnosis and Treatment* chapter.)

What the treatment for it is and how it works.

How fast they can expect their body to heal itself.

What they can do themselves to help speed up the healing process.

You may also have specific questions in addition to these general ones.

If your doctor fails to clear your doubts or fears, tell them so. If they are still unable to help you, or if they refuse to answer your questions, see another doctor or talk to the head of the clinic about this problem. Since it is your body, you have every right to be allowed to participate as fully as possible in healing yourself.

Your participation will depend, also, on your trust in your doctor and your acceptance or rejection of the treatments your doctor prescribes. Understand, however, that *there are often many different ways to treat any one disease.* For example, one doctor may choose to surgically remove a lump in the breast of a young woman, while another may choose to follow it and see that it does not change. There is debate among medical authorities as to what method is the best; neither is wrong, and both methods are used.

If you do not feel good about the treatment your doctor suggests, tell them so. They may be able to suggest alternative healing methods that are equally valid and which would work better for you. It would work better for you because you would trust your doctor more and you would be participating in the treatment and following your body's signals. The fact that you make the choice involves you more fully in the act of healing. If your doctor is unable to suggest a method that makes you feel good, feel free to seek out other methods. The search in itself is an important part of healing. At this time there are many innovative and effective healing techniques available, both Western and non-Western — everything from acupuncture to faith healing, surgery, or bio-feedback training.

If people make known to their doctors the kinds of treatment they want, they can better influence the course of healing. For example, if women want to have their babies out of the hospital, and they communicate this strongly and directly to their doctors, eventually other obstetrical methods, such as midwifery, will develop. In the paragraphs below we suggest additional methods to get the kind of treatment you want from the doctor.

WHEN TO GO TO THE DOCTOR

People go to doctors for many reasons. The basic reason is when you are worried or need help. More specific reasons are:

You get an illness then diagnose it yourself, but your body does not get well at the rate you think it should. This worries you and you go to the doctor for help.

You get an illness, diagnose it yourself, but instead of getting better you get worse. So you go to the doctor for help.

You get an illness but are completely unable to diagnose what you have. You go to the doctor for help in diagnosis and treatment.

You get an illness, diagnose it, but you know that you need the resources of a doctor to treat it: x-ray, cultures, a prescription, surgery, etc.

The Well Body Book will help you greatly in diagnosing and treating yourself. Use the above guidelines to help you decide when you need more help than the book provides.

PATIENT'S LIB: VANISHING SYMPTOMS

Let's say that you go to see the doctor about a cough you have been having. You get an appointment for 10 o'clock, you wait for an hour in the outer office, then when you finally get into the examination room your cough has vanished. You feel apologetic for having bothered *the busy doctor*. You leave feeling frustrated, embarrassed, and more than a little angry for having spent your time on a wild goose chase. In addition, by the time you get back home your cough has started up again.

Understand that is not unusual for this to happen. People often feel better the moment they get into the examining room — at least temporarily better. Perhaps it is nervousness, perhaps it's involved with wanting to *perform* for the doctor, perhaps it's your body responding to the fact that you are doing something concrete to make it feel better. Whatever it is, the fact remains that many people have this response, and because they feel better they fail to ask the doctor the questions which they came to have answered.

To solve this problem or to completely prevent it from occuring, write down what you want answered on a piece of paper before you leave to see your doctor. Also list your fears. The person with a cough might write, "My cough has lasted so long I'm afraid I might be getting pneumonia." When you get to the office, take out your written list and actually read the doctor what you have written down. Remember, you have gone to the doctor, and are paying them to get this kind of help. Quelling your fears about disease is at least as important as getting a prescription for a new *miracle drug*. Don't feel apologetic about this, and don't allow your doctor to intimidate you into feeling that you are being foolish. If they continuously do so, change doctors. You may also wish to write a letter stating your complaints and send it to the local American Medical Association, whose address you will find in the phone book. Send one copy of the letter to the Association and another copy of the letter to the doctor about whom you are complaining. This is one of the few ways open to the patient for demanding the kind of medical attention they want. Change is needed, and though it will come slowly in any case, patients must make their demands clearly known before those changes will ever become possible.

PATIENT'S LIB: WAITING ROOM DOLDRUMS

Few doctors feel they have the time to do very much to make their waiting rooms comfortable. Fewer still consider the waiting room important to the healing process. As a result most waiting rooms are antiseptic and impersonal, not at all conducive to the kinds of healing energy which we describe in this book.

If your doctor's office feels cold and uncomfortable to you we suggest that you do this: next time you find yourself there, look around and figure out ways to improve the atmosphere. A warmer color for the walls, a carpet on the floor, more comfortable furniture, pictures on the walls, living plants, etc., are all ways to bring more healing energy to the environment. The more relaxed and at ease you feel the closer you will be to a healing attitude.

Explain your feelings to the doctor. Tell them that the waiting room brings you down, makes you feel sicker than when you came, and that you feel that coming there should make you feel better. Suggest specific changes that can be made to improve the situation. Clearly explain that the waiting room can actually become a health aid by helping to create a pleasant, alive and healthy association with coming to see the doctor.

Change begins with single people making positive suggestions for change. Most doctors never give a second thought to their waiting rooms. It is up to you to bring this facet of healing to their attention. (Bring your doctor a plant, painting, or other decoration for their office.)

PATIENT'S LIB: WAITING AND WAITING

Many times you have probably found yourself waiting at the doctor's office for an hour or more after having rushed around to keep your appointment. *The unspoken message is that your time is less valuable than the doctor's.* In truth everyone's time is of equal value: the doctor's, the janitor's, the writer's, the unemployed person's, the house person's, the student's, etc. No one has the right to "waste" another person's time. You give the doctor the right to make you wait by:

Making an authority figure of them.

Feeling in yourself that their time is more important than yours.

Neglecting to tell your doctor that you do not like to wait.

In most cases the only excuse the doctor has for making you wait is that they have booked more appointments than they can possibly handle in the time they have allowed themself. They do not have to do this. Many doctors do the same thing day after day and year after year. They continue to get away with it only because few patients ever complain. *The doctor's crowded schedule* aggravates you, brings negative energy to the whole office, overworks the doctor causing them to become ill, and actually is at the root of many early deaths in the medical profession. The only possible *benefit* could be economic — that the more patients the doctor sees in one day the more money they make. Only in rare situations are disease or other medical emergencies the causes of such a crammed appointment schedule.

Understand that your doctor is in the business of selling you a service. They are selling their medical knowledge to you. You pay for these services, regardless of whether you pay for them in cash or through medical insurance policies which you have purchased, or through taxes if you are going to a tax-supported clinic. You have every right in the world to demand what you consider to be good service. If you come away from your doctor's office angered and resentful because you have had to wait for an hour or more, your doctor has been responsible for this. You should be able to come away with positive healing energy — not anger, frustration, and resentment.

If long waits in your doctor's office annoy you, tell your doctor so. We suggest that a wait of no more than ½ hour from your appointment time is reasonable, and allows the doctor enough leeway to make up for unforeseen changes in his or her schedule. Tell your doctor clearly that you will wait for no more than ½ hour. Then stick to it. When the times goes over, tell the receptionist that you are leaving, and then leave. Be sure that your doctor gets the message. Write it down and ask the receptionist to give it to the doctor, if necessary. The chances are that they will not pass along a verbal message.

If this doesn't work, change doctors. There are a few doctors around who keep reasonable appointment schedules and who don't keep their patients waiting. If you change doctors, by all means tell your old doctor why you are leaving. Only then will the message get through to them. And by all means send a letter to the AMA (and a copy to your old doctor) recounting your waiting experiences.

PATIENT'S LIB: UNCOMFORTABLE EXAMS

Some examinations the doctor does are uncomfortable, often *because the situation under which they are given is tense.* The vaginal examination is a classic example of this. However, there is no reason in the world why the pelvic exam has to be uncomfortable. Many factors contribute to the discomfort of this and other exams. Among them are:

The person being examined is treated abruptly or coldly, making them tense.

The doctor guards his or her true feelings behind *objectivity* and *abruptness,* instead of being out front about their own emotional discomfort about the situation. (Remember, doctors are human.)

The person being examined does not know what the examiner is doing or why they are doing it. These unknowns breed fear, fear breeds tension, and tension makes the exam more difficult for the examiner and more painful for the person being examined.

The doctor labors under the illusion that they must be in *full control* of the situation at all times, or else they're not a good doctor. Thus they refuse to ask the patient for participation and help in the exam, making the exam more difficult than it has to be.

If you are going to have an examination which you have never had before, or if you are going to be examined in a way that has been uncomfortable for you in the past (as with a vaginal exam), consider the following ways to improve the situation:

Tell your doctor that the exam is uncomfortable for you, and that it makes you very tense. If you have any suggestions for making the exam more comfortable, tell your doctor these suggestions for change, and ask if they are possible. For example, if your doctor does a pelvic exam with a cold speculum, ask if they can warm it up first. (A great many doctors do this.)

If your doctor is cold and abrupt, understand that this attitude is not necessarily directed toward you as a person. Doctors are human and are just as prone to embarrassment and fear as the rest of us. The only difference is that doctors often mask their emotional discomfort behind "scientific objectivity," because they believe that the public expects that is the way they should be. (In spite of all the technical preparation doctors receive in medical school, there is *no* preparation for dealing with the emotions of being a doctor.) If you suspect this to be the case with your doctor, try to respond to the part that is masked rather than to the mask itself. You may even wish to tell your doctor that they are acting as if the exam made them uncomfortable. Do it kindly, and leave yourself open to discussing the situation fully with them. (If the truth were known, many patients would discover that they are more skillful in emotional things than their doctors.)

If there is any part of the exam which you don't understand, by all means ask about it, and expect to get a satisfying answer. Ask how the exam is done, what kinds of instruments, if any, are used, how the instruments work, and what is accomplished by doing the exam. Understand that there is no reason in the world why such information should not be willingly given to you.

Ask the doctor to explain to you what they are doing and why they are doing it as they go through the exam.

If tension is a problem for you, tell your doctor that you can relax your muscles at will if they will give you a chance. For example, some women find pelvic exams uncomfortable because they tense up their pelvic muscles and the doctors, who are often men, don't know what to do to help the woman relax. At home you can practice relaxing your pelvic muscles, or even practice doing the pelvic exam, as described in the *Physical Examination* chapter, then you will be fully able to do it during your pelvic exam. When the time comes it may help you to tell your doctor to wait until you have relaxed the muscles before inserting the speculum.

Putting the doctor in the position of being a high authority, and exalting them, as is usually the case in our culture, inevitably puts the patient in a subservient role. This is especially true for women with male doctors. The situation robs the patient of the benefit of his or her own healing energies, and makes the doctor's job, in both diagnosis and treatment, more difficult. Both the doctor and the person coming to them for medical services, will benefit when we all, as patients, begin to take more active roles in the whole process.

PATIENT'S LIB: PRESCRIPTION DRUGS

If your doctor prescribes a drug to help your body get well, be sure to ask them all of the following:

What does the drug do?

What are the possible side effects? (All drugs have side effects.)

Can they prescribe a *generic* drug?

For more on this, read our chapter *Drugs Are Helpers.* Understand that there are reasonable answers to all of these questions and your knowledge of the answers (at least the first two) are absolutely essential to help you help your body heal itself.

PATIENT'S LIB: THE RUSHED DOCTOR

Many doctors give the impression of being too busy to bother with you. The chances are that they treat every one of their patients in this way, and each comes away with the feeling of having been an imposition on the doctor. The doctor often has no time for anyone in their life — sometimes wife and family included. The point is this: the doctor is selling you a service. Part of that service must be to answer your questions and put your mind at ease about your body. If they are not giving you the time to accomplish this, then they are not providing you with the services for which you are paying them. There is no difference between the abrupt doctor who will not take the time to talk to you and the mechanic who fails to do the auto repairs for which you have paid.

If your doctor is this way, tell them that they make you feel as though you are imposing on them. Tell them that you don't think this is right, that you want to feel free to ask questions and discuss health concerns with them. Tell them that if these things really are impositions, or if you are taking up too much of their time, that you will gladly change doctors. Understand that many doctors are not fully aware of their personal effect on their patients. Since doctors seem to be such powerful authority figures few people feel that they have the right to tell them these things. But you may very well be helping such doctors get more in touch with both their patients and themselves.

TRUST AS A HEALING TOOL

Through the *patient's lib* sections in this chapter you can get in touch with your feelings about your doctor and can do specific things to improve the kind of medical care you are getting. All of these are aimed at helping you to create a situation where you can feel good and where your internal feelings are positive, so that you are most able to use available healing energy. Your conscious decision to trust your doctor is a valuable tool; it enables you to actively participate (through making the choice to trust) in the healing process, and the energy previously used in worry and doubt are released to be used in healing. If you feel good about the kind of care you are getting, if you trust your doctor and all your questions have been answered, then you are receiving the best medical care for you.

DRUGS ARE HELPERS

DRUGS ARE HELPERS

Most drugs are potent herbs or organic substances. They come from natural sources — plants, animals, and earth minerals. *Penicillin* comes from bread mold, *digitalis* from the Foxglove plant, and *hormones* or *steroids* from the glands of certain animals. They're foods that give us a specific substance to open a blood vessel, shrink a mucous membrane, kill a bacteria, etc. They treat the *symptoms* of diseases to make you feel better, regain your trust in your own body and allow your body to heal itself.

Sometimes drugs are very valuable in healing, as in the case of an antibiotic used for treating a serious infection. The antibiotic cuts the number of bacteria in the body down to a quantity your own antibodies can fight. It's almost indispensable when the number of bacteria gets higher than your own antibodies can handle on their own.

We think it's important to look upon drugs as allies, as helpers, the way your imaginary doctor, or your real doctor, or this book are helpers. They can all assist your three-million-year-old healer to heal you.

MYSTIQUES AND SIDE EFFECTS

There's nothing mystical about drugs. The scrawls that your doctor puts down on the piece of paper that you take to the drugstore to get a healing drug are not mystical at all. There's a book called *Physicians' Desk Reference,* (P.D.R.) which tells all about drugs. P.D.R. is given free to all doctors. Unfortunately this book is not easily available to the general public but if you have a friendly doctor they may be willing to give you their last year's edition when they're done with it. P.D.R. contains the whole story about each drug manufactured and sold in the United States. It has color codes and pictures of each drug so that they can be identified visually. It has stories about the actions of drugs, what they do in your body — the affects and general effectiveness, as well as descriptions of their chemical ingredients.

The Foxglove

In P.D.R., side effects are discussed in detail because if a person suffers one of these side effects and it's not listed either by the manufacturer or in the book, the drug company can be sued. Your doctor may or may not explain side effects to you when they prescribe a drug for a disease you might have. But every drug has side effects: nausea, vomiting, dizziness, sleepiness, extra-alertness, constricting blood vessels, hot flashes, cold flashes, rashes, etc.

Most drugs affect the whole body. For example, *antihistimines* don't affect just the mucous membranes of the nose. They affect *every* mucous membrane in your body, and every blood vessel in your body. It's certainly worth thinking about this whenever you consider taking an antihistamine.

DRUGS AS BIG BUSINESS

Drugs are made by giant corporations who send out people called "detail men," whose sole job it is to go to doctors' offices and clinics and hospitals and make people interested in their company's drugs. Many doctors own stock in these companies. Although drugs are manufactured and sold under brand names, each drug also has a *generic* name (generic being the chemist's name for the chemical molecule itself.) For example, there are many different brand names of *tetracycline,* and each drug company has its own name for that same substance. These drugs are identical, as tested by the Federal Drug Administration (F.D.A.).

Each drug company tries to tell the doctors, through their detail men, that their particular brand of drug is better than all the others. They often give doctors gifts, sometimes expensive gifts, to make the name of their particular brand of drug easier to remember. And the generic names are often so difficult to remember that doctors don't even know them. The name "Pen Vee K Tabs," for example, is one company's name for the drug *phenoxymethylpotassiumpenicillin.* Doctors get into habits. They'll write easily remembered brand names on their prescription orders, not even knowing that the drug they've prescribed may cost several times as much as the same drug produced under a different name.

Doctors, druggists, and drug manufacturers all participate in the drug industry. Remember that drug manufacturers are huge, multi-million dollar corporations with enormous advertising budgets and detail men to push their products. In essence, they keep the pharmacists' shelves stocked, and try hard to keep this stock selling. When you get a prescription, all the pharmacist does is count out and bottle the drugs you need, and then charge you anywhere between 50 and 500 percent over their cost of the drug for this service. Not that I'm against a druggist making a living. But the point is that many brand name drugs are excessively expensive, and are sold to you at high profit even though you could get the exact same chemical substance at a fraction of the cost, if the doctor would prescribe by using the *generic* rather than the *brand* name.

Many things contribute to this situation: pressure from pharmacist lobbies, ignorance or lack of interest on the part of the general public as well as doctors, and the absence of anyone's making such information broadly available to the public. What all this means to you is that other people are making a great deal of money because you get sick.

KARMA AND HEALING DRUGS

Drugs come to you the same way that most other products come: through the American mega-corporations and conglomerates. That may be alright in buying a car. That may be alright in buying a television set. But in buying a healing herb I think that the *karma* (or attitude toward life) of the whole industry comes through with the herb: the *karma* of the executive sitting in the market square scheming on ways to make more money; the *karma* of the chemist being paid to find another rare herb for another rare disease to make more money; the doctor not caring, or too busy to care; the pharmacist's lobby; the huge drugstore chains selling the stuff to you. You get the picture of an herb that comes to you the most expensive way it can. We don't feel all this is good *karma* for healing.

What can you do about this? **Ask your doctor to prescribe only generic drugs,** and to find out which pharmacy near you sells generic medications (not all of them do), and which carry the least expensive generic medications. Drugs can be priced at the pharmacy by your doctor, *if they are interested.* They can call on the phone and find out which pharmacy carries the less expensive medications as easily as you can call a department store to get the price of some article that you may want to buy. There is no reason in the world that your doctor shouldn't do this for you. It could put an end to the exploitation of disease by companies whose main goals are wealth.

Some drug companies may argue that profit goes into research for the invention of new healing drugs. But it is interesting to note that, in addition to their high profits, both private foundations and government grants provide drug researchers with millions of dollars each year for necessary medical research, including pharmacological research.

INFORMATION ABOUT DRUGS

There are thousands of different kinds of drugs which doctors prescribe and people use in the United States each year. But for the most common medical problems these fall into the following categories: aspirin and aspirin containing drugs, antacids, laxatives, antihistimines, antibiotics, hormones, tranquilizers, barbiturates, amphetamines and other "speed" drugs, caffeine, and nicotine.

I feel that if you ever have to take any of these drugs, you would do well to know what you are putting into your body: how the drug works on you; the way it affects your *whole* body rather than just the part where you feel the present symptom; and all about the potential side effects. I believe that there are times when drugs are necessary and helpful, but *they are just as often over-used.* Many of the things that drugs do, you can learn to do without them — with no side effects and probably with much better karma. Other parts of this book will tell you about alternatives to drug therapy; in this chapter we'll tell you what some of the more commonly prescribed drugs do. Then you can make your own choices about healing therapies that you may need now or in the future.

STORIES OF COMMON DRUGS

Aspirin: (Acetylsalicylic Acid) This is the most commonly used drug for relieving fever and mild pain. It is the major ingredient in many "over-the-counter" drugs (drugs that you can buy without a prescription). It is used by itself or mixed with caffeine, antihistimines, buffers such as *aluminum hydroxide* or *magnesium hydroxide* (to neutralize acids in your stomach), and sometimes chemicals made from coal tar, called *phenacetin* or *acetaminophen* which act on the body in ways similar to aspirin.

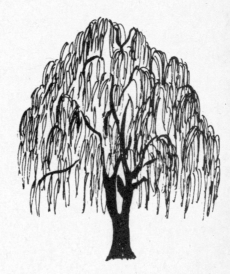

The active ingredients of aspirin itself are found in willow bark, and have been known and used by man for perhaps thousands of years. Willow bark is a natural herb. It lowers fever by acting directly on your body's thermostat in your brain, to cause an increase in sweating and in blood flow to skin surfaces where the blood is cooled more quickly. It alleviates low intensity pain by acting as a mild depressant on the brain. Aspirin is known to have no influence on the course of a cold; it only treats the symptoms of fever and pain that go along with a cold. It can actually cause your disease to get worse because it allows you to be active instead of paying attention to your symptoms — your body's messages to you — and getting some rest.

Aspirin is a relatively safe drug with few serious side effects. The major side effect is stomach upset. One aspirin per day for three days results in a small amount of blood appearing in the stools since it causes small ulcerations in the stomach mucosa.

We emphasize that all drugs have some side effects, and aspirin is considered one of the safest drugs you can take. But when you take drugs of any kind, it is interesting to realize that they will do many things to your body other than relieve the sometimes minor complaints for which you took them. (See the *Diagnosis and Treatment* section of this book, page 195, for alternative ways to reduce fever and pain without the use of drugs.

The American Medical Association has recently stated that plain aspirin is just as effective as aspirin combined with other drugs, and that no brand of aspirin works any better than any other. So if you wish to use aspirin, and drugs containing aspirin, buy the cheapest, generic, least-complicated aspirin you can find, rather than a more expensive, highly-advertised brand. To reduce the side effects of aspirin, take it on a full stomach.

Antacids: Studies have shown that *placebos* — harmless pills with no active ingredients whatsoever — work just as well as most antacids in controlling minor stomach upset.

Contrary to the impression created by the advertising world, man is *not* constantly fighting a battle against acidity in the stomach. Most belching and minor gastrointestinal upsets are not even due to excess acids, so are not affected by the use of antacids. Advertising by large drug firms has convinced a great many people that antacids are necessary for very minor stomach upset. This type of upset is almost always due to diet: overeating, eating foods that are difficult to digest, drinking beverages with or without alcohol that overtax the digestive system, or simply eating "on the run" and not giving the stomach the time and energy it needs to do its part of the digestive process.

Normally your three-million-year-old healer — your body — keeps the acid balance in your stomach in the right range for digestion. The cells in your stomach that secrete hydrochloric acid, necessary for digestion, are controlled by the *vagus* nerve which receives impulses from your mind. Conscious control of the acidity of your stomach, done by learning to relax and tell your stomach to balance out, is possible and is a much better way of controlling stomach acids than by using chemicals. A *placebo* works because you take it with the faith that it will work; in essence, you send your *vagus* nerve a positive message to balance things out. There's no reason you can't do the same without the *placebo*.

Antacids are needed only in peptic ulcer conditions diagnosed by a doctor, or for true hyper-acidity of the stomach in rare conditions. Belching, gas, and minor stomach discomfort are no reasons to take antacids. You can easily correct these discomforts by getting in touch with your diet — the foods you are attempting to incorporate into the living cells of your body. (See our *Preventive Medicine* chapter on diet.) Doing it this way will save you the discomfort of the symptoms and the energy ripoffs caused by the antacids you feel you have to take to reduce those discomforts.

If you overeat, the discomfort that you experience is usually because your stomach is stretched by all the food. Antacids will not help relieve this. If you believe in an antacid strongly enough, you will no doubt feel better in a very short time, partly because your stomach will just normally empty in that same length of time, and partly because your vagus nerve will reestablish the proper acid balance in your stomach, aided by your faith in the drug.

Sodium bicarbonate is widely used as a gastric antacid in popular over-the-counter "selzer-type" preparations. The disadvantages of sodium bicarb probably outweigh its advantages. It does neutralize hydrochloric acid in the stomach while it is there, but promptly leaves the stomach and is absorbed from the intestinal tract, doing nothing to correct the cause of the hyper-acidity. Acid is, of course, normal in the stomach and is absolutely necessary for digestion. Whether or not you want to disrupt that acid balance is certainly a question worth considering.

When sodium bicarbonate reacts with the hydrochloric acid in your stomach, carbon dioxide is produced. This causes a further stretching of your stomach and often makes your symptoms worse. It may cause you to belch, which you may find somewhat pleasurable when your stomach is overfilled, but it is nothing more than a side effect of a chemical reaction which you have induced in your stomach by mixing sodium bicarbonate with hydrochloric acid. Furthermore, the sodium bicarbonate left unused by your stomach is quickly absorbed into your blood stream where it disturbs the normal and necessary acid balance of all your body fluids.

We believe that by getting in touch with your body's food needs as we describe in the *Preventive Medicine* chapter, and by learning to relax your body during periods when you are digesting what you have just eaten, you can wholly do away with the need to ever use antacids.

Laxatives: It is more common for doctors to treat people for "laxative abuse" than for them to prescribe a laxative. The fact is that laxatives are very rarely prescribed by a doctor.

Deluded by the advertising world, many people take laxatives when they have missed one bowel movement, and once the laxative has been taken, it causes *complete* evacuation of the bowels. It then takes several days to have a normal bowel movement again, so the person will become concerned all over again and take yet another laxative. This results in "laxative habit," where the person's normal bowel patterns are completely disrupted by chemicals. They are unable to move their bowels without a laxative, and thus have become dependent on the drug.

The advertising world has been paid by drug firms to convince Americans that it is essential to have a bowel movement every day for their mental well-being. This is simply not true. For some people, a daily bowel movement may not be normal to their particular life rhythm. Furthermore, it is not serious to miss a bowel movement.

Serious gastrointestinal disturbances, such as irritation of the colon and stomach, can result from laxative abuse. Potassium deficiency can also be a side effect. **Laxatives should never be taken for abdominal pain, colic, cramps, nausea, vomiting,** because of the risk of rupturing an appendix.

It is easy to correct your constipation by correcting your diet, your intake of fluids, and by doing body relaxation and exercise. It is so easy to correct constipation by these means that there is no real reason to ever take laxatives, except if prescribed by a doctor for special situations. (See page 252, *Diagnosis and Treatment,* for more on this.)

Antihistamines: These synthetic drugs block the action of natural substances, called *histamines,* found throughout your body. Histamines are one of the natural healing substances in your three-million-year-old healer; they act on smooth muscle, causing dilation of tiny blood vessels. If you want to see histamine work, take a pin and scratch it lightly over the skin of your arm. Rapidly the area becomes red and raised. What happens is that the peripheral vessels dilate, a little swelling occurs, and blood flows to the area.

Antihistamines block the action of the histamine, and they do nothing about what caused the histamines to be there in the first place. So when you take an antihistamine for a cold, all you do is block the swelling of certain membranes. The antihistamine does not influence the course of the cold.

Sometimes antihistamines can be helpful in that they can help to open up the *Eustachian tubes* — the tubes running from your ears to the back of your throat — and allow the ear to drain normally. In this case, your body is helped toward taking over the job of healing itself.

Antihistamines should not, I believe, be looked upon as necessary in treating all minor colds or allergies, since they can rob more energy from you than they provide.

Antihistamines act on your whole body, not just the mucous membranes in your nose, sinuses, or throat. *Side effects* seen while taking an antihistamine may include drowsiness, confusion, nervousness, nausea, blurring of vision, dizziness, headache, insomnia, dryness of mouth, nose, and throat, and tingling and weakness of the hands. Prolonged use of over-the-counter antihistamines has been known to cause permanent damage to the mucosa of nose, sinuses, throat, and other areas of the body, robbing the body of its necessary defenses against infection.

Antibiotics: These are substances produced naturally by micro-organisms which kill bacteria or prevent their multiplication, and thus lower the number of bacteria in an infection, so that *your own antibodies* can handle the remainder and cure you of the infection. There are over 100 different antibiotics on the market. The first recorded use of an antibiotic was over 2500 years ago when people in China learned that they could reduce boils by dressing them with fermented soybeans.

Our modern day penicillins stop the synthesis of the protein in the cell wall in a bacteria. Since the bacteria are dependent on this protein cell wall for their existence, they die when this happens. But penicillin, like all other antibiotics, has no affect on viruses; it only stops the growth of bacteria. **Therefore it is of no use for curing the common cold.**

But antibiotics are very discriminating — they will attack only certain kinds of bacteria. The reason for this is that each bacteria is sensitive to only certain antibiotics; penicillin works against some, tetracycline against others, etc. Amphicillin, a *broad spectrum* antibiotic, kills many different types of bacteria.

Antibiotics kill all bacteria — of the type sensitive to it — in your body. This means helpful bacteria as well as harmful bacteria. After taking an antibiotic it takes your body a while to restore the ecological balance of the helpful bacteria to your mouth, bowels, and vagina. Some people say that you can assist your body in restoring this balance by eating yoghurt and other *acidophilus* foods.

A doctor must choose an antibiotic based on his or her knowledge that a specific illness is caused by certain types of bacteria. For example, a doctor knows that ear infections are usually caused by *streptococci* bacteria, and they are usually sensitive to penicillin. Sometimes the doctor will take a culture from the sight of your infection, to identify the bacteria causing the illness and its sensitivity to antibiotics. From this he can tell what kind of antibiotic will work best for that particular disease.

In general you should use antibiotics, when you use them at all, for a sufficient period of time (usually five days minimum) so that many generations of bacteria will be destroyed. If the drug is used for a shorter period of time, or is used in insufficient amounts, only a low number of bacteria will be destroyed and the remaining ones will often times become resistant to the antibiotic. The ones that are left, being stronger in their resistance, will continue growing and the infection will get worse. It should be obvious that antibiotics be used in sufficient dosages, and for effective lengths of time. A doctor is very valuable in providing you with the specifics of this kind of information.

Antibiotics can be dangerous. There are some people who are allergic to them. Side effects of antibiotics can be nausea, vomiting, stomach distress, and diarrhea. A less common, allergy related side effect involves a person's breathing. If you have ever had any kind of reaction to an antibiotic, at any time in your life, you should tell your doctor about it before they write you a new antibiotic prescription.

Many people are under the impression that their body can become resistant to an antibiotic. The truth is that your body does not become resistant, but bacteria living in your body do. So don't worry about taking antibiotics many times except if you happen to be allergic to them.

Hormones: Hormones are substances released by the endocrine glands of your body such as your thyroid, pituitary, pancreas, adrenal, ovaries, testes, etc. Ordinarily these normal secretions regulate vital functions such as respiration, heart beat, rate of metabolism, sexual activity, etc. Estrogen, birth control pills, thyroid, insulin, and adrenalin are some of the more commonly used hormones given for "medical" reasons.

Sometimes hormones are given as medication when a person's own glands fail to secrete the right amount of that substance on its own. These *artificial* hormones are usually derived from animal glands. Because the endocrine system is a delicate system of sympathetic balances it is easy to disturb it by introducing these substances artificially. All the vital functions of your body may well be affected.

Any of the relaxation exercises which we describe in this book will be an aid to you if you want to help increase the normal responsiveness of any or all of your endocrine glands. (See page 342 for a drawing of these glands).

Steroids are one kind of hormone, and are potent substances ordinarily produced by the adrenal glands of your body. These substances work on your whole body, almost every cell of you. They affect metabolism, water balance, the nervous system, blood, lymph, and immunity systems.

Steroids are sometimes prescribed to treat rheumatoid arthritis, asthma, eczema, and severe allergic reactions such as poison oak and some antibiotic reactions. They are often found in skin ointments, creams, lotions, and sprays, used on the skin to reduce inflamation, swelling, and itching. In these cases they are used purely to treat symptoms, not the causes of the discomforts. Steroids also come in the form of pills and injections.

Because of the profound affect that steroids can have on your body, I believe they should only be used when judged absolutely necessary. I believe that the body can usually release sufficient amounts of steroids for most situations, if directed to do so by the mind.

Birth control pills are probably the most commonly used hormones. They are made of normal body hormones, *estrogen* and *progesterone;* the first inhibits the growth of the egg, and the second brings on the flow of menstrual period blood. These are the same hormones that are secreted by the ovaries within the normal steps of a woman's reproductive cycles.

Birth control pills act on the entire body; they cause changes in the lining of the person's uterus, and they cause abnormally thick cervical mucous. The most frequent side effects are nausea, vomiting, dizziness, and discomfort in your breasts. It is now believed that with time your body gets used to birth control pills and these side effects are reduced.

We feel that it is useful for women to know that birth control pills are made up of normal ovarian hormones given in doses and times to control the menstral and ovulation cycles in a rhythm that you body would not normally follow.

Doctors now consider birth control pills relatively safe.

Tranquilizers: One of the most commonly prescribed type of drugs in the United States is the tranquilizer. The effects of some tranquilizers are actually unknown (as to whether they work or not!) Two such drugs, *meprobamate* and *chlordiazepoxid*, (generic names), with millions of users in the United States, were found to have no measurable psychological effect on the people who used them. They seemed to work best when prescribed by a doctor who felt very positively about them; they worked not at all when prescribed by a doctor who felt negatively about them.

In my medical experience, I have found that tranquilizers are the ultimate way to deal with the *manifestation* of a disease rather than the *idea* which leads up to the person getting that disease, or the *cause* of the disease. The "idea" that precedes a disease and makes the person get a disease, is generally a habit, a thought pattern, a philosophy, which doesn't work out for that person. It may be a job which causes tension, a boss who causes tension, a marriage which causes tension. The thing is to solve the problem, at the idea end of it, not just treat the manifestation. In the case of most of the tensions for which tranquilizers are prescribed, these are most easily treated by doing relaxation exercises, such as those we describe all through this book.

Tranquilizers are usually synthetic substances whose ill side effects are not wholly known. An example of this, now known by most people, is the German-produced tranquilizer, *thalidomide*, which caused a tremendous number of birth defects in the children of women who took them during pregnancy.

In the busy, expanding mega-clinic, the doctor sees you for ninety seconds, or three minutes if you're lucky. You look tense and upset. You are obviously carrying around a lot of anxiety. So the doctor writes you a prescription for a tranquilizer — one tab three times a day. The detail men for producers of tranquilizers have been to this doctor's office and have said, "Hey, this stuff works terrific. It'll get all these people off your back." They lay a hundred samples on the doctor to try on patients. The patients take them, and probably get better either because of the doctor's bedside manner or because they would have gotten better anyway.

Especially where tranquilizers are concerned, I'm saying that many people get better due to their own body's healing itself, and due to faith in their doctor. And the point is that for a great many diseases you can do these things for yourself, using relaxation exercises and other methods that we describe in this book, without using drugs or doctors or

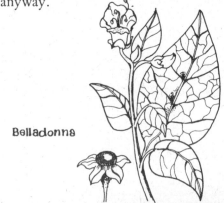

Belladonna

clinics, with fewer side effects, less cost to you, and probably a lot better karma all around.

Barbiturates: These drugs depress everything in your body, *every cell of you.* They reduce the oxygen consumption in all cells, depressing nerve activity, skeletal muscle, heart muscle — they'll even shut off the glow of a firefly. In the central nervous system, these drugs can produce sedation or coma. The sleep they produce differs radically from normal sleep, in that it sharply lowers the amount of RE.M. dreaming (see page 128), which is a phase of sleeping which has been demonstrated to be necessary for health. Barbiturates depress the respiratory drive, the desire to breath, so that you can literally stop breathing from an overdose.

Doctors prescribe barbiturates for sleeping medication, sedation, and as an anti-convulsion medicine for people who are epileptic. These drugs are truly addictive, in that they create definite physiological dependency.

I feel that depressing your whole body in this way cuts you off from your body entirely. Relaxation exercises get you to a much better place than barbiturates could ever do, without addiction or danger of poisoning. (See chapters on sleep, relaxation, and meditation, in the *Preventive Medicine* chapter, for more information about alternatives to the use of this drug.)

Amphetamines, Benzadrines, Dexadrines, and other "Speed" Drugs: These drugs act on your central nervous system and on virtually every cell of your body, causing a complete disruption of your normal life rhythms. We feel that they put you wholly out of touch with your body since they mask your normal energy levels and distort sensory and emotional impressions. In spite of all this the drug industry spends thousands and thousands of dollars every year convincing doctors that these drugs are effective in treating "depression," and other common emotional complaints.

Amphetamines (a generic name) cause tremors, restlessness, sleeplessness, mood elevation, unpredictable feelings of agitation, confusion, and often a generalized feeling of apprehension. They upset your normal rest-work cycles, blinding you to necessary signals of fatigue, raising your blood pressure, relaxing bronchial muscle, depressing appetite, and increasing your oxygen consumption. In addition, the drug is addictive.

Amphetamines have been widely prescribed as diet (weight-loss) pills, which is just another example of treating symptoms without paying attention to their causes.

Manufacturers of amphetamines list the side effects as "psychotic episodes, diarrhea, impotence, changes in sex drive, dizziness, and headache."

Everything we say about the use of tranquilizers to treat symptoms without paying attention to causes can also be said about these "speed" type drugs. (For more information on alternatives to the use of speed drugs, see the entire chapter on *Preventive Medicine*.)

Caffeine: This is a powerful, central nervous system stimulant. Apparently, man has used it since earliest recorded history. Presently it is contained in *coffee, tea, cocoa, cola drinks,* and is also mixed with aspirin, antihistimines and other symptom-treating drugs. Caffeine stimulates all portions of the brain. It stimulates thought and masks fatigue, stimulates breathing, stimulates the heart muscles directly, dilates some blood vessels and constricts others. It stimulates gastric secretions, and has unpredictable effects on your blood pressure. It can result in restlessness, disturbed sleep, heart palpitations, and diarrhea.

The popularity of beverages containing caffeine is undoubtedly due to their stimulant effect, but if you use caffeine regularly you may become quite unaware of its effects on you. If you are taking caffeine in any amount, you are taking a drug which affects your entire body as potently as many powerful prescription drugs, and the effects of it are *not under your conscious control.* To get in touch with your body, and its messages to you, it is useful to be able to separate the effects of your next cola drink, or your next cup of coffee, from your normal life rythyms.

If you use caffeine to give yourself more energy it is possible for you to get even more energy than it supplies by doing breathing exercises (page 103) which increase the amount of oxygen, and thus energy, going to each cell in your body.

Nicotine: This drug produces complex and unpredictable changes in your whole body. It is both a stimulant and a depressant, and it affects nerve transmission at the junctions between cells in the body. It stimulates the central nervous system, excites respiration, and can cause tremors and vomiting in some people. In some people, too, smoking one cigarette inhibits urination for two to three hours!

The more you use nicotine, the more you get out of touch with your body. In addition to the well-publicized relationship between nicotine and lung cancer, nicotine seems to be the cause of many minor upper respiratory infections: difficult breathing, lack of normal response to hunger, increased salivation, heart palpitations, skin blood-vessel constriction, and increased blood pressure. Nicotine is a potent drug which affects your entire body, every cell of you, in a way that you can't control and which puts you out of touch with your body and its messages to you.

The benefits of the relaxation exercises and other things in this book will be difficult for you to perceive or enjoy if you are stimulated by caffeine, nicotine, or other drugs affecting the central nervous system. It is impossible to take full control of your own body, and your health, as long as chemicals which you ingest are messing with the life rythyms of every organ of your body.

If you consciously choose what you do with drugs, and know what you are doing, drugs can be allies. But we think that caffeine and nicotine are too difficult to control and predict. They are simply not very promising allies.

A REFLECTION ON DRUGS

The affects of drugs very often prevent you from understanding your body's messages. In many cases they simply confuse you. Most drugs affect your whole body in ways that you can't control or predict. But they can be potent friends and helpers, giving you healing energy from the earth, from Nature, to help you get your body together to heal your illness. In themselves, most drugs are neither all good nor all evil, but like all other things in our Universe, must be understood before they can be used toward either of those ends. Once a drug and its effects are understood, the choice is yours.

318

INCREASING THE POSITIVE ENERGY OF DRUGS

We feel that a ritual to increase the positive energy of healing drugs, and to overcome some of the karma we told you about, makes the drug you need work better for you. If you feel positive about a drug you relax your muscles, allowing small blood vessels to open, thus increasing the circulation of the drug to the areas that need it. You will be helping your three-million-year-old healer heal you.

If the drug you are going to use is derived from an herb, you might want to try this ritual:

Close your eyes and try to imagine that herb in its most natural, most vital, most living form. If necessary, you might first find a picture of that herb at the library. Picture it growing in a field, bathed in bright sunshine, alive and healthy, producing within its stems, leaves, and flowers potent substances to heal you. Concentrate on this source. Know in your mind that this life force, in itself, is absolutely positive and pure. As you take the pill, say to yourself, "I am taking the source, and its positive energy and healing power will help heal me."

Another ritual to do this is to close your eyes, relax, and imagine each pill that you take, a moment before you take it, bathed in white light, carrying pure healing energy to your body. Say to yourself, "I am taking the source and its positive energy and healing power will help heal me."

Yet another way is to do the exercise for getting your imaginary doctor. Discuss the drug with them. Ask them how they would bring positive healing energy to it. There are as many answers and rituals as there are imaginary doctors. The main thing is for you to *take a drug with an absolutely positive attitude, and with total confidence that it will help heal you.* However you get to that point is your own choice.

☆ ☆ ☆

Prepare your body to receive the healing energy of a drug by first relaxing the body part that is sick and telling that part to be open and ready to receive the healing energy which you are sending it in the form of the drug and your positive feelings about it.

Cascara
Sagrada

RARE DISEASES, HEART DISEASE AND CANCER

When I was in medical school an elderly, distinguished professor of medicine, who was thought to be a renegade by his younger staff members, pointed out to us that *rare diseases are rare*. This was at a time when my entire medical school training had been involved with studying the molecular structures of antibodies, and studying the molecular structure of a disease that had affected only five people in the whole world. (As far as I could tell the only reason to study this rare disease was that the professor I had had "discovered" or "invented" it.)

When the distinguished professor of medicine said to us that *rare diseases are rare*, he meant that if a disease had a low incidence, say it affected about 1 person in 200,000, the average doctor would *never* see that disease. This was probably the most valuable lesson I learned in medical school. When I went into private practice I found, indeed, that no matter how hard I tried to diagnose an illness as a rare disease, people just weren't that sick. The diseases they did get were common, everyday diseases.

The Television Diseases:

Hospital and medical dramas on television dupe the American public into dwelling on rare diseases. Each week you can see people dying of rare diseases, and then miraculously saved by Medical Science on these shows. All the medical shows I've seen on television have shown people with diseases so rare that I have *never* seen them in private practice, in medical school, or in hospitals where I have worked. The only contact I ever had with them was by reading about them in medical textbooks during my second year of medical school. What does it do to people who watch these shows? Probably they get a symptom such as a sore throat, and they know, from past experience, that it's a cold. They idle along with it for a while and if it doesn't get better in the time they think it should, the spector of the rare disease that they saw on television the night before pops into their mind. *"Do I have multiple myeloma? Do I have fibrasomatosis? Do I have a strange, rare tumor of the respiratory system?* Soon the worry constricts blood vessels leading to that part of the body, changes the hormonal balance, changes the acid balance, the temperature, and lo and behold the little cold indirectly produces a perfect area for bacteria to grow.

People then go to the doctor with (in the back of their minds) fear that the doctor will discover something terrible. They feel: *I am prey to a rare disease that the doctor will discover in me. I must keep it a secret.* For this reason people often don't tell their doctors the truth about what's going on, and their state of tension and fear is parallel to that of a small animal about to be devoured by a tiger. The reality of the situation probably is that the person has a very common disease, in an average form, compounded slightly by tension or fear. This attitude, these negative feelings,

320

will not help the person's body to heal. The negative feelings will do just the opposite. On the other hand, the best healing attitude is: *I trust my body. It is doing the right thing. I'm sick because I am fatigued. I have ideas in my head that probably need changing in order to make my life better.*

One of the things that we talk about in this book is the fact that your body is different from any other body in the universe, and a cold will behave a little differently in your body than it does in anyone elses. Trust your body, relax, let your three million year old healer heal you, and you will be cured with no problem. If you do become afraid or have a constant worry, go to the doctor with the attitude that they will be able to help you get better. You have 99.99% chances that your disease is a common ailment your body can easily handle, either by itself or with a little help from the doctor.

Perspectives On Heart Disease and Cancer:

With the United States Senate heavily influenced by people in their 60's, it is not so surprising that most of the federal health money in the U.S. goes toward research in cancer and heart disease. These are the two largest causes of death in the United States, especially among older people. But these claims warrant closer scrutiny.

In part, heart disease and cancer have taken their places as major causes of death in the U.S. because many diseases which used to cause numerous deaths no longer do. Previously fatal diseases such as Smallpox, Diptheria, Polio, Tuberculosis, and even Pneumonia, are no longer listed among the top fatal diseases, because they can now be easily prevented or cured through immunization and antibiotics. You should also recognize that heart disease is perhaps overemphasized because the heart stopping is the last event of *every* terminal illness, just as it is the last event in death because of old age. There is great room for question whether old age or other diseases are in fact the causes of many "heart attack" reports that get written in on county death certificates, from which medical statistics are drawn.

The Prevention of Rare Diseases:

Cancer and Heart Disease may be the culmination of the lack of skill or knowledge necessary for early prevention of health problems. Cancer and Heart Disease are what I call "end-stage diseases." Sometimes, earlier in a person's life, a minor problem comes up, and years pass without the person heeding the signals of that problem. They do not listen to their body telling them to change. Over the years this produces chronic tension states in certain areas of their body, changes tissue in those areas so that they are more susceptible to viruses and more susceptible to different tissue growths. Then over a period of forty or fifty years they slowly create diseases to end their lives — resulting in the "end-stage diseases."

There is a choice: a person can, through worry and tension, restrict blood flow to an organ for a number of years and thereby set up the perfect situation for disease; or they can learn to change their life, relax and allow normal blood flow throughout the body.

In the United States, we *attack Cancer* rather than putting our energy and money into *discovering the reasons why people get it;* we attack the *manifestation* rather than the *idea* that makes the manifestation possible. Modern medicine has had rather mixed luck with this approach. It does cure many cancers and has made remarkable strides in treating heart disease, but at a cost tremendously great to the rest of the medical structure — especially in the field of *prevention.*

The average doctor sees most of his patients for problems not related to cancer or heart disease, yet most of everyone's research budgets go to cancer and heart disease. There's got to be something wrong here. Cancer and heart disease, through television and other media, have spread to be major terrors in the lives of most Americans. For that reason the symptoms of common diseases often become, in people's minds, the symptoms of cancer and heart disease. People will go to the doctor with a small lump, pains in their chest, pains in their arm, some extra heart beats, irregular heart rhythm, and they're sure that they have cancer or heart disease. People come to me looking frightened. I examine them and find a simple explanation for their problem and ask them, "What did you think you had?" And they say, "Doc, I was sure I had cancer," or "Doc, I was sure I had a heart attack." In such cases I enjoy telling them how wrong they are.

The American Cancer Society publishes a list of symptoms which include: discharge from the nipples, change in weight, change in bowel habits, sores that don't heal, changes in moles, a growing mass in one part of the body or another, etc. All these things, it's true, can be signs of cancer. But *most* of the time they are not. Instead they are symptoms of more common diseases: small infections, moles, and numerous early conditions that a body manifests long before the rare or serious disease is actually present.

The businessman who has some extra heart beats becomes sure that he's going to have a heart attack. But extra heart beats are often caused by tension and anxiety, not by heart disease. The businessman becomes afraid to tell his doctor. Or he tells the doctor and the doctor puts him through several hundred dollars' worth of tests. The greatest likelihood is that these tests will show a normal heart. But the fact that the doctor has him go through these tests makes the man suspect that a heart condition is imminent. After all this, the doctor diagnoses an anxiety state and probably gives the man a prescription for tranquilizers — one of the most commonly prescribed drugs in the United States. The tranquilizer drug treats the tension, but not the situations which cause the tension. So that person's anxiety threshold is *lowered by a drug, not by a change in the man's life to remove the stimulus that causes the anxiety.* The man no longer has the extra heart beats themselves, but the tension-creating situations in the man's life are still there. The tension on the heart muscles is still there. The changed acid/base balance to the heart tissue is still there. And slowly, over 40 years of popping tranquilizers, the person creates the perfect environment for heart disease in their body.

In this book we advocate a different approach to health. We believe that people *can* have complete control over their body, that though they can create an extra heart beat due to anxiety, they can also learn to change that anxiety state, to return the heart beat to normal. The fact that you can create an extra heart beat is proof that you can control your heart for more positive health goals as well. One way to do this is by relaxation. Another way is to examine your external environment. Examine where you are going with your life. Examine your diet and sleep patterns. All these are techniques basic to preventing disease. Each is discussed in our *Preventive Medicine* chapter.

Arrangements And Changes:

In this book we advocate the treatment of *causes*. We advocate changes to improve your life in order to prevent disease. We're interested in treating the common diseases for which most people seek the help of a doctor. If you know how to seek change for improvement, and you understand how to treat the common diseases that often are messages from your body telling you to change, the chances of your ever becoming seriously ill are, indeed, greatly reduced. Understand, though, that the responsibility for these changes lies with you, not with the doctor, and not with this book. Your body is *yours* and *only you* can read your body's early messages. Understand, too, that your doctor may or may not have the inclination or the knowledge to help you in this.

When I was in medical school I was taught that it was really not worthwhile to go into private practice, that it was really uninteresting and boring out there, that all the real "intellectual challenge" was in medical research, in the structure of molecular antibody formation and such. I was told that 75% of the diseases seen by local medical doctors (LMD's, as they were derisively called) were psychosomatic and 23% were "uninteresting" simple problems, and the real meat of medicine was in the 2% of rare diseases found in medical centers.

Now that I am an LMD I feel that the real health care is going on *outside* the medical centers. Some medical center discoveries are fascinating, some are useful, but unfortunately they are not creating a world of health. The real work going on now, I believe, is in bio- feedback research occuring often in small, informally-arranged clinics; and in yogin monasteries in India, and elsewhere around the world, where people are learning to control their vital functions; and in small independent health centers dedicated to providing actual patient care rather than research into rare diseases.

We believe that people can take full responsibility for their own health. This does not mean that you have to be your own doctor if you really don't feel that's what you want to do. You can, however, take responsibility for choosing your own doctor, for understanding the doctor's decisions and treatments, and then helping that doctor to help your body heal itself.

The *Diagnosis and Treatment* section of this book will give you the knowledge to participate more fully in the healing process when you are ill with one of the diseases we list there. In that chapter we give many of the secrets that have kept the medical doctor a mysterious and aloof figure since the beginning of time. If this book accomplishes nothing else but to demystify the doctor for you, it will have been a real benefit. It will enable you to go to your doctor with your eyes open, understanding what the medical arts are really about.

The Incidence Of Rare Communicable Disease:

The television and news media play up certain communicable diseases as fearful spectors about to strike each of us down at any moment. To put things in perspective, we looked at communicable disease incidence charts for California, between the years 1967 and 1972. The figures here are taken randomly from 1970 figures put out by the public health services. Keep in mind that the year these figures were taken the total population of California was nearly 20 million people (19,953,134).

Name of Disease	Number of Cases	Incidence	Number of Deaths
Botulism	2	(1 case per 10 million people)	1
Diptheria	6	(1 case per 3-1/3 million people)	0
Leprosy	55	(1 case per 363,636 people)	0
Meningitis	420	(1 case per 47,618 people)	62
Plague	3	(1 case per 6-2/3 million people)	0
Polio	2 new cases since innoculation began		
Rabies	0		0
Rocky Mountain Spotted Fever	2	(1 case per 10 million people)	0
Tetanus	9	(1 case per 2-2/9 million people	3
Trichinosis	19	(1 case per million people)	1
Typhoid Fever	62	(1 case per 322,580 people)	0

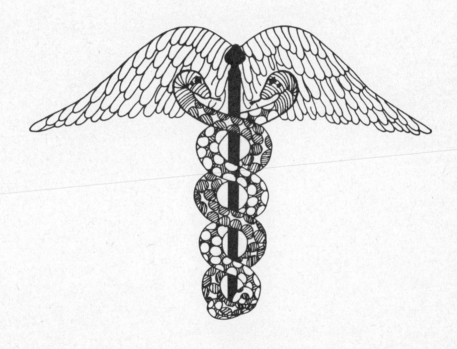

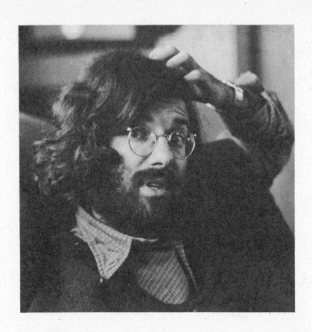

HOW I CAME TO WRITE THIS BOOK — by Mike

When I entered Medical school I was interested in Immunogenetics — the study of the inheritance of body defenses. I enjoyed working with the people in the research lab, but the subject and the methods did not apply to my life. During medical school I thought that I would be a Psychiatrist but sitting indoors listening to people didn't make me feel good. After my internship I was sent to an Indian reservation by the Public Health Service. I liked the Indians but not the medicine we practiced.

When I left the Indian reservation I moved to a small town on the California coast and decided to do photography, which I had enjoyed all my life. I walked on the beaches, took pictures of rocks and light and was really happy. During this time people in the town heard that I was a doctor and would call me asking about their health problems. The problems were for the most part simple to solve but made me realize that people had been taught very little about their bodies.

Then Nancy and I bought some land and began building our own small house. I enjoyed working outdoors, seeing a day's work standing when we left each day. I started counting my breaths and relaxing to help me build our house. That kept me from worrying about our lack of knowledge of housebuilding, and kept me from getting tired after a day's work.

I also started doing medicine again at the county venereal disease clinic. I had always liked free medical care and liked the young people I was doctoring. They taught me about the questions people had about how their bodies healed themselves.

About this time two oil tankers collided off our coast and the oil came up on our beach. I started a clinic to treat and keep well the thousands of volunteers who helped clean up the oil. At this clinic I again realized how little most people knew about their bodies. A friend who lived in a commune asked if I would teach him how to take care of his people. I rapped out a story something like the diagnosis and treatment section of this book, which he was going to mimeograph and mail out to other communes, but never did.

Another Doctor in town, whom I had met at the oil slick clinic, and I decided to set up a clinic which would help people treat themselves, and that we would enjoy. We had massage people, faith healers, Indian medicine men, color healers and three M.D.'s on the staff. It was fun to do; it did itself. It was like a clubhouse where people learned how to take care of their own health problems, with us as their helpers. The clinic tried to write the book but was too busy being a clinic.

After a while I went back to being a builder/farmer. We moved into our house and made vegetable gardens, chicken coups etc. I was back outdoors working on the land.

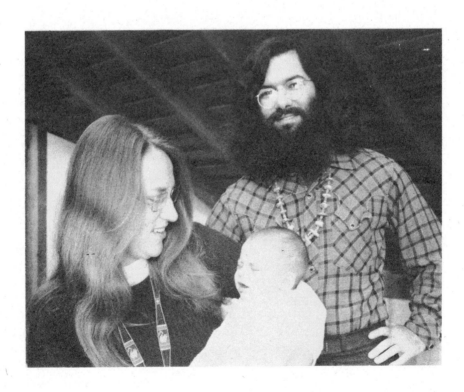

One day Hal showed up. I had met him when he taught in a day care center with Nancy. He had just finished a book with Don at Bookworks. Years ago I had told Hal about the mythical doctor-yourself book. Hal now said that Don wanted to publish it if I would finally write it. We talked about it and decided to write it together. We set a deadline for six months and started working.

From the beginning the book had a life of its own. Hal and I had ideas based on our experiences as people but the book chose the ones it wanted. This is the book that we birthed.

Yesterday with about ten pages left to write I went outside and cut firewood for the afternoon. That felt really good, so its time to work outdoors again.

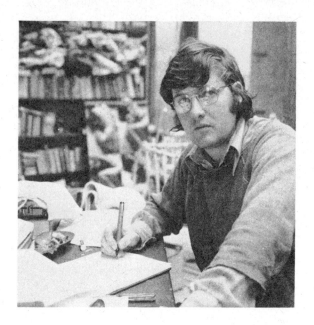

HOW I CAME TO WRITE THIS BOOK — by Hal

I met Mike and Nancy several years ago while I was running a children's day care center in the county where they lived. Nancy was a teacher and from time to time she did substitute work for me. Through her I got to know Mike, and the friendships which developed between our families grew.

I don't remember when we first started talking about writing *The Well Body Book.* But Mike and I often talked about healing and the need for radical changes in the medical profession and in patient-doctor relationships. The first book project we ever discussed was a book to present a very workable understanding of common diseases for the non-medical person. It seemed to me a good step toward greater patient participation. But we never got started on that book.

Mike went about his business and I went about mine. I was in the middle of writing a book about education (*No More Public School*), while Mike and Nancy were in the midst of building their own house. So our medical book wasn't ready to be born yet. Other things seemed more important for the time being.

Then one day an oil tanker split open off the Pacific coast, and it spilled oil over the bay and across the beaches of the town where Mike and Nancy live. Wildlife was threatened, the sea life was threatened, and several miles of beautiful California beaches were marred by a black viscous goo. The townspeople rallied together to save what they could. Mike and Nancy were among them.

Mike set up a free clinic and first aid station. From that point he and others directed the mop-up project. They had every human and technological resource at their fingertips: several hundred people cleaning the beaches and the birds, helicopters bringing in supplies, and the nearly unlimited finances of a large oil company. A huge amount of very positive energy was focused on this tiny town. In the end the people succeeded. They restored what could not be claimed as the property of any one man: the birds, the beaches, and the life in the sea.

One by-product of this near tragedy was the continuation of the first aid station, and its transformation into a free clinic which came to be known as the *Headlands Clinic*. This clinic continued to draw positive energy from all over the country: M.D.s, Yoga masters, Psychic healers, bio-feedback experts, Indian medicine men, massage healers, etc. Some succeeded more than others. But it soon became apparent that Western medicine had no monopoly on healing. Other forms of healing were succeeding where Western medicine failed.

The book once again became a real possibility in my mind. My imagination was inspired by stories about the *Headlands Clinic* and by my visits to it. The clinic was the kind of place where you could walk in, feel very comfortable being there, and even be asked to participate in a healing session. Sometimes it was just a lot of people discussing what they thought might be causes and cures for illnesses which seemed to have no cures in Western medical terms. Patient and doctor were equals here.

Some time after the formation of the *Headlands Clinic*, Mike and I found ourselves with the time and the spirit to write the book. We began with a modest, simple book. But it grew. It took on its own life in a way that I have never had a book do. Linda agreed to do the illustrations, which would be a considerable undertaking, and Nancy agreed to help with the editing. We had little difficulty selling Don Gerrard at *Bookworks*, and then *Random House*, on the idea of publishing it.

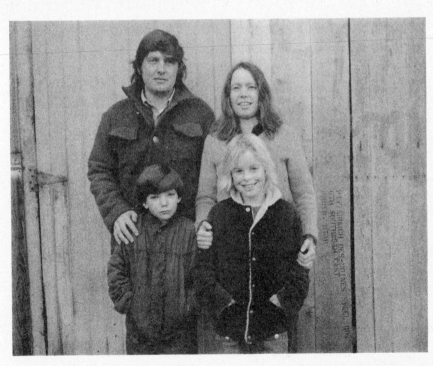

My feeling about the finished *Well Body Book* is that it is more complete than I could have ever imagined it could be. This may sound like a commercial, but the truth is that the book has literally changed our lives. My attitudes toward illness and the healing arts have radically changed for the better. Our health, and thus our lives, continue to improve as a result of the exercises and attitudes we have discovered in the process of doing the book.

☆　☆　☆

We would enjoy hearing from you — how you feel about the book, how you have used it, and about any ideas for healing that you may have. Write us:

C/O Random House
201 E. 50th Street
New York, New York
10022

GOING FURTHER

In this chapter we tell you about books which have been important to us in writing and researching *The Well Body Book*. It is more than a bibliography in that we tell you, for each entry, what the book or resource offers in the way of health information.

You will notice that we have arranged the books under subject headings relevant to *The Well Body Book*. For example, books which will be useful to you in going further than we have taken you in our chapter on *Preventive Medicine* are found under the heading of *Preventive Medicine* here.

You will probably notice that we don't list books on childbirth or pediatric medicine. We feel that childbirth is a learned skill rather than a health problem, and books such as Dr. Jacobsen's *How To Relax and Have Your Baby,* or Lester Hazell's *Commonsense Childbirth* are good. There's also an excellent photo essay on the subject called *Two Births,* published by our publishers. For pediatric medicine, you still can't do much better than Dr. Spock.

Use this chapter for putting together your own home medical library.

CREATING YOUR IMAGINARY DOCTOR

Castaneda, Carlos. *A Separate Reality.* New York; Simon and Schuster, 1971. Amazing stories of imaginary beings.

Simmons, Leo. *Sun Chief.* New Haven; Yale University Press, 1942. Chapter 6 contains an account of healing by an imaginary doctor.

A Resource: *mind control* courses such as Silva Mind Control, EST, Mind Dynamics. This is *not* an endorsement; you have to check the courses carefully to see if they are what you want. Silva Mind Control teaches you how to get your own spiritual advisor.

GENERAL INFORMATION

Most city or county health departments have counciling available for immunizations and communicable diseases. Some also have genetic counciling clinics to help you with questions about inherited disease. University hospitals (connected with medical schools) may also have such services.

MIRROR, MIRROR

Downing, George. *The Massage Book.* New York; Random House — The Bookworks; 1972. This book tells about getting in touch with your body through massage. We consider massage a primary healing tool.

Esalen Institute, 1776 Union St., San Francisco, Calif. 94123. Write for their catalog of workshops, and list of Esalen publications.

Arguelles, *Mandala*, Berkeley, California, and London, England; Shambala, 1972. Mandala is a method which man has used for thousands of years to conceptualize his relationship to the universe. It is an extension of the *Health Colors* chart concept which we present in *The Well Body Book*. It is a beautiful book, with many full-color reproductions of mandalas, and instructions on how to do your own.

PREVENTIVE MEDICINE

Davis, Adele. *Let's Eat Right To Keep Fit.* New York; Harcourt, Brace, Jovanovich, Inc.; 1954. An enormous amount of information about how nutritional deficiencies relate to specific symptoms and diseases. It really makes you think about what you eat, but it has a heavy disease consciousness. A valuable book. Contains charts on the nutritive value of foods.

Lappe, Frances M. *Diet For A Small Planet.* New York; Friends of the Earth/Ballantine; 1971. A book about how to combine foods to get complete protein and save the environment. Very useful because she has put together information which would not otherwise be readily available.

Luce, Gay Gaer, *Body Time,* New York, Pantheon Books, 1971. This book tells you about the latest scientific research on the physiological rhythms of life. The book is very readable and is a valuable reference to help you get in harmony with your natural body rhythms. Contains a long list of books for going further.

Mishra, Rammurti. *Fundamentals of Yoga.* New York; Lancer Books; 1959. A how-to-do-it book, written by an M.D., that links all kinds of yoga with medicine. A totally positive book whose goal is to unite you with Nature in a simple manner. A valuable book. It has specific information on relaxation, exercises, breath control, etc.

Watt, B. and Merrill, A , *Composition of Foods,* Washington, D.C., Superintendent of Documents, U.S. Government Printing Office, Washington, D.C., 1963. This is a 190 page collection of food charts, telling you the nutritional contents of foods. Probably the most comprehensive resource of its kind. Sells for $2.00, and is available from the U.S. Government Printing Office.

Huxley, Laura, *You Are Not The Target,* New York, Farrar, Strauss, and Co., 1963. This is an excellent book which describes practical exercises to do to relieve tension and better cope with everyday affairs. It will help you get more in touch with yourself in a very pleasant way.

Satchidananda, *Integral Yoga Hatha,* New York, Holt Paperback, 1970. This book is a course in Yoga. Yoga positions are described with words and excellent photos.

Kapleau, Philip. *The Three Pillars of Zen.* New York; Harper and Row; 1961. Contains excellent instructions for *counting your breaths* (meditation) and relaxation.

Lama Foundation. *Be Here Now.* New Mexico, 1971. Its "Cookbook, Part 3" contains spiritually-orientated information about sleeping, eating, exercise, getting straight, etc., all of which are good healing techniques.

"Organic Gardening and Farming." Published monthly by Rodale Press, Emmaus, Pa. Contains information on how to grow your own food, plus much about *Where You Be.*

Jung, Carl. *Memories, Dreams, and Reflections.* New York, Random House, 1963. Jung's autobiography; contains fascinating journeys into his dream world. Useful to find out about dreams, spiritual advisors, and the collective unconscious.

Casteneda, Carlos. *Journey To Ixtlan.* New York; Simon and Schuster; 1972. Specific information on ego loss, controlling dreams, and becoming a man of knowledge.

Wilhelm, Richard, translator. *The I Ching.* New York; Princeton University Press; 1950. A method for making decisions without anxiety. Also profound Chinese philosophy. Especially important to Westerners because it takes you out of the bounds of cause and effect.

Maltz, Maxwell. *Psycho-Cybernetics.* New York; Prentiss-Hall; 1960. The book deals with self-image, imagination, and positivity as keys to success, happiness, etc.

Yogananda, Paramahansa. *Autobiography of A Yogi.* Los Angeles; Self-Realization Fellowship; 1969. Stories of miracles, the astral plane and healings.

PHYSICAL EXAMINATION

Hopkins, M.D., Henry, *Leopolds Principles and Methods Of Physical Diagnosis,* Philadelphia, W. B. Saunders Co., 1966. A medical school textbook on how to do a physical exam, this book talks a lot about disease and for that reason is somewhat negative. If you can get through pages of photos, drawings, and verbal descriptions of diseases, you will get a very complete picture of what's involved in doing physical diagnosis according to Western medicine. We cite it only because it is one of the few books available on the subject — through medical school bookstores, and sells for about $10.00.

DIAGNOSIS AND TREATMENT

Krupp, Marcus, and Chatton, Milton. *Current Diagnosis and Treatment.* Los Altos; Lange Medical Publications; 1972. It contains the symptoms, physical signs, stories, and treatments for most diseases. It is intended for the practicing doctor as a desk reference. It is written in technical language, but is *fairly* understandable to a layman, especially with the help of a medical dictionary. The rarest diseases known can appear to be identical to the most common in this book, since it does not tell the non-medical person how to distinguish between them. $10 - $12 in medical school bookstores.

The Merck Manual of Diagnosis and Therapy. Rahway, N.J.; Merck, Sharp & Dohme. Another doctor's desk reference; sometimes easier to understand than the one above. Contains some home remedies. Almost 2000 pages long. At medical school bookstores, the cost is around $12.

McGuire, Thomas. *The Tooth Trip,* New York; Random House — Bookworks; 1972. Information on examining and taking care of your teeth. A true *preventive* dentistry handbook for non-medical people. Has ideas for preventing cavities and how to "survive" in the dentist's office. $3.95.

Medical school bookstores are open to the public. They are usually arranged by medical school course. For example, Internal Medicine, Pediatrics, Surgery, etc. The biggest pile of books in each section is probably the one recommended by the professor of the course; it's usually the standard for the whole country. The books cost around $20 a piece and are extremely difficult even for medical students to use. They are highly technical, poorly written, and are filled with scientific research and rare diseases. Medical school libraries have these books; you may be able to read them there. If you wish to learn about one disease in tremendous detail, you can start with general textbooks.

Current Diagnosis and Treatment, mentioned above, has an excellent technical bibliography after each disease. By looking up these periodical articles in a medical library you can read about the most recent research and ideas about the disease. This may help you participate in the treatment. It is no more difficult than doing research for a term paper in college. Information about diseases is not secret; it is available in medical school libraries and bookstores.

DRUGS AS HELPERS

Physicians' Desk Reference. Oradell, N.J.; Medical Economics, Inc.; up-dated yearly. It contains the manufacturer's instructions that are packaged with all drugs. It has a description of the drug, what the drug contains, how it acts, indications for usage, contra-indications to usage, precautions for usage, side-effects, and the dosages usually prescribed. Your doctor probably gets one every year; it is possible that they might give you an old one. Also check medical school libraries. It is extremely useful if you wish to know more about drugs.

EMERGENCY MEDICINE — FIRST AID

Kodet, Russel, M.D. and Angier, Bradford, *Being Your Own Wilderness Doctor,* published by Stackpole Books, Harrisburg, Pa. This is probably the mellowist first aid book around. It is very readable and covers everything from suturing wounds to transporting people with broken bones. In the back is a list of prescription drugs to take with you whenever you will be a great distance from medical help. The book is written for people who are living miles from a doctor or a hospital.

American National Red Cross, *First Aid*, New York, Doubleday and Co. This is the old standby first aid book that practically everyone has either seen or now owns. The Red Cross keeps it updated.

CATALOGS OF HEALING TECHNIQUES

Portola Institute, *The Last Whole Earth Catalog*, Portola Institute/Random House, 1972. A good place to look up books for specific health concerns. Lists and gives short descriptions of books covering everything from prescription drugs to childbirth and nutrition.

Canadian Whole Earth Research Foundation, *Canadian Whole Earth Almanac* on *Healing*, Canadian Whole Earth Research Foundation, 341 Bloon Street West, Toronto, Canada, 1971. This catalog lists and tells about healing techniques and books about healing.

BOOKS ON HEALING ENERGY

Since the first printing of this book friends have told us about various published materials which explain in scientific terms what we call "healing energy." Some of the information brought to us deals with how people can learn to direct this energy to improve their lives. Another kind of information deals with electrically measuring and photographing this energy at work in plants, animals, and in human beings. The following are just a few of such books.

Krippner, S. *Galaxies of Life*, New York; Interface 1973. Technical scientific info on aura, acupuncture and Krilian photography. Great help in developing your own ways of directing healing energy. $12.50.

Oyle, I. *Magic, Mysticism and Modern Medicine*, California, Headlands Healing Press 1973. The author, a doctor, and director of the Headlands Clinic, has put together an amazing book of healing experiences and techniques.

Ostrander, S. & Schroeder, L. *Psychic Discoveries Behind The Iron Curtain*, New York, Bantam 1970. Reports on parapsychology, psychic healings, and allied research.

Carter, M. & McGary, W. *Edgar Cayce On Healing*, New York, Paperback Library 1972. Personal narratives about psychic healings.

Yogi Ramacharaka, *The Science Of Psychic Healing* (and other books on healing) Shambala Publishers, 1409 Fifth Street, Berkeley, Ca.; This yogin has written several books describing healing techniques. Valuable how-to material for developing your skills.

HOW THINGS WORK

In the following seven pages you will find drawings showing some basic actions that take place in your body. Look upon this chapter as a resource for understanding how your body nourishes, maintains, protects, and heals itself, as well as for locating the positions of various organs and systems.

There are numerous ways to use these pages. You may find the labeled body charts, as well as the endocrine system drawing, helpful to you when you are working on your color charts, or when you are doing a physical examination, or when you are using the diagnosis and treatment chapter and you want to know more about the locations of organs. The drawings of lymph, blood, and antibodies will provide you with information about how your body uses energy for healing whenever you are ill.

We suggest that you acquaint yourself with these pages enough to know what they contain. Later you may want to adapt this information to your own needs, such as visualizing in your mind the *How Things Work* drawings while relaxing a part of your body that is ill, allowing healing energies to move naturally to the areas that need them.

WHAT BLOOD DOES

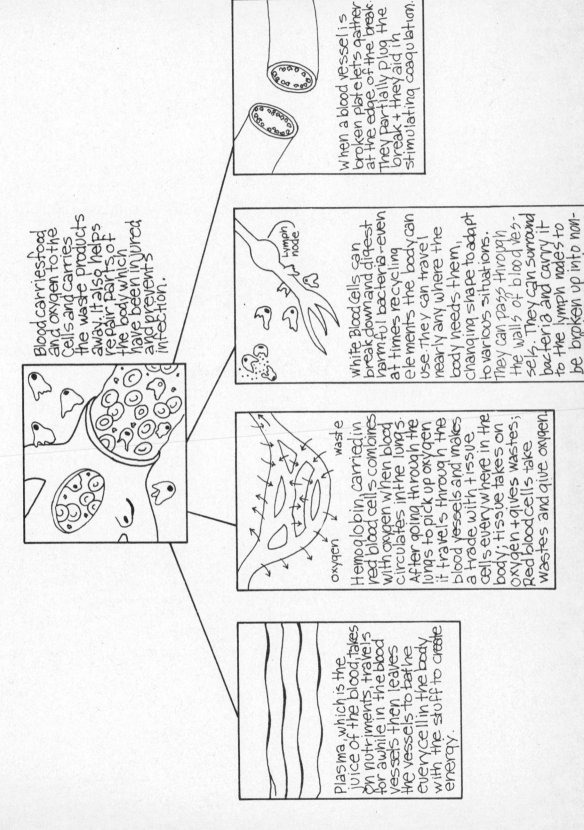

Blood carries food and oxygen to the cells and carries the waste products away. It also helps repair parts of the body which have been injured and prevents infection.

When a blood vessel is broken platelets gather at the edge of the break. They partially plug the break + they aid in stimulating coagulation.

White blood cells can break down and digest harmful bacteria-even at times recycling elements the body can use. They can travel nearly any where the body needs them, changing shape to adapt to various situations. They can pass through the walls of blood vessels. They can surround bacteria and carry it to the lymph nodes to be broken up into non-harmful elements.

Hemoglobin carried in red blood cells combines with oxygen when blood circulates in the lungs. After going through the lungs to pick up oxygen it travels through the blood vessels and makes a trade with tissue cells everywhere in the body; tissue takes on oxygen + gives wastes; Red blood cells take wastes and give oxygen.

waste

oxygen

Plasma, which is the juice of the blood, takes on nutriments, travels for awhile in the blood vessels then leaves the vessels to bathe every cell in the body with the stuff to create energy.

lymph node

WHAT HAPPENS WHEN YOU CUT YOURSELF

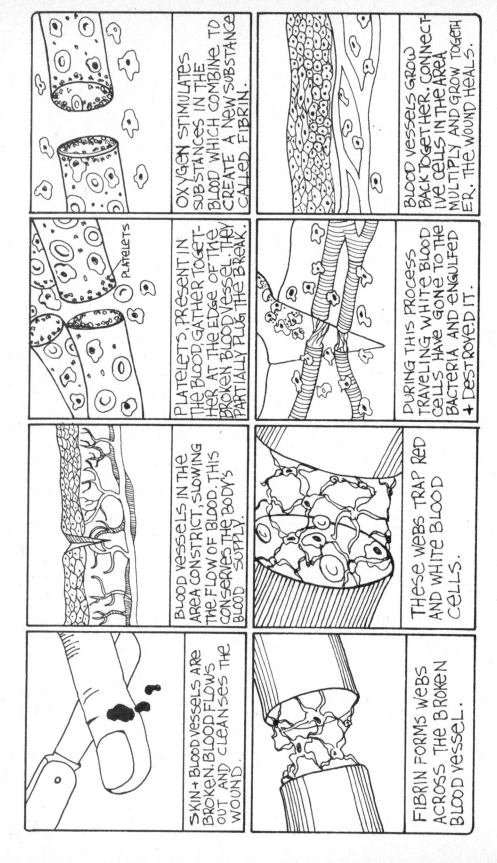

OXYGEN STIMULATES SUBSTANCES IN THE BLOOD WHICH COMBINE TO CREATE A NEW SUBSTANCE CALLED FIBRIN.

BLOOD VESSELS GROW BACK TOGETHER. CONNECTIVE CELLS IN THE AREA MULTIPLY AND GROW TOGETHER. THE WOUND HEALS.

PLATELETS, PRESENT IN THE BLOOD, GATHER TOGETHER AT THE EDGE OF THE BROKEN BLOOD VESSEL. THEY PARTIALLY PLUG THE BREAK.

DURING THIS PROCESS TRAVELING WHITE BLOOD CELLS HAVE GONE TO THE AREA. BACTERIA AND ENGULFED + DESTROYED IT.

BLOOD VESSELS IN THE AREA CONSTRICT, SLOWING THE FLOW OF BLOOD. THIS CONSERVES THE BODY'S BLOOD SUPPLY.

THESE WEBS TRAP RED AND WHITE BLOOD CELLS.

SKIN + BLOOD VESSELS ARE BROKEN. BLOOD FLOWS OUT AND CLEANSES THE WOUND.

FIBRIN FORMS WEBS ACROSS THE BROKEN BLOOD VESSEL.

HOW LYMPH FIGHTS INFECTION

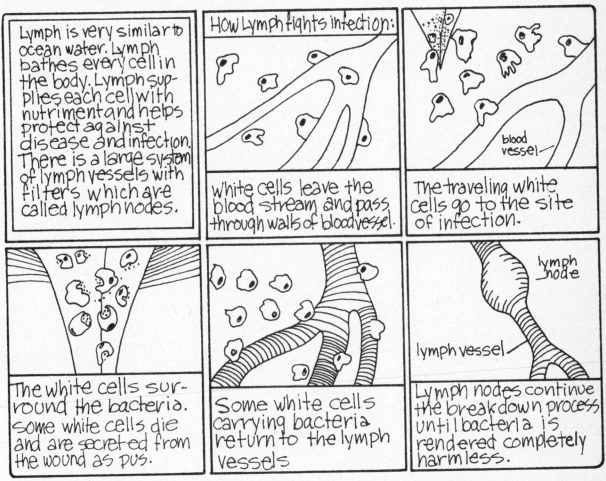

Lymph is very similar to ocean water. Lymph bathes every cell in the body. Lymph supplies each cell with nutriment and helps protect against disease and infection. There is a large system of lymph vessels with filters which are called lymph nodes.

How Lymph fights infection:

White cells leave the blood stream and pass through walls of bloodvessel.

blood vessel

The traveling white cells go to the site of infection.

The white cells surround the bacteria. Some white cells die and are secreted from the wound as pus.

Some white cells carrying bacteria return to the lymph vessels

lymph node

lymph vessel

Lymph nodes continue the breakdown process until bacteria is rendered completely harmless.

Each group of lymph nodes protects a particular area of your body: neck nodes protect the head, nodes at the tops of your thighs protect legs and genitals. etc. Lymph nodes can become enlarged due to any type of infection in the area they protect - pimples, boils, sore throat, ear infection Herpes, etc. Enlarged lymph nodes indicate that your Three Million Year Old Healer is at work to protect and heal your body. (See page 280 for a map of the lymph system.)

THE ENDOCRINE SYSTEM

THYROID GLANDS
Secrete a protein substance containing iodine. It regulates respiration - the speed at which body cells use oxygen.

PARATHYROID GLANDS
are located within the thyroid glands. The parathyroids regulate the amount of calcium in the blood. Calcium is necessary for healthy bones + teeth. A particular calcium level regulates nerve and muscle responsiveness.

STOMACH + DUODENUM
Food coming into stomach stimulates gastrin which helps in digestion of food.

PANCREAS
Little islands of tissue in the pancreas secrete insulin which regulates the amount of sugar in the blood.

OVARIES or TESTES
Determine sex characteristics, body hair distribution, voice differences, amount of fat under the skin, sex drive, mental vigor and blood circulation.

OVARIES ♀

PITUITARY GLAND (The Master Gland)
Located in the very center of the head; it is about the size of a bean. It secreates hormones which in turn regulate the rate of secretions of other glands: thyroid, testes or ovaries and adrenal glands. It in turn responds to the secretions of the glands it helps to regulate. This is a true bio-feedback system. It secretes a substance which plays a role in the production of milk. It secretes "growth" hormones for growth + regeneration. It regulates water balance, and the contraction of smooth muscles and blood vessels in the uterus during child birth.

ADRENAL GLANDS
Secrete steroid, such as cortisone, which regulate metabolic processes in cells: level of water, ions, carbohydrates, fats + amino acids. Hundreds of other compounds are produced here to regulate the storage of sugar in the liver, skin coloration + sex hormones. A portion of the adrenal gland produces epinephrine which regulates dilation of eyes, blood, pressure, sugar in the blood + goose bumps.

342

ANTIBODY CREATION

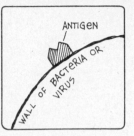

1. A bacteria or virus enters the human body through the mouth, a break in the skin, a mucous membrane, etc. Then lymphocytes - a type of white blood cell - discover the bacteria or virus + recognize a protein substance on the wall of the virus or bacteria (called antigen) as foreign, or as not normally belonging in the body.

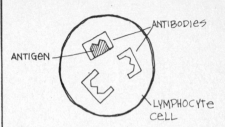

2. The lymphocyte cells create proteins (called antibodies) which are structured in such a way as to join with the specific antigen.

Note: Scale is purposefully distorted. Understand that a lymphocyte is many thousands of times larger than a bacteria or a virus.

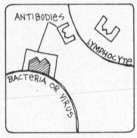

3. The lymphocyte releases the antibodies, which it has created, into the fluids of the body, to combine with the foreign proteins on the surface of the bacteria or virus. When combined this renders the virus or bacteria harmless to your body.

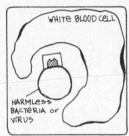

4. Another type of white blood cell engulfs the now harmless bacteria or virus and carries it to other parts of the body to get rid of it.

5. This process makes immunization possible. With immunization, virus or bacteria are first rendered harmless though the antigen on their walls remains intact. A small amount of this substance is introduced to your body. Then your body creates antibodies to combine with that specific antigen. Your body has then developed a large stock of those specific antibodies so that if the live virus or bacteria were to come into your body you would already have the "knowledge" and/or the antibodies to easily protect yourself from the infection.

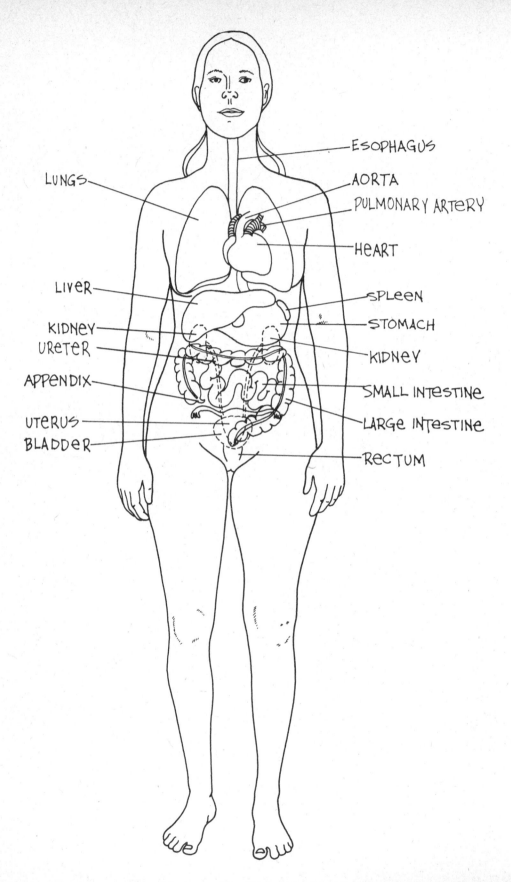

ESOPHAGUS

LUNGS

AORTA

PULMONARY ARTERY

HEART

LIVER

SPLEEN

STOMACH

KIDNEY
URETER

KIDNEY

APPENDIX

SMALL INTESTINE

LARGE INTESTINE

UTERUS
BLADDER

RECTUM

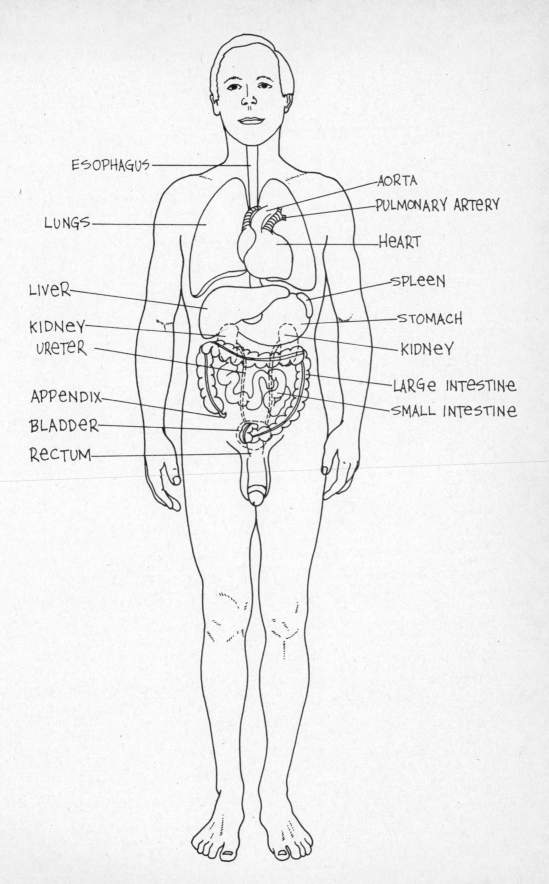

ESOPHAGUS

AORTA

PULMONARY ARTERY

LUNGS

HEART

LIVER

SPLEEN

KIDNEY

STOMACH

URETER

KIDNEY

LARGE INTESTINE

APPENDIX

SMALL INTESTINE

BLADDER

RECTUM

USE THIS PAGE FOR YOUR NOTES

INDEX

HOW YOU CAN BE THE AUTHOR OF THIS BOOK

After you have read this book, imagine yourself as the author. You are fully justified in claiming this feeling. Once you have read the whole book and have it fully in your possession, you have all the knowledge the authors put into it. Fully accept yourself as the author of what you know as a result of your life, of which reading this book is a part.

Imagine now that you are your own three million year old healer.

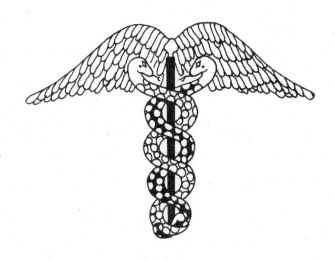